This report contains the collective views of an international group of experts and does not necessarily represent the decisions or the stated policy of the United Nations Environment Programme, the International Commission on Non-Ionizing Radiation Protection, or the World Health Organization.

Environmental Health Criteria 160

ULTRAVIOLET RADIATION

An Authoritative Scientific Review of Environmental and Health Effects of UV, with Reference to Global Ozone Layer Depletion

Published under the joint sponsorship of the United Nations Environment Programme, the International Commission on Non-Ionizing Radiation Protection and the World Health Organization

World Health Organization
Geneva, 1994

The **International Programme on Chemical Safety (IPCS)** is a joint venture of the United Nations Environment Programme, the International Labour Organisation, and the World Health Organization. The main objective of the IPCS is to carry out and disseminate evaluations of the effects of chemicals on human health and the quality of the environment. Supporting activities include the development of epidemiological, experimental laboratory and risk-assessment methods that could produce internationally comparable results, and the development of manpower in the field of toxicology. Other activities carried out by the IPCS include the development of know-how for coping with chemical accidents, coordination of laboratory testing and epidemiological studies, and promotion of research on the mechanisms of the biological action of chemicals.

WHO Library Cataloguing in Publication Data

Ultraviolet radiation

(Environmental health criteria; 160)

1.Ultraviolet rays 2.Radiation effects
3.Environmental exposure I.Series

ISBN 92 4 157160 8 (NLM Classification: WD 605)
ISSN 0250-863X

PRINTED IN FINLAND
93/9908 - VAMMALA - 5500

CONTENTS

PREFACE

The World Health Organization (WHO), in collaboration with the United Nations Environment Programme (UNEP) and the International Non-Ionizing Radiation Committee (INIRC) of the International Radiation Protection Association (IRPA), published the first Environmental Health Criteria (EHC) monograph on Ultraviolet Radiation in 1979. At the United Nations Conference on the Environment and Development (UNCED) in 1992 it was declared under Agenda 21 that there should be activities on the effects of ultraviolet radiation. Specifically:

"(i) Undertake, as a matter of urgency, research on the effects on human health of the increasing ultraviolet radiation reaching the earth's surface as a consequence of depletion of the stratospheric ozone layer;

(ii) On the basis of the outcome of this research, consider taking appropriate remedial measures to mitigate the above-mentioned effects on human beings".

Within the United Nations mandate, and that of the 1993 WHO Global Strategy for Health and Environment, this monograph has been drafted to provide the essential authoritative review on which future research programmes in UV can progress.

IRPA initiated activities in NIR by forming a Working Group on Non-Ionizing Radiation in 1974. This Working Group later became the INIRC at the IRPA meeting held in Paris in 1977. In May 1992 the INIRC was chartered as an independent scientific commission called the International Commission on Non-Ionizing Radiation Protection (ICNIRP). ICNIRP continues the work of the IRPA/INIRC by reviewing the scientific literature on NIR and making assessments of health risks of human exposure to such radiation. Using the Environmental Health Criteria monographs, developed in conjunction with WHO, ICNIRP recommends guidelines on exposure limits, drafts codes of practice, and works in conjunction with other international organizations to promote safety and standardization in the non-ionizing radiation fields.

A UNEP/WHO/ICNIRP Task Group to review the final draft of the updated Environmental Health Criteria on Ultraviolet (UV) Radiation met in Geneva from 8-11 December, 1993. Dr W. Kreisel, Executive Director, World Health Organization opened the meeting on behalf of WHO. Dr H. Gopalan and Mr R. Matthes welcomed the participants on behalf of UNEP and ICNIRP respectively.

The first revision of this publication was compiled by members of the IRPA/INIRC and more recently by members of ICNIRP. Chapters were prepared by Drs B. Armstrong, J-P. Cesarini, L. Court, P. Dolan, G. Johnson, A. Kricker, A. McKinlay, M. Repacholi, M. Selgrade, D. Sliney and R. Tyrrell. These chapters together with the report of an informal consultation held in Geneva, in August 1993 on "The Effects of Solar UV Radiation on the Eye", the International Agency for Research on Cancer (IARC) report of the meeting on "Health, Solar UV Radiation and Environmental Change " held in Lyon in October 1992, and the meeting on Immunotoxicology held in Bilthoven in July 1993, were used by Drs M. Repacholi and D. Sliney to compile the review draft in September 1993. Comments were received from a broad cross-section of specialists in the UV fields and their reviews were gratefully received. These comments were then incorporated for Task Group review. Final scientific editing of the text was completed by Drs J-P. Cesarini, A. McKinlay, M. Repacholi and D. Sliney. Sincere thanks to Christine Cornish and Nancy Smith for their assistance in the preparation of this text. An editorial group consisting of Drs M. Repacholi, H. Gopalan and T. Kjellström coordinated the preparation of this monograph.

This monograph comprises a review of the data on the effects of exposure on biological systems pertinent to the evaluation of human health risks. Its purpose is to give an overview of the known biological effects of UV, identify gaps in knowledge and provide direction for further research. This monograph will assist health authorities, regulatory and similar agencies to provide guidance on health risks from exposure to UV and limits for occupational and general public exposure.

Earlier reports were not necessarily included, as they were reviewed in the 1979 monograph. Every effort has been made to distinguish clearly between established biological effects and those that have been reported as preliminary or isolated results, or as hypotheses proposed to explain observed results. The conclusions are based on established knowledge of interactions of UV with biological systems.

Subjects reviewed include: the physical characteristics of UV; measurement techniques; applications and sources of exposure; mechanisms of interaction; biological effects; guidance on protective measures; and recommendations on exposure limits.

This monograph will also serve as a scientific database for the planned WHO/UNEP/IARC/ICNIRP International Research Programme on Health, Solar UV Radiation and Environmental Change (INTERSUN). The general objectives of INTERSUN are to:

(i) evaluate the quantitative relationship between solar UV at the surface of the earth and human health effects, develop reliable predictions of the health consequences of changes in UV, provide baseline estimates of the incidence of health effects of UV in representative populations around the world, and develop practical ways of monitoring change in these effects over time in relation to environmental and behavioural change;

(ii) provide essential input into the development of environmental and public health policies and actions in relation to depletion of stratospheric ozone; and

(iii) provide a framework for monitoring the effects of solar UV and the impact of prevention programmes.

Health agencies and regulatory authorities are encouraged to set up and develop programmes that ensure effective protection against the health effects of UV. It is hoped that this criteria monograph will provide useful information for such endeavours.

TASK GROUP MEETING ON THE REVISION OF ENVIRONMENTAL HEALTH CRITERIA ON UV RADIATION

Members

Dr J.P. Cesarini	LRTPH, Fondation Rothschild, Paris, France
Dr L. Court	Centre de Recherches du Service de Santé des Armées, La Tronche Cédex, France
Dr A. McKinlay	National Radiological Protection Board, Didcot, United Kingdom
Dr D. Sliney	US Army Environmental Hygiene Agency, Aberdeen Proving Ground, MD, USA
Dr M.J. Selgrade	Immunotoxicology Branch, USEPA, Research Triangle Park, NC, USA
Dr G. Johnson	Institute of Ophthalmology, University of London, London, United Kingdom
Dr B. Armstrong	International Agency for Research on Cancer, Lyon, France
Dr H. Van Loveren	National Institute of Public Health & Environmental Protection, Bilthoven, Holland
Dr A. Koppikar	Office of Health & Environmental Assessment, USEPA, Washington DC, USA
Dr R.M. Tyrrell	Swiss Institute for Cancer Research, Epalinges/Lausanne, Switzerland
Dr J.C. van der Leun	Academisch Ziekenhuis Utrecht, CX Utrecht, Holland
Dr I.A. Badr	King Khaled Eye Specialist Hospital, King Saud University, Riyadh, Saudi Arabia
Dr G. Kulandaivelu	School of Biological Sciences, Madurai Kamaraj University, Madurai, India

Dr E. Turowski	Institute for Water, Soil and Air Hygiene, Berlin, Germany

Observers

Dr B. Weatherhead	Surface Radiation Research Branch, Boulder, Colorado, USA
Dr H. Gopalan	United Nations Environment Programme (UNEP), Nairobi, Kenya
Dr A. Kulmula	World Meteorological Organization (WMO), Geneva, Switzerland
Dr A. Kricker	International Agency for Research on Cancer, Lyon, France
Dr U. Feister	Deutscher Wetterdienst, Potsdam, Germany
Dr W.H. Weihe	President, International Society of Biometeorology (ISB), Brannenburg, Germany
Dr R. Matthes	Bundesamt fur Strahlenschutz, Ingolsädter, Oberschleissheim, Germany
Dr C. Remé	Professor of Ophthalmology, Universitätsspit, Zurich, Switzerland

WHO Secretariat

Dr W. Kreisel	Executive Director, Health and Environment
Mr G. Ozolins	Manager, Prevention of Environmental Pollution
Dr T. Kjellström	Prevention of Environmental Pollution
Dr M. Repacholi	Prevention of Environmental Pollution (Secretary)
Dr B. Thylefors	Manager, Programme for the Prevention of Blindness
Dr P.-H. Lambert	Chief, Microbiology and Immunology Support Services
Dr A.-D. Négrel	Programme for the Prevention of Blindness
Dr V. Koroltchouk	Cancer and Palliative Care

NOTE TO READERS OF THE CRITERIA MONOGRAPH

Every effort has been made to present information in the criteria monographs as accurately as possible without unduly delaying their publication. In the interest of all users of the Environmental Health Criteria monographs, readers are kindly requested to communicate any errors that may have occurred to the Director of the International Programme on Chemical Safety, World Health Organization, Geneva, Switzerland, in order that they may be included in corrigenda, which will appear in subsequent volumes.

1. SUMMARY AND CONCLUSIONS

This monograph is concerned with the effects of ultraviolet (UV) radiation exposure on human health and the environment. Such a review of the scientific literature is considered timely in view of the consequences of increased levels of UV at the surface of the earth resulting from depletion of stratospheric ozone.

1.1 Physical Characteristics

Exposure to UV occurs from both natural and artificial sources. The sun is the principal source of exposure for most people. Solar UV undergoes significant absorption by the atmosphere. With depletion of the stratospheric ozone people and the environment will be exposed to higher intensities of UV. The consequences of this added UV exposure are considered so serious that it was a major topic for discussion at the World Environment Conference, held in Rio de Janeiro in 1992. In Agenda 21, adopted by the Conference, it was specifically recommended to "undertake, as a matter of urgency, research on the effects on human health of the increasing ultraviolet radiation reaching the earth's surface as the consequence of depletion of the stratospheric ozone layer." It is this issue that underscores the current need to better understand the potential health and environmental risks of UV exposure.

UV is one of the non-ionizing radiations in the electromagnetic spectrum and lies within the range of wavelengths 100 nm (which corresponds to a photon energy of approximately 12 eV) to 400 nm. The short wavelength limit of the UV region is often taken as the boundary between the ionizing radiation spectrum (wavelengths < 100 nm) and the non-ionizing radiation spectrum. UV can be classified into UVA (315 - 400 nm), UVB (280 - 315 nm) and UVC (100 - 280 nm) regions, although other conventions for UVA, UVB and UVC wavelengths bands are in use.

Most artificial sources of UV, except for lasers, emit a spectral continuum of UV containing characteristic peaks, troughs and lines. These sources include various lamps used in medicine, industry, commerce, research and the home.

UV-induced biological effects depend on the wavelengths of the radiation. It is necessary for a proper determination of hazard to have spectral emission data. These consist of spectral irradiance (W m^{-2} nm^{-1}) measurements or calculations of emissions from the source. The total irradiance (W m^{-2}) is obtained by summing over all wavelengths emitted. The biological or hazard weighted irradiance (W m^{-2} effective) is determined by multiplying the spectral irradiance at each wavelength by the biological or hazard weighting factor (which quantifies the relative efficacy at each wavelength for causing the effect) and summing over all wavelengths. Such factors are obtained from action spectra.

1.2 Action Spectrum and Minimum Erythemal Dose

An action spectrum is a graph of the reciprocal of the radiant exposure required to produce the given effect at each wavelength. All the data in such curves are normalized to the datum at the most efficacious wavelength(s). By summing the biologically effective irradiance over the exposure period, the biologically effective radiant exposure (J m^{-2} effective) can be calculated. For UV induced erythema, the action spectrum adopted by the International Commission on Non-Ionizing Radiation Protection (ICNIRP), International Commission on Illumination (CIE), the International Electrotechnical Commission (IEC) and various national bodies, is a composite curve obtained by statistical analysis of many research results on the minimum radiant exposure of UV at different wavelengths necessary to just cause erythema.

The most commonly used quantity for describing the erythemal potential of an exposure to UV is the number of minimum erythemal doses (MEDs) represented by the exposure. An MED is the radiant exposure of UV that produces a just noticeable erythema on a previously unexposed skin. It corresponds to a radiant exposure of monochromatic radiation at the maximum spectral efficacy for erythema (around 300 nm) of approximately 150 to 2000 J m^{-2} effective, depending on skin type. In this text 200 - 300 J m^{-2} effective is used as the value of 1 MED for comparative safety purposes for white skin.

1.3 Cellular and Molecular Studies

To produce any change, UV must be absorbed by the biomolecule. This involves absorption of a single photon by the molecule and the production of an excited state in which one electron of the absorbing molecule is raised to a higher energy level. The primary products caused by UV exposure are generally reactive species or free radicals which form extremely quickly but which can produce effects that can last for hours, days or even years. DNA is the most critical target for damage by UVB and UVC radiations. While a considerable amount of knowledge is available concerning the interaction of UV with nucleic acids, controversy exists as to which lesion constitutes the most important type of pre-mutagenic damage.

Cell death, chromosome changes, mutation and morphological transformations are observed after UV exposure of procaryotic and eucaryotic cells. Many different genes and several viruses (including HIV) are activated by UV exposure. The genes activated by UVB and UVC are different from those activated by UVA. Studies of DNA repair defective disorders have clearly established a link between UV induced DNA damage in skin and various types of cancer.

1.4 Animal Studies

Solar UV has been shown to produce cancers in domestic and food animals. In experimental animals UV causes predominantly squamous cell carcinomas. UVB is most effective at producing SCCs, although they are produced by UVA but at much higher intensities, similar to the levels needed for erythema and tanning. The effectiveness of UVC is unknown except at one wavelength (254 nm). At this wavelength the effectiveness is less than UVB.

Melanomas are much less common and only two animal models have been found for induction of melanoma by UV alone. An initial action spectrum determined for a type of hybrid fish indicates a peak in the UVB range but also shows a high level of effectiveness in the UVA. Basal cell carcinomas are rare in animals.

Exposure to suberythemal doses of UV have been shown to exacerbate a variety of infections in rodent models. UV affects infections both at the site of exposure and at distant sites. Recent work indicates that systemic infections without skin involvement may be affected. Enhanced susceptibility appears to result from T-helper cell activity. The mechanisms associated with this suppression appear to be the same as those identified with suppression to contact and delayed type hypersensitivity responses. Suppression of these immune responses appears to be mediated by release of soluble mediators from UVB exposed skin which alters the antigen presentation by Langerhans and other cells so that they fail to activate TH 1 cells. The resulting immune suppression is antigen specific, can occur regardless of whether or not antigen is applied at the site of exposure, and is relatively long lasting. UV exposure also prevents the development of protection immunity to a variety of infections in mice and rats.

Many studies in experimental animals have demonstrated that UV exposure can cause both acute and delayed effects such as cataract, photokeratitis, damage to the corneal epithelium and various retinal effects. Studies of photochemical retinal injury in aphakic monkeys have shown that the retina is six times more vulnerable to photochemical damage from UV than the visible wavelengths.

1.5 Health Effects on Humans

1.5.1 Skin

Acute effects on the skin consist of solar erythema, "sunburn", which, if severe enough, may result in blistering and destruction of the surface of the skin with secondary infection and systemic effects, similar to those resulting from a first or second degree heat burn. Although UVC is very efficiently absorbed by nucleic acids, the overlying dead layers of skin absorb the radiation to such a degree that there is only mild erythema and, usually, no late sequelae, even after repeated exposures. Much less is known about the biological effects of UVA. However, doses of UVA, which alone may not show any biological effect, can, in the presence of certain environmental, consumer and medicinal chemical agents, result in injury to tissues (phototoxicity, photoallergy, enhancement of photocarcinogenesis).

Chronic skin changes due to UV consist of skin cancer (both melanoma and non-melanocytic), benign abnormalities of melanocytes (freckles, melanocytic naevi and solar or senile lentigines), and a range of other chronic injuries resulting from UV exposure to keratinocytes, blood vessels and fibrous tissue, often described as "photoaging" (solar elastosis). The much increased rates of skin cancer in patients with xeroderma pigmentosum, who have a deficiency in the capacity to repair UV-induced DNA damage, suggest that direct UV damage of the DNA may be a step in the cause of these cancers. This suggestion has also been supported by the observation of UV specific mutations of the p53 tumour suppressor gene in a proportion of patients with non-melanocytic skin cancer. Oxidative and immune suppressant effects may also contribute to the capacity of UV to cause skin cancers.

Cancer of the lip is much more common in fair than dark skin populations and is associated with outdoor work. However possible confounding with tobacco and alcohol use has not been adequately controlled in any study.

The worldwide incidence of malignant melanoma has continued to increase. Strong epidemiological evidence exists that sun exposure causes cutaneous melanoma and non-melanocytic skin cancer. Their incidence is less in darker than light skin groups living in the same geographical area. Risk of skin cancer decreases with increasing pigmentation. The anatomical site most seen for squamous cell carcinoma (SCC) is the head and neck, areas most exposed to the sun. Incidence of both melanoma and non-melanocytic skin cancer are increased in areas of high ambient solar UV radiation. Melanoma is strongly related to frequency of recreational exposure to the sun and to history of sunburns.

There is suggestive evidence that exposure to sunlamps may increase the risk of melanoma, but the studies conducted so far have not consistently controlled confounding factors.

1.5.2 Immune system

A number of studies suggest that UV exposures at environmental levels suppress immune responses in both rodents and man. In rodents this immune suppression results in enhanced susceptibility to certain infectious diseases with skin involvement and some systemic infections. Mechanisms associated with UV-induced immunosuppression and host defence mechanisms which provide for protection against infectious agents, are similar in rodents and man. It is therefore reasonable to assume that exposure to UV may enhance the risk of infection and decrease the effectiveness of vaccines in humans. However additional research is necessary to substantiate this.

1.5.3 Eye

The acute effects of UV on the eyes consist of the development of photokeratitis and photoconjunctivitis, which are unpleasant but usually reversible and easily prevented by appropriate eyewear. Chronic effects on the eye consist of the development of pterygium and squamous cell cancer of the conjunctiva and cataracts. A review of the studies suggests that there is sufficient evidence to link acute ocular exposure to photokeratitis but our knowledge of the effects of chronic exposure is less certain. While there is sufficient evidence that cortical and posterior subcapsular cataracts (PSC) can be caused by UVB in laboratory animals, there is limited evidence to link cortical and PSC cataracts in humans to chronic ocular exposure to UVB. Insufficient information is available to separate out the other factors contributing to cataract formation, or to state the proportion of cataracts which can be attributed to UVB exposure. There is also limited evidence to link the development of climatic droplet keratopathy and pterygium, but insufficient evidence to link uveal melanoma with UV exposure.

1.6 Environment

Increased levels of UV due to ozone layer depletion may have serious consequences for living organisms. A 10% reduction in ozone could lead to as much as a 15-20% increase in UV exposure depending on the biological process being considered. While the impact on human health, crop production, fisheries etc. is largely unknown, adverse effects of increased exposure to UVB have been reported on plant growth, photosynthesis and disease resistance. Further, the impact of increased UV levels on aquatic ecosystems (the major contributor to the earth's biomass) may be substantial. Phytoplankton, at the base of the aquatic food chain, serves as food for larvae of fish and shrimp. These in turn are consumed by fish, which subsequently provide an essential food source for many human beings and other animals. A significant reduction in phytoplankton from increased UVB exposure will directly affect the human and animal marine food source.

1.7 Guidelines on Exposure Limits and Protective Measures

Guidance on exposure limits for UV are described in chapter 13. International guidelines define exposure limits (ELs) below which it is expected that nearly all people may be repeatedly exposed without adverse effects. The ELs are intended to be used to evaluate potentially hazardous exposures from, for example, solar radiation, arcs, gas and vapour discharges, fluorescent lamps and incandescent sources. The ELs are generally below levels which are often used for the UV exposure of patients required as part of medical treatment and below levels associated with sunbed exposure. ELs are not intended to apply to exposure of pathologically photosensitive individuals, to people concomitantly exposed to photosensitising agents or to neonates.

Finally this monograph describes protection and control measures such as the containment of UV sources, and methods for personal protection including the use of sunscreen preparations, clothing, eye and skin protection, and behavioural modifications.

While topical application of sunscreen is a preferred method of absorbing UVB, some preparations do not absorb the longer wavelength UVA effectively. Moreover, some have been found to contain ingredients that are mutagenic in sunlight. There is still much research necessary before the impact on health of increased levels of UVA will be known. In the meantime people using sunscreens should use only those with the highest sun protection factor (SPF) and be aware that they are for their protection from the sun and not for tanning purposes. Use of wide brimmed hats, protective clothing and UV absorbing eye glasses is still the best personal protection against the adverse effects of UV exposure.

With increasing levels of solar UV resulting from depletion of the ozone layer, and the continuing rise in the level of melanoma worldwide, people should become more aware of their UV exposure and take appropriate precautions. These precautions include staying out of the sun during the period around noon (the period when the UV levels are highest), or wearing UV protective clothing, hats and sun glasses. Broad spectrum (UVB and UVA protective) sunscreens should be used when other means of protection are not feasible. These sunscreens should be used to reduce exposure rather than lengthen the period of exposure to the sun. Protection of young children is particularly important for the prevention of long-term consequences of UV exposure. In general behavioural patterns must change to protect against increasing solar UV levels.

2. PHYSICAL CHARACTERISTICS

2.1 Electromagnetic Spectrum

Oscillations of electromagnetic fields can cause energy to be transported in the form of electromagnetic radiation. Examples of this type of radiative transport of energy include radiofrequency waves, light and x rays. Ultraviolet (UV) radiation is one form of electromagnetic energy in the optical region of the electromagnetic spectrum. All electromagnetic radiation is characterized by frequency f and wavelength λ. These two quantities are linked through the relationship:

$$f = c/\lambda$$

where c is the speed of light ($3\ 10^8$ m s^{-1}). The energy of a single photon is determined by the wavelength of the photon as described by the relationship

$$\text{(photon energy)} = hf = hc/\lambda \quad \text{where } h = 1.24 \text{ eV nm}$$

Non-ionizing radiation (NIR) is the term generally applied to all forms of electromagnetic radiation whose primary mode of interaction with matter is other than by producing ionization. NIR refers to electromagnetic fields and radiation with wavelengths exceeding 100 nm, which is equivalent to quantum (photon) energies below 12.4 eV, the minimum energy needed to break the weakest macromolecular bonds. The non-ionizing spectrum encompasses all fields of radiation from UV to DC fields.

For purposes of health protection, the optical portion of NIR can be subdivided into several wavelength ranges, as shown in table 2.1. The nomenclature was standardized by the International Commission on Illumination (CIE) however, some scientists use a modification of this system by shifting the 315 nm break point between UVA and UVB to 320 nm; the reader should always check the definition given in each publication. For the purposes of this document, the CIE convention is followed.

Table 2.1 Optical Radiation Spectral Bands

Ultraviolet radiation	100 - 400 nm
UVA	315 - 400 nm
UVB	280 - 315 nm
UVC	100 - 280 nm
Visible radiation (light)	400 - 760 nm
Infrared radiation (IR)	760 - 10^6 nm = 1 mm

UV of wavelengths less than 180 nm has no direct biological effect on humans since it is effectively absorbed in a few centimetres of air. For this reason, the spectral region below 180 nm is frequently referred to as the *vacuum ultraviolet region.*

2.2 Radiometric Quantities and Units

Radiometric quantities are absolute physical quantities used to describe the characteristics of a source or radiation field. For UV, ten generic radiometric terms are summarized in table 2.2. Each of these quantities can be defined for a certain wavelength or frequency range, or can be integrated over the whole spectrum of a given source. Since UV is normally absorbed over a surface, with very limited penetration depth, the most common quantities used to describe exposure dose and dose rate to UV are: radiant exposure (incident energy divided by the receptor surface area) and irradiance (incident power divided by the receptor surface area) respectively. Radiant exitance is the power per area of the emitted radiation *at the emitting surface.* The receptor surface is most often considered as a flat plane. However, for some biological and chemical purposes, the radiation incident on a cylindrical or spherical surface may also be considered.

For the purpose of radiation protection, physical quantities are needed to describe sources and fields of radiation as well as the interaction of this optical radiation with matter. These are described in IRPA/INIRC(1985).

2.3 UV Production

Sources of electromagnetic radiation can be categorized in several different ways; for example they can be grouped according to the type of material or the type of equipment that produces the radiation. At the submicroscopic level, the manner in which the radiation originates can be described in terms of nuclear, electronic or molecular transitions between

Table 2.2 Radiometric terminology for UV: Useful radiometric quantities and units

Quantity	Symbol	Defining equation	Unit and abbreviation
Radiant energy	Q_e	$Q_e = \int \Phi_e \, dt$	joule (J) = 1 watt second
Radiant energy density	W_e	$W_e = \frac{dQ_e}{dV}$	joule per cubic metre ($J\ m^{-3}$)
Radiant flux (radiant power)	Φ_e , P	$\Phi_e = \frac{dQ_e}{dt}$	watt (W)
Radiant exitance	M_e	$M_e = \frac{d\Phi_e}{dA} = \int L_e \cos\theta \, d\Omega$	watt per square metre ($W\ m^{-2}$)
Irradiance or Radiant Flux Density	E_e	$E_e = \frac{d\Phi_e}{dA}$	watt per square metre ($W\ m^{-2}$)
Radiant intensity	I_e	$I_e = \frac{d\Phi_e}{d\Omega}$	watt per steradian ($W\ sr^{-1}$)
Radiance[1]	L_e	$L_e = \frac{d^2\Phi_e}{d\Omega \, dA \cos\theta}$	watt per steradian per square metre ($W\ sr^{-1}\ m^{-2}$)
Radiant exposure (dose in photobiology)	H_e	$H_e = \frac{dQ_e}{dA}$	joule per square metre ($J\ m^{-2}$)
Radiant efficiency[2] (of a source)	n_e	$n_e = \frac{P}{P_i}$	unitless
Optical density[3]	D_e	$D_e = -\log_{10}(\tau_e)$	unitless

NOTE: All terms in this table are radiometric terms and should not be confused with photometric terms. The symbol A represents surface area, Ω is solid angle, θ is the incident (zenith) angle, V represents volume, t is time. The units may also refer to narrow spectral bands in which the term is preceded by the word *spectral* and the unit is then per wavelength interval and the symbol has a subscript λ. For example, spectral irradiance E_λ has units of $W\ m^{-2}\ nm^{-1}$ or $W\ cm^{-2}\ nm^{-1}$. While the metre is the preferred unit of length, the centimetre is still commonly used for many of the above terms and the nm or µm are most commonly used to express wavelength.

1. At the source $L = \frac{dI}{dA \cos\theta}$ and at a receptor $L = \frac{dE}{d\Omega \cos\theta}$
2. P_i is electrical input power in watts
3. This formula applies only to situations where the radiation is not scattered, but only absorbed. In this case τ represents the fraction of transmitted energy.

energy states or by the acceleration of charged particles. Common sources of UV emission involve energy transitions between electronic states of molecules in materials.

2.3.1 *Thermal emitters*

When the temperature of a material increases, electrons in the molecules are raised to higher energy states, a variety of energy transitions take place and photons are emitted. The higher the temperature the greater is the fraction of these photons at higher energies. Matter at temperatures above 2500 K emits a significant number of photons in the UV spectral range. The emission spectra of such incandescent sources are characteristically smooth - so-called "continuum", possibly with superimposed spectral emission lines.

The spectral emission of a heated material is governed by basic physical laws. The Stefan-Boltzmann Law expresses the total radiation emitted by a heated material as a function of its temperature. The total radiant power emitted by a theoretically perfect radiator, a so-called black body, is proportional to the fourth power of its temperature (in kelvin, K). Any practical thermal emitter in equilibrium emits less radiant power than its equivalent black body at the same temperature and unlike a black body the amount depends on the nature of its surface. The spectral distribution of black body radiation is described by the Planck Radiation Law. Wien's Displacement Law is illustrated in figure 2.1, and describes mathematically the spectral distribution of emission from a black body and the wavelength of the maximum emission shift to shorter wavelengths as temperature increases. When a material is heated so that incandescence occurs, it first appears red and, with increasing temperature, progresses to white or blue.

2.3.2 *Electrical gaseous discharges*

Radiation may be produced when an electric current is passed through a gas or vapour. Atoms may be ionized if sufficient energy is transferred from a moving electron. Alternatively the moving electron may not impart sufficient energy for ionization, but instead may impart energy to raise the electrons of the gas to an excited (higher) energy level. When they return to a lower energy level, or their ground state, radiation of one or more characteristic wavelengths is emitted. The wavelengths of emission are determined by the type of gas or vapour present in the discharge and appear as spectral emission lines. The width of the lines and the amount of radiation in the interval between them depends on the pressure of the discharge. At low pressure, fine lines with little or no continuum are

Figure 2.1 Black-body spectra. Line AB shows Wien's Displacement Law for the shift of the peak wavelength with change in absolute temperature (in K) (from Sliney & Wolbarsht, 1980).

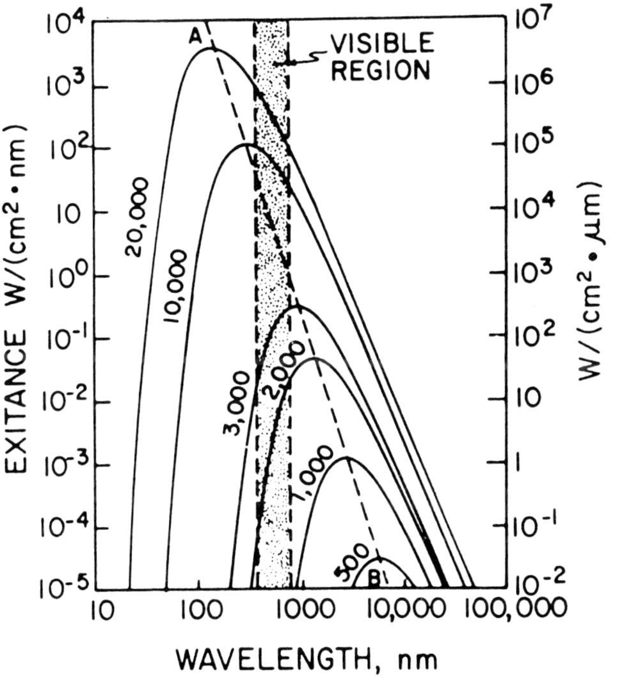

produced. As the pressure of the discharge is raised the lines broaden and their relative magnitudes alter. The magnitude of the continuum increases. The electrical gaseous discharge is the basis of operation of many UV emitting lamps.

2.3.3 *Stimulated emission*

Radiation can be produced by the specific electronic transition process of stimulated emission. This depends on the ability of the radiating medium to undergo "population inversion", i.e., achieving a condition where there are more atoms or molecules in a higher energy excited state than in a lower one. Once population inversion occurs an avalanche of photons can be generated by stimulated emission. Initially, spontaneously emitted photons stimulate other excited atoms to emit photons of the same energy in phase with one another. This is the basis of operation of the laser.

2.4 Summary

UV is a part of the non-ionizing region of the electromagnetic spectrum. Its position in the spectrum can be characterised by wavelength and it is quantified using radiometric quantities and units. Production of UV is possible by different mechanisms that are all based on atomic or molecular excitation. Excitation in a medium can be achieved by thermal, electrical or optical energy absorption. Emission of radiation is caused either by de-excitation or by stimulated synchronised processes.

3. UV SOURCES

3.1 The Sun

The sun is the main source of UV. The broad spectrum and intensity of UV from the sun are due to the high temperature at its surface and its size. The intensity of solar UV reaching the earth's atmosphere would probably be lethal to most living organisms on the earth's surface without the shielding afforded by the atmosphere. Solar UV undergoes absorption and scattering as it passes through the earth's atmosphere with absorption by molecular oxygen and ozone being the most important processes. The ozone layer prevents almost all UV of wavelengths $\lambda < 290$ nm and a substantial fraction (in excess of 90% of the total energy) from 290 - 315 nm from reaching the earth's surface. Thus the terrestrial environment is exposed to UV between 290 nm and 400 nm. The spectrum, both before passage through the atmosphere and at sea level, is shown in figure 3.1

The solar radiation reaching the top of the earth's atmosphere is affected by the solar output and the earth-sun distance. Variations in solar output are much smaller than the variations caused by atmospheric attenuation factors. The irradiance incident on the top of the earth's atmosphere is summarised in table 3.1, but will vary with the exact distance of the earth from the sun at a particular time. The extreme values associated with this variation are approximately $\pm$ 3.3% above and below the annual mean and occur in January and July respectively.

Table 3.1 Spectral distribution of solar radiation prior to attenuation by the earth's atmosphere (Frederick et al., 1989).

Wavelength band	Irradiance (W m^{-2})	Percent of total
UVC	6.4	0.5
UVB	21.1	1.5
UVA	85.7	6.3
Total UV	113.2	8.3
Visible and IR	1254	91.7

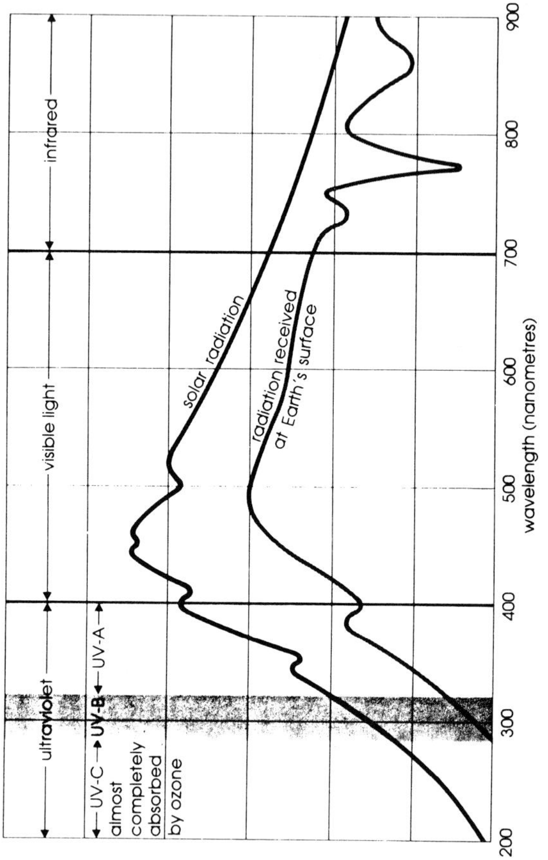

Figure 3.1 Solar optical radiation attenuation by the earth's atmosphere. (from UNEP, 1987).

The atmosphere has a profound effect on the irradiance which reaches the surface of the earth. In January (in the northern hemisphere) or July (in the southern hemisphere) when the solar elevation is low, direct UV travels a longer path through the atmosphere and a large amount of scattering occurs. In addition, much of the resultant scattered UV propagates downwards to the earth's surface at angles to the horizontal that are larger than the solar elevation, hence travelling a shorter and less absorptive path. This results in large ratios of scattered to direct UV. During the summer the ratio of diffuse to direct UV is smaller.

3.1.1 *Factors affecting solar UV levels*

The total solar UV reaching the earth's surface, termed global UV can be divided into two components: direct and diffuse. Global UV reaching a horizontal surface is the quantity most often measured. For biological entities such as people and trees, UV hitting cylindrical or spherical surfaces may be more important.

The amount and spectral distribution of solar UV irradiance reaching the earth's surface depends on a number of factors, including

(a) wavelength of the UV
(b) solar zenith angle, which depends on latitude, date of the year and time of day
(c) solar source spectrum incident at the top of the atmosphere
(d) ozone column thickness and vertical distribution
(e) molecular absorption and scattering (including localized gaseous pollutants)
(f) aerosol absorption and scattering (including anthropogenic aerosols)
(g) absorption, scattering and reflection by clouds
(h) reflectance characteristics (albedo) of the ground
(i) shadowing by surrounding objects
(j) altitude above sea level

The presence of cloud cover, air pollution, haze, or even scattered clouds, plays a significant role in attenuating UV. UVB and UVA irradiances are reduced due to scattering by water droplets and/or ice crystals in the clouds. Clouds can block a significant portion of the UV which would have otherwise reached the surface.

Cloud cover and type are highly variable. The transmission of UV radiation through clouds depends on cloud height, type and optical density.

The resultant effect on UV transmission is difficult to assess particularly in the case of partial cloudiness. The effect of cloudiness on the solar irradiation of a horizontal plane can be approximated by

$$F = 1 - 0.056\ C$$

where C is the total cloud index in tenths of sky covered from 0 to 10, 10 being complete sky cover. Thus for complete cloud cover, the transmitted UV irradiance would decrease by 72% and for half cloud cover by 44%. In extreme cases cloud cover can decrease UV irradiance by over 90%. Estimates of the average reduction of UVB due to clouds (relative to cloudless skies) based on satellite measurements of backscattered solar UV are 30% at 60 degrees latitude, 10% at 20 degrees latitude and 20% at the equator.

3.1.2 *Ozone depletion effects*

Over 90% of the total atmospheric ozone resides in the stratosphere (the upper atmosphere). The total ozone column is important for filtering solar UV. Only UVB is affected by changes in the ozone column. UVC is almost completely absorbed by ozone and oxygen in the atmosphere; even with severe ozone reduction UVC would still be effectively absorbed by the remaining oxygen.

As stratospheric ozone levels decrease, the resulting higher levels of solar UVB could increase the production of reactive OH radical molecules, potentially increasing the chemical reactivity of the troposphere. In polluted areas with sufficient concentrations of oxides of nitrogen (NO_x) (above 0.5 ppb by volume) and hydrocarbon compounds this enhanced reactivity is calculated to result in greater levels of tropospheric ozone and other potentially harmful oxidized products, such as hydrogen peroxide and acids.

The amount of ozone in the free troposphere is increasing for example over central europe and other parts of the globe. The effect of these trends on UV radiation needs to be studied further (WMO, 1993). For high sun angles, tropospheric ozone is a more effective absorber of UV radiation than stratospheric ozone because of the increased path length of scattered radiation in the lower atmosphere (Brühl & Crutzen, 1989).

The total ozone column is not uniform but varies with latitude and time of year. At the same latitude, away from the equator and tropics, the total ozone column tends to be greater in spring than in autumn. Thus, even though the sun angles are the same on March 21 and September 21, the differences in total ozone column result in more UVB in early autumn than in early spring. If cloud cover and atmospheric pollution are not taken into account, in the tropics, the relatively constant ozone column and the similar solar angles throughout the year, result in little variation in solar UVB with season.

Changes in total column ozone were observed by both ground based and satellite based instruments from the WMO Global Ozone Observing System. The measurements show pronounced ozone depletion over Antarctica in months 9-12 (local early spring) (UNEP-WMO, 1989). Increases in biologically effective UVB were observed during this same time period (NSF, 1993). Over representation of UVA in the common broad band meter action spectrum, relative to most biological action spectra, produces less pronounced relative and absolute changes in assessed UVB. Therefore under cloud free conditions common broad band meters are less sensitive in assessing the ground level UVB effects of ozone depletion than detectors with a steeper action spectrum response such as for DNA damage or for erythema.

3.1.3 *Trends in UV*

There have been no significant changes in ozone at the equator. Total column ozone over the Northern mid-latitudes has decreased by several percent over the past two decades. Efforts to detect changes in UV over long time periods have failed due to changes in column ozone.

Besides the problems indicated in the interpretation and comparison of measurement data from different sites and sources, there are also insufficient direct solar terrestrial UVB measurements for constructing a global climatology or trend assessment due to some of the following (Driscoll 1992):

(a) problems in establishing appropriate instrumentation: either highly sophisticated and reliable spectral instruments or broad band instruments which fairly represent the sensitivities of different biological and chemical targets (with different wavelength dependencies and sensitivity to different orientations),

(b) difficulty of maintaining accurate field instrument calibrations over many years, and

(c) practical limitations in establishing a global monitoring network especially with the potential for disturbance from locally polluted areas.

With insufficient spectral measurement data collected over long periods, data from the more extensively used broad-band measurement systems have been scrutinised. UV data from eight stations in the US showed decreases in UVB between 0.5% and 1.1% per year during the time period of 1974-1985 (Scotto et al., 1988). However, this result does not agree with theoretical predictions and may be due to problems in the long-term calibration of meters or local pollution in mainly urban or semi-urban sites (Munkata, 1993; Smith & Ryan 1993). In Russia, a 12% decrease of UVB was observed in Moscow between 1968 and 1983 with a concurrent 15% increase in turbidity and a 13% increase in cloudiness. At the Jungfraujoch observing station in the Swiss alps (3.6 km above sea level), increases of $0.7 \pm 0.2\%$ per year in UVB were observed under clear sky conditions between 1981 and 1989. A comparison of summer spectral data weighted with the CIE erythemal action spectrum using the same instrumentation at Lauder, New Zealand (45°S) and Neuherberg, Germany (48°N) showed weighted UV irradiances were 1.6 times larger in New Zealand due to decreased ozone column thickness (24% lower than in Germany). Spectral filter measurements at 39° N between 1976 though 1990 showed large increases in monthly maximum values which were not statistically significant (Correll et al., 1992).

3.1.4 *Theoretical models*

To overcome some of the deficiencies in interpreting the results from solar UV measurements, theoretical models have been used to predict UV levels. However, the theoretical determination of the spectral distribution of global UV including the effects of cloud cover and ground reflection is extremely complex. There are three categories of models to predict UV transmission. Empirical and semi-empirical models are useful for assessing daily or annual erythemal doses as a function of latitude, solar zenith angle, cloud cover and ground albedo. These models have been used for a long time at a variety of locations. Two of the most common examples are the models of Green et al. (1974) and Diffey (1977)

Two stream models simulate the radiative transfer through the atmosphere. They have been well verified with field data from Antarctica as well as mid-latitudes (e.g. Frederick et al., 1989).

Multistream models allow for the angular distribution of UV transmission. This is useful for more detailed dosimetry (Stamnes et al., 1988).

The maximum erythemally effective UVB irradiances, calculated by the Diffey model, are shown in table 3.2 for the Northern Hemisphere, as a function of latitude and time of year at sea level (Driscoll 1992). There are strong seasonal and latitudinal variations in UVB. Under cloudless skies, the UVB is more intense in summer and at all times of year is greater at lower latitudes. The solar elevation angle determines the length of the path of the sun's rays as they penetrate the atmosphere. When the sun is low in the sky, the path through the atmosphere is longer and the filtering action of the air is therefore increased. When the sun is directly overhead, the sun's rays have the shortest path through the atmosphere. Approximately 50% of the daily UV is received during the middle four hours around noon when the sun is high in the sky (Sliney, 1987).

The number of minimum erythemal doses (MEDs) in a 3 hour exposure period around noon for fair skin is shown as a function of latitude and time of year in table 3.3 for the Northern Hemisphere. For example, at 55°N (Newcastle), a calculated value of 6 MED would be received for a sensitive skin type in a 3 hour exposure around noon on a clear day in July (1 MED per half hour exposure).

Comparing the values in table 3.2 with the results of calculations using the model developed by Frederick et al. (1989) for clear sky conditions at noon, the latter are typically 50% higher. This may be due to differences in the biological action spectra used or in the spectral irradiance data calculated. The R-B meter response characteristic used by Frederick et al. (1989) does not follow the CIE reference erythema action spectrum used in the model developed by Diffey (1977) at wavelengths greater than 300 nm.

3.1.5 *UV monitoring*

Recent public and scientific concern about ozone depletion and increased UV have lead to the establishment of many UV monitoring centres in the last few years. Five years ago less than fifty UV monitoring stations were operating around the world. Today more than 250 monitoring centres are underway for a variety of reasons. Governmental agencies, scientific institutions, universities and private groups have begun to monitor UV. The World Meteorological Organization (WMO) has established a global network called Global Atmosphere Watch (GAB). It presently has eight observatory stations that make continuous spectral and broad band UV measurements. The Global Environment Facility is supporting the creation of 10-15 additional stations in developing countries. Various national and multi-national agencies are also operating and establishing UV monitoring networks.

Table 3.2 Calculated clear sky noontime erythemally effective UVB irradiances (mW m^{-2} CIE erythemally weighted) on a horizontal surface as a function of latitude (°) and time of year for the sea level in the Northern Hemisphere using typical ozone values (Driscoll, 1992).

	Jan	Feb	Mar	Apr	May	Jun	Jul	Aug	Sep	Oct	Nov	Dec
0	229	251	260	229	210	207	214	233	278	248	226	221
5	212	232	242	235	214	213	220	241	258	227	207	206
10	203	220	229	248	226	225	232	255	244	215	198	175
15	155	199	201	227	221	226	234	240	223	198	155	135
20	127	183	191	215	234	239	247	227	212	184	127	111
25	95	134	165	185	203	227	219	200	194	143	101	84
30	79	110	157	176	192	215	208	190	186	117	85	56
35	42	80	114	146	160	188	182	166	148	93	50	31
40	28	61	93	139	152	178	172	158	121	73	33	21
45	16	33	66	105	126	158	153	128	93	42	21	13
50	12	22	54	85	119	150	145	104	77	28	15	8
55	6	14	33	65	92	130	114	81	48	18	8	4
60	4	10	21	53	75	105	93	67	31	12	5	2
65	0	6	14	35	59	85	76	42	21	7	2	0
70	0	3	10	23	48	70	62	29	15	4	0	0
75	0	0	6	15	30	53	39	20	9	0	0	0
80	0	0	3	11	20	33	26	14	5	0	0	0
85	0	0	2	7	14	23	18	9	2	0	0	0
90	0	0	0	4	10	16	13	5	0	0	0	0

Table 3.3 Number of MEDs in a 3 h exposure period for a sensitive skin type (1 MED = 200 J m^{-2} effective) for the erythemally effective UVB irradiances given in table 3.2 as a function of latitude (°) and time of year for the Northern Hemisphere (Driscoll 1992).

	Jan	Feb	Mar	Apr	May	Jun	Jul	Aug	Sep	Oct	Nov	Dec
0	12	14	14	12	11	11	12	13	15	13	12	12
5	11	13	13	13	12	12	12	13	14	12	11	11
10	11	12	12	13	12	12	13	14	13	12	11	9
15	8	11	11	12	12	12	13	13	12	11	8	7
20	7	10	10	12	13	13	13	12	11	10	7	6
25	5	7	9	10	11	12	12	11	10	8	5	5
30	4	6	8	10	10	12	11	10	10	6	5	3
35	2	4	6	8	9	10	10	9	8	5	3	2
40	2	3	5	8	8	10	9	9	7	4	2	1
45	1	2	4	6	7	9	8	7	5	2	1	1
50	1	1	3	5	6	8	8	6	4	2	1	0
55	0	1	2	4	5	7	6	4	3	1	0	0
60	0	1	1	3	4	6	5	4	2	1	0	0
65	0	0	1	2	3	5	4	2	1	0	0	0
70	0	0	1	1	3	4	3	2	1	0	0	0
75	0	0	0	1	2	3	2	1	0	0	0	0
80	0	0	0	1	1	2	1	1	0	0	0	0
85	0	0	0	0	1	1	1	0	0	0	0	0
90	0	0	0	0	1	1	1	0	0	0	0	0

The reasons for monitoring UV are generally divided into the following four areas:

(i) to provide information to the public on UV levels and variations,

(ii) establishing a basic UV climatology,

(iii) studying cause and effects of UV transmission, and

(iv) detecting long term variability.

While these reasons are not mutually exclusive they can often dictate the type of care taken with instrument maintenance. The quality and care needed for trend detection requires a great deal more effort than for UV measurements to provide public information.

There are many difficulties in making accurate field measurements of ambient UV. Care must be taken that no part of the instrument is shaded from either direct or indirect sun; nearby surfaces must not change during the time period of monitoring; and routine maintenance such as snow and debris removal must be conducted systematically to avoid trend bias. The value of the measurements for trend detection rely on diligent maintenance of the site including co-located measurements. The data must have spectral, temporal and angular resolution appropriate for validation of model calculations and for evaluation of biological effects (spectral resolution better than <1 nm). Broad band instruments are useful for establishing climatology and operations where spectral instruments are not practical.

Frequent and reliable calibration of the instrumentation is necessary. UV monitoring for the detection of trends is difficult and failure to detect a trend may be due to lack of awareness of changes in instrument behaviour and correction of it. Intercomparison of different types of UV monitoring instruments have shown that individual instrument characteristics can cause substantial differences in measurements. Further intercomparisons are necessary to understand and reduce the uncertainties of measurements.

3.1.6 *Analysis of UV data*

Atmospheric UV data are difficult to analyze. To date all UV data have been analyzed separately by each investigator and in a different manner. This variation in analysis makes the interpretation and comparison of results difficult. Unfortunately, the data are normally not easily obtained and re-analyzed for comparative studies.

UV data pose difficult problems because they are not generally independent and normally distributed, therefore robust time series techniques should be used to analyze the data correctly. Standard techniques, depending on how they are applied, can greatly over or under estimate the confidence in the observed trends, as well as supply spurious trends when used on UV data. Bishop (1992) has suggested that using proper statistical techniques, at least ten years of data will be necessary to correctly detect a trend of 5% per decade. This estimate was made based on analysis of a single station's data independently. However, analysing groups of data may allow trend detection in less time.

3.1.7 *Conclusions*

The earth's atmosphere has a profound effect on the UV irradiance reaching the earth's surface. It absorbs a large fraction of the incident UV and changes part to diffuse radiation. Variations in UV intensity depend on solar zenith angle, atmospheric ozone, cloudiness, aerosol load and other factors.

One of the most important tools to determine climatological values and long-term changes in solar UV radiation is the monitoring of solar UV. Atmospheric parameters which modulate UV need to be observed in parallel to help explain the changes observed in the measurements. The existing data base is much too scarce to derive climatological values and trends on global or regional scales. Efforts are being made to establish national and international networks for measurements of solar UV radiation.

Models that simulate typical values and predictions of changes in UV radiation for different atmospheric conditions are also used. The results from these models need to be compared with measurements.

3.2 Artificial Sources

Artificial sources of UV are commonplace. There are few artificial sources that result in human exposure to UV greater than that from the sun. However, exceptions are those used for medical therapy and diagnosis, cosmetic tanning. Industrial sources are generally effectively enclosed, but accidental exposure may occur. There are very few non-laser sources of optical radiation that emit UV solely.

Any unfiltered optical source, whose emissions are due to the heating of a material e.g. a filament lamp, that emits significant quantities of UV will also emit visible and infrared radiations. In the case of high temperature tungsten halogen lamps biologically significant amounts of shorter wavelength UVB are also emitted. Essentially the same holds true for high intensity (gaseous) discharge (HID) lamps. Some incandescent and HID lamps have sufficient intrinsic filtration in the glass envelope of the lamp. However, additional filtration, afforded by incorporation of the lamp in a suitably filtered luminaire, may be necessary.

Most man-made sources of UV can be grouped together in the categories shown below. The spectrum of the UV emitted varies from one source to another.

Incandescent sources
- tungsten lamps

Gas discharges
- mercury lamps (low-, medium- and high-pressure)
- mercury lamps with metal halides
- xenon lamps
- hydrogen and deuterium lamps
- flash tubes

Electric discharges
- welding arcs
- carbon arcs

Fluorescent lamps
- fluorescent lighting tubes
- fluorescent sunlamps (UVB emitters)
- fluorescent UVA tubes

Lasers
- excimer laser
- dye laser
- gas laser

3.2.1 *Incandescent sources*

When a material is heated a large number of energy transitions occur within its molecules and optical photons are emitted. An ideally efficient emitter (radiator) is termed a black body radiator. The total radiant power and its spectral distribution depend only on the temperature of the black body. The spectral emissions in terms of spectral radiant exitance of a black body radiator for different temperatures are illustrated in figure 3.2

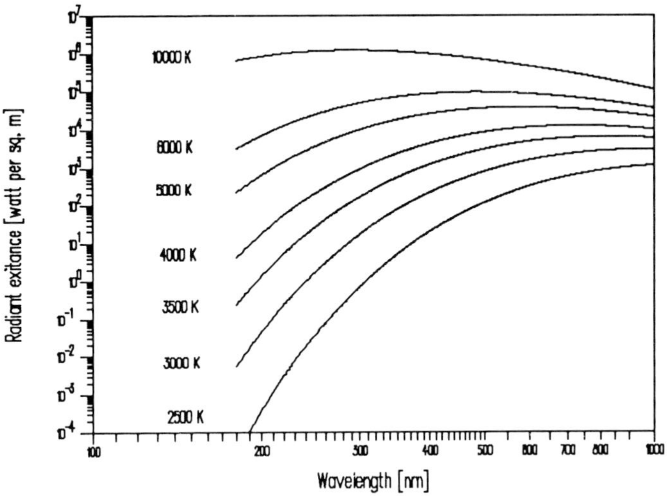

Figure 3.2 Spectral emissions of black body radiators at different temperatures (McKinlay et al., 1988)

and tabulated in table 3.4 (McKinlay et al., 1988). The wavelength corresponding to the peak of the spectral emission of a black body radiator varies inversely as its temperature and as the temperature increases an increasing amount of UV is emitted. Incandescent sources whose temperatures are greater than about 2900 K emit significant amounts of UV with respect to possible effects on human health. The optical emission of the sun corresponds approximately to that of a black body radiator at a temperature of around 6000 K.

By integrating over all wavelengths the area under an absolute plot of spectral radiant exitance against wavelength, the total radiant exitance M can be determined by the formula:

$$M = \sigma T^4$$

where σ = Stefan-Boltzmann constant (5.67×10^{-3} W m^{-2} K^{-4})
and T = absolute temperature (K).

Table 3.4 Approximate radiant exitances of black body sources at different temperatures

Temperature K	UVB/C 200-315 nm [W m^{-2}]	UVA 315-340 nm [W m^{-2}]	UVA 340-400 nm [W m^{-2}]
1500	8.6×10^{-5}	5.6×10^{-4}	2.7×10^{-2}
2000	2.4×10^{-1}	7.9×10^{-1}	14.2
2500	29	62	634
3000	760	1147	8095
3500	8050	9220	5×10^{4}
4000	4.8×10^{4}	4.4×10^{4}	2×10^{5}
5000	6.3×10^{5}	4×10^{5}	1.4×10^{6}
6000	3.6×10^{6}	1.7×10^{6}	5×10^{6}
10000	1.4×10^{8}	3.2×10^{7}	6.9×10^{7}

In practice no material emits radiation with a black body spectrum. However, tungsten at high temperatures (such as used for the filaments of ordinary and tungsten halogen incandescent lamps) and molten metals approximate to theoretical black bodies. Such sources are termed grey bodies. The ratio of the actual spectral radiant exitance to the theoretical black body spectral radiant exitance is a measure of how closely the grey body approximates in its spectral emission at a particular wavelength to a black body and is termed the spectral emissivity (ε_λ). Similarly, by summation over all wavelengths, the total radiant exitance M of a material is given by

$$M = \varepsilon\sigma T^4$$

where ε is the emissivity.

The emissivity depends on the material and on its surface structure, and is a function of wavelength. For example, for tungsten at 3000 K (typical of a tungsten halogen lamp filament), the emissivity varies from an average of about 0.45 in the UVA region to about 0.2 in the IRB (1.4 - 3.0 μm) region.

The incandescent lamp is the oldest type of electric lamp still in common use. The optical radiation from incandescent lamps results from the heating of tungsten filaments which, with the exception of lamps for some photographic and graphic arts applications, are not heated to temperatures in excess of about 3000 K. Typical gas-filled incandescent filament lamps operate between 2700 and 3000 K with electrical input powers up to 500 W and the peaks of their spectral emissions are in the infra-red (IRA) region. The emissions of UV by tungsten filament lamps are generally negligible with respect to human health.

In applications where greater power (up to 5 kW) is required, tungsten-halogen (often called quartz-halogen) lamps are often used. These are quartz envelope tungsten filament lamps to which a halogen vapour (usually iodine) is added. The presence of the vapour enables operation at an increased gas pressure compared with conventional incandescent lamps, and evaporation from the filament is minimized. These features result in improved luminous efficacy and longer life. In order to operate efficiently, the temperature of the wall of the bulb must be maintained at not less than 260 °C. The majority of the bulbs of tungsten-halogen lamps are made from silica (quartz) whose thermal properties are most suitable. The combination of filament temperatures which are likely to be in the range 2900 to 3450 K and quartz bulbs results in a significantly higher level of emission of potentially harmful UV compared with ordinary tungsten filament lamps. The incorporation of suitable secondary filtration to reduce UV emissions to an acceptable level is an important feature of the design of any illumination system using tungsten halogen lamps (McKinlay et al., 1989).

3.2.2 *Gaseous discharge sources*

The electrical excitation of a gas or vapour is a typical mechanism for generating optical radiation. An electric current is passed through a gas or a mixture of gases ionized to produce electrons and positive ions. Emissions are the result of electronic transitions in the atoms of a material from low to high energy states (absorption and excitation) followed by transitions from the high to low energy states (de-excitation and emission). This process is often combined with the process of luminescence, whereby the characteristic (line) photon emissions of the gas are absorbed by a luminescent material (luminophor or phosphor) which in turn emits optical radiation, typically as a continuum over a range of longer wavelengths. The 253.7 nm UV emission from a low pressure mercury vapour discharge is used as a source of excitation in low pressure fluorescent lamps. By raising the pressure of the discharge to a few atmospheres the emission lines increasingly broaden effectively forming a continuum. In some cases the 253.7 nm line emission will be self-absorbed by the vapour of the discharge.

Low pressure discharge lamps

Germicidal lamps

The low pressure mercury-discharge lamp is often used for the purpose of germicide and disinfection. Such lamps are very efficient emitters of UV. Approximately 50% of the electrical power is converted to UV of which up to 95% is emitted at a wavelength of 253.7 nm (see figure 3.3). Germicidal type lamps are available in a range of sizes, shapes and powers. Small, low-wattage (5-10 W) germicidal lamps are often used as fluorescence-inducing lamps for the purposes of, for example, chromatographic analysis and the fluorescence identification and authentication of documents. The quartz envelopes of some lamps in this category transmit 185 nm wavelength radiation characteristic of mercury vapour.

Fluorescent lamps

The most common application of the low-pressure discharge is fluorescent lamps. These operate by means of a discharge between two electrodes through a mixture of mercury vapour and a rare gas, usually argon. Light is produced by conversion of 253.7 nm mercury emission to longer wavelength radiations by means of a phosphor coating on the inside of the glass envelope of the lamp. Lamps are available with many different phosphors and envelopes to produce a wide range of spectral emissions covering the visible (light), UVA and UVB regions. While the continuum emissions of fluorescent lamps are characteristic of the phosphors the narrow peak, spectral emissions are dominated by the characteristic line emission spectrum of the low-pressure mercury vapour discharge.

General lighting fluorescent lamps

These lamps are available in a range of physical sizes, powers and phosphors. The range of phosphors includes a large selection of "near white" and "special colour" lamps. In relation to other light sources the fluorescent lamp is particularly efficient, with about 20% of the input energy resulting in useful light. Detailed spectral analysis of the UV emissions of different general lighting fluorescent lamps have shown that in general UVB and UVC emissions are extremely low due to the marked attenuation of wavelengths < 320 nm afforded by the glass envelope.

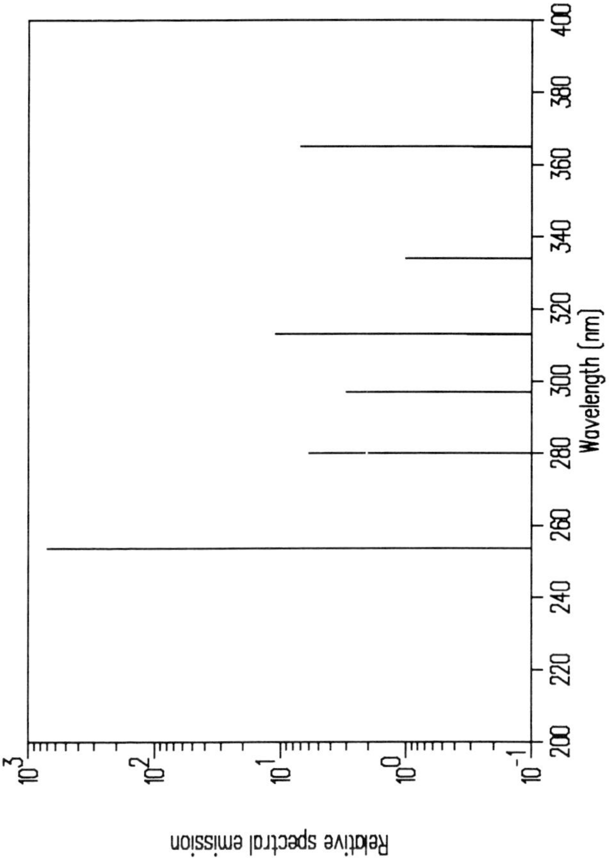

Figure 3.3 Spectral emissions from a low pressure (germicidal) mercury discharge lamp.

Frequently in office and industrial environments where fluorescent lamps are used, the luminaire assembly incorporates a diffuser or controller. Three materials are commonly used in the construction of diffusers; opal acrylic, opal styrene and opal polycarbonate. Controllers are luminaire covers that are configured with small prisms or lenses. Two commonly used materials are clear acrylic and clear styrene. Some luminaires incorporate opal (diffusing) sides and a clear figured [controller] base. The use of diffusers and controllers results in the absorption and reflection of the radiation emitted by the associated lamp. The UV-attenuating properties of different diffusers is demonstrated by the measurement data in table 3.5.

During the past few years the further development and improved design of general lighting fluorescent lamps have been evident in the production of compact fluorescent lamps. These lamps are essentially low power small diameter fluorescent tubes folded in a compact form. They are most readily available commercially with cool white phosphors but other phosphors are also available. For a given illuminance their spectral emissions of UV are essentially no different from those of full size tubular fluorescent lamps as shown in table 3.6.

"Special" applications fluorescent lamps

Apart from a number of colour-rendering fluorescent lamps, which are essentially variations of general lighting fluorescent lamps, a number of special applications fluorescent lamps have been developed.

A common example of a UVB emitting fluorescent lamp is the FS type lamp with spectral emission shown in figure 3.4. Such lamps were previously used for cosmetic tanning and are now often used as a source of UVB in biological experiments. The blacklight lamp uses a nickel/cobalt-oxide (Woods glass) envelope that is almost entirely opaque to light. The phosphor chosen for this type of lamp emits around 370 nm in the UVA. Such lamps are used for a number of commercial, scientific and industrial fluorescence purposes as well as for display and entertainment. Three types of fluorescent lamps that emit UVA in printing and copying merit mention viz; lamps suitable for diazo printing with a principal emission around 360 nm; those intended for modern fast diazo printing with a main emission around 420 nm; and those used for photocopying with predominantly green emissions.

A medical treatment for hyperbilirubinaemia in neonates (neonatal jaundice) consists of irradiating the newborn child with phototherapy lamps emitting in the wavelength range approximately 400 to 470 nm. Some

Table 3.5 Measurements of UV irradiance from various diffusers/controllers with a white fluorescent lamp as the source. Irradiance totals in each waveband in mW m^{-2} (percentage in parentheses), (McKinlay et al., 1988).

Diffuser Type	UVA mW m^{-2}	UVB mW m^{-2}	UV_{ACGIH}** $[mW\ m^{-2}]_{effective}$
Bare lamp	22.32 (100)	3.45 (100)	59 x 10^{-3} (100)
Clear acrylic+	16.35 (73)	2.91 (84)	48 x 10^{-3} (81)
Clear styrene+	2.87 (13)	0 (0)	0 (0)
Opal styrene*	0.92 (4)	3 x 10^{-3} (< 0.1)	0.02 x 10^{-3} (< 0.1)
Opal polycarbonate*	0.20 (< 1)	12 x 10^{-3} (< 1)	0.09 x 10^{-3} (< 1)

+ Surface figured with small prisms

* Reeded surface

** ACGIH occupational hazard weighted irradiance: 1 maximum permissible exposure for an 8 h working day is equivalent to 10^{-3} $[W\ m^{-2}]_{effective}$ ..

Table 3.6 Measurements of UV from compact fluorescent lamps, normalised to an illuminance of 500 lux (Whillock et al., 1990)

Lamp type	UVA mW m^{-2}	UVB μW m^{-2}
Luma (7 W) LC7	47 x 10^{3}	0
Luma (7 W) LC7 with diffuser	197	0
Osram (11 W) Dulux EL	38 x 10^{3}	0.1
Philips (9 W) SL9	37 x 10^{3}	0
Sylvania (13 W) Lynx CFD	43 x 10^{3}	30.81
Thorn (16 W) 2D	54 x 10^{3}	2.48
Tungsram (16 W) Globulux	663	0

Figure 3.4 Spectral emission of an FS type UVB fluorescent lamp.

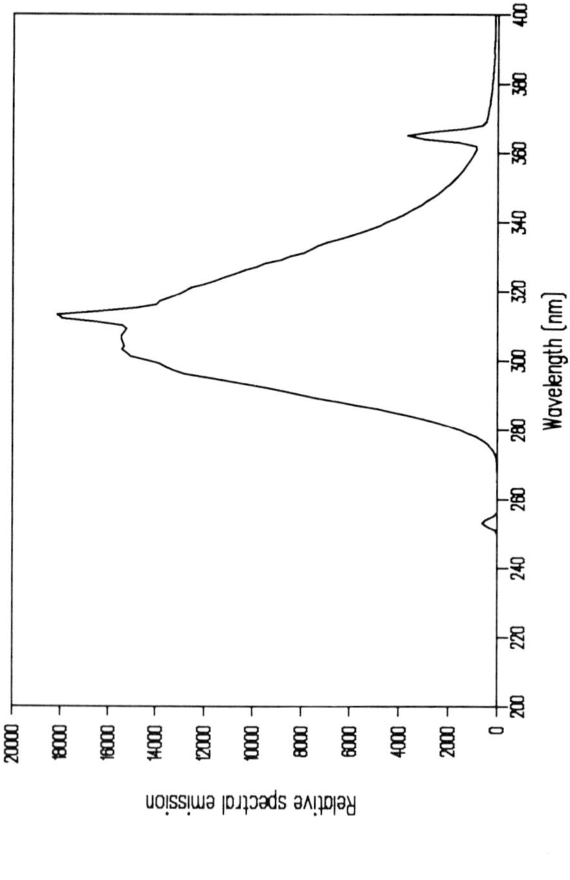

lamps used for this purpose have emission spectra that extend into the UV region. Fluorescent lamps in printing and copying include lamps for diazo printing with a principal emission around 360 nm.

The development of a range of phosphors with enhanced UVA emissions has led to the widespread use of fluorescent lamps in sunbeds, solaria and PUVA (Psoralen + UVA) treatment cabinets.

High pressure discharge lamps

The designation "high pressure discharge" lamps is taken in this monograph to include the families of lamps often called high intensity discharge (HID), such as mercury vapour or metal halide lamps, where an electric arc is not created. At still higher pressures, arcs may be produced, e.g., the xenon or mercury compact (short-arc) lamps.

Mercury and metal halide lamps

High-pressure mercury vapour lamps are widely used for lighting in commerce, streets, displays, floodlighting and a large number of printing, curing and other industrial applications. The spectral emissions of the discharge are in the blue, green and yellow regions of the spectrum and a large amount of UV is also generated. The general construction of high-pressure mercury lamps is a fused silica (quartz) discharge tube containing the mercury/argon vapour discharge mounted inside an outer envelope of soda-lime or borosilicate glass.

The outer glass envelope effectively absorbs most residual UV. Consequently the quantity of potentially harmful UV emitted by such lamps depends critically on the integrity of this envelope. In the USA, but apparently not in Europe, it is a legally enforceable manufacturing requirement that breakage of the outer envelope must either cause the lamp to fail to operate, in which case the lamps are described as "self-extinguishing" and are marked with the letter "T", or if not "self-extinguishing" they should be marked with the letter "R". In the latter case a warning notice must be included with the packaging of the lamp (FDA., 1988). Data from measurements made at 2 m from a mercury HID lamp with the outer envelope removed illustrate the importance of this aspect of safety design, as shown in table 3.7.

The family of metal halide lamps encompasses a number of different types of high pressure mercury lamps whose discharges all contain additives. The additives are most typically metal halides chosen to produce either a strongly coloured emission (usually a single halide), to produce a

Table 3.7 UV emissions from HID mercury vapour general lighting (USA) lamps; effective irradiance in mW $m^{-2}_{effective}$, (ACGIH), (Piltingsrud et al., 1978).

Test condition	A		B		C		D	
Lamp type	With outer bulb	Without outer bulb	With outer bulb	Without outer bulb	With outer bulb	Without outer bulb	With outer bulb	Without outer bulb
General Electric H400 A33-1 Clear	2.5	110*	< 0.1	160	12.5	3640	0.2	0.2
Westinghouse H33 GL 400/DX White	< 0.1	1040	< 0.1	190	0.2	3680	< 0.1	0.3
General Electric H400D x 33-1 White	< 0.2	75*	< 0.1	180	0.5	3900*	< 0.1	< 0.1*
General Electric MV400/BUH [Metal halide]	< 0.3	122*	< 0.1	6*	1	510*	< 0.1	< 0.1*

Test Conditions:
A: Lamp mounted vertically - measurements at 2 m on mid-line axis of lamp.
B: Lamp mounted horizontally - measurements at 2 m on central axis of lamp.
C: Lamp mounted horizontally in reflector shield with no face plate - measurements at 2 m on central axis of lamp.
D: Lamp mounted horizontally in reflector shield with glass face fitted - measurements at 2 m on central axis of lamp.

* Lamps did not operate at normal intensity.

more broadly spectrally uniform emission (multi-halide) or to enhance the UV (most often UVA) emission. Compared with ordinary high pressure mercury lamps the luminous efficacies of metal halide lamps are high. They are used for a range of industrial and commercial applications that include photochemical processing, graphic and photographic illumination, studio lighting, reprography and are also used for UVA cosmetic tanning equipment, for some medical applications and for solar radiation simulation. The UV irradiances of some metal halide lamps used in filtered industrial applications requiring an activating range of wavelengths between 320 and 440 nm, e.g. lithographic platemaking and printed circuit photo-resist etching, are shown in table 3.8 (McKinlay et al., 1988).

Table 3.8 UV irradiances measured at 1 m from typical graphics arts metal halide mercury lamps (McKinlay et al., 1988)

Lamp type	Power [W]	UVC [W m^{-2}]	UVB [W m^{-2}]	UVA [W m^{-2}]
HPA 400	400	0.5	3.2	9.0
HPA 1000	930	2.3	9.0	23.0
HPA 2000	1750	4.5	19.0	48.0

The emission of a device incorporating iron additive halide lamps for phototherapy is illustrated in figure 3.5. The importance of incorporating filtration in such devices in order to remove unwanted components of the UV spectrum is illustrated.

Xenon, compact and linear arcs

Where an optical source of very high radiance is required and of small size a very high pressure arc lamp may be used. These have a filling gas of mercury vapour, mercury vapour plus xenon gas or xenon gas. Metal halide types are also available. Two physical types are commonly used; the compact (short) arc and the linear arc. The spectral emission of xenon lamps, which at wavelengths shorter than infra-red, closely matches that of a black-body radiator at about 6000 K. This enables their use in photography and as solar radiation simulators.

The spectral emission of xenon lamps, which at wavelengths shorter than infrared closely matches that of a black body radiator at about 6000 K, enables their use as solar radiation simulators. Their emission spectrum is continuous from the UV through to the IR regions. Large amounts of UVA, UVB and UVC are emitted by unfiltered lamps to the extent that

Figure 3.5 Spectral emissions of a phototherapy system incorporating metal halide lamps. The system is fitted with 2 filters and the measurement data illustrated are for; none, one or both filters in place (McKinlay 1992, measurement data kindly provided by Diffey).

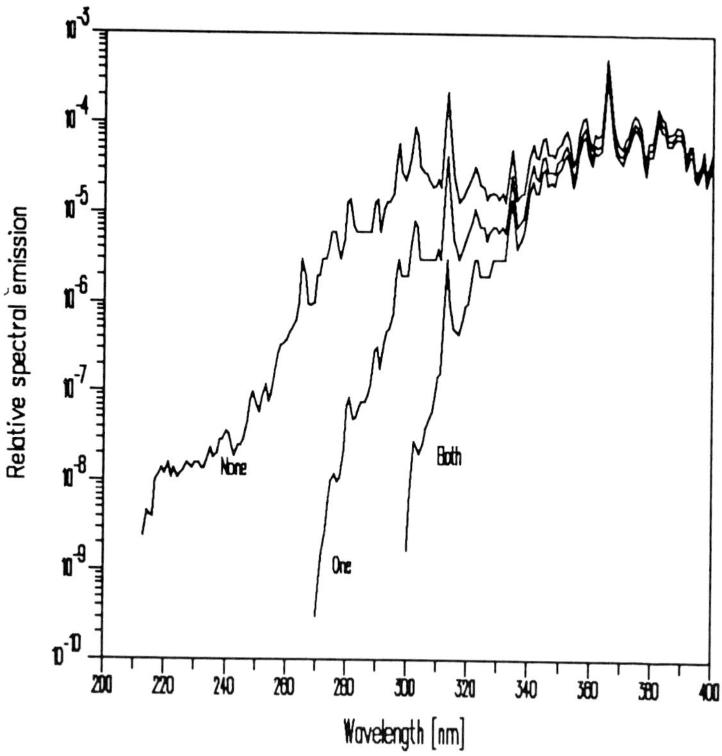

they can present a significant health hazard if incorrectly used. The luminance of compact xenon arcs may approach that of the sun and in some lamps with greater than 10 kW rating the luminance may exceed that of the sun. They therefore present a potentially severe retinal hazard if viewed.

3.2.3 *Gas welding*

Oil, coal and gas flames normally operate at temperatures below about 2000 K and consequently emit virtually no UV. Oxyacetylene and oxyhydrogen flames burn at much higher temperatures and emit UV mostly in the UVA region.

3.2.4 *Arc welding*

By comparison with gas flame processes, the emissions of UV from arc welding are very high (see figure 3.6) and many data on the optical radiation emissions associated with a variety of electric arc welding processes have been published (e.g., Sliney & Wolbarsht, 1980).

3.2.5 *Lasers*

All lasers have three basic components (see figure 3.7): (a) a laser (active) medium; (b) an energy source (pumping system) and; (c) a resonant optical cavity. A pumping system is necessary to provide energy to electrons to raise them to excited states and achieve population inversion. Optical pumping, using an intense source of light such as a xenon flashtube; electron-collision pumping, using an electrical discharge and; chemical pumping, using the energy released from making and breaking chemical bonds, are all used for this purpose. A resonant optical cavity is formed by mirrors placed at each end of the laser medium. The construction is such that the beam passes through the laser medium several times and the number of emitted photons is amplified during each transit. One of the mirrors is chosen to be partially transmitting thus enabling part of the beam to be emitted from the cavity (figure 3.7). Examples of lasers that emit UV are presented in table 3.9.

Figure 3.6 Emission spectrum from gas tungsten arc welding. The spectral emissions of all kinds of arc welding processes varies with the composition of the electrodes and the metals being joined, the plasma that is created and the shielding gas used (Sliney & Wolbarsht, 1980).

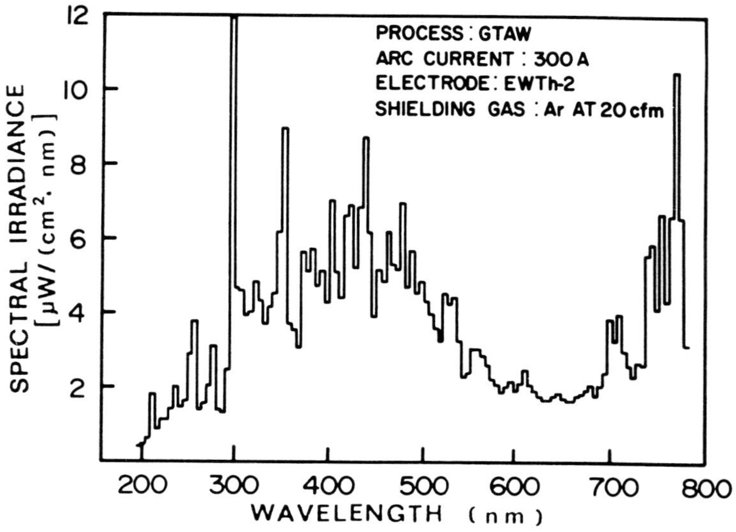

Figure 3.7 Simplified diagram of a laser. All lasers consist of a resonant cavity (generally two mirrors, one partially transmitting), an energy source and an active medium. The diagram here illustrates an optically pumped crystal laser (Sliney & Wolbarsht, 1980).

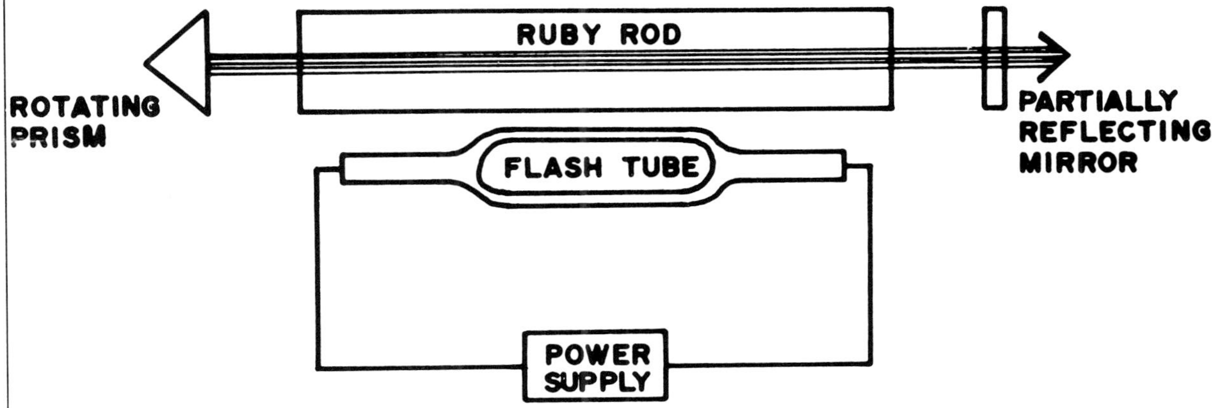

Table 3.9 UV laser emissions and characteristics, (McKinlay, 1992)

Type	Name	Spectral emissions
Excimer	Argon fluoride [(ArF)	193 nm
	Krypton fluoride (KrF)	248 nm
	Xenon chloride (XeCl)	308 nm
	Xenon bromide (XeBr)	282 nm
	Xenon fluoride (XeF)	351 nm
	Krypton chloride (KrCl)	222 nm
Dye	Excimer-, Nitrogen-,	300 nm-
	Flash lamp pumped	340 nm-
Gas	Nitrogen (N_2)	337 nm
	Helium cadmium (He-Cd)	325 nm
Gas ion	Argon (Ar^+0	333 nm-
		357 nm
		363 nm
	Krypton (Kr^+)	337.5 nm
		350.7 nm
		356.4 nm

A recent generation of UV lasers are the excimer lasers. The active media used are rare gas halides such as ArF, KrCl, XeBr or XeF. The molecules of those gases have only a short lifetime in the ground state, however they are very stable in the excited state. As a buffer medium, helium is often used. Population inversion is easily achievable because the ground state is very unstable.

3.2.6 Sunbeds

Sunbeds are broadly used for cosmetic tanning purposes. The expression "sunbed" includes tanning equipment consisting of a UV emitting lamp or a number of such lamps incorporated in a bed, canopy or panel, or any combination thereof. There are four distinct types of lamps in use, each with different UV emission characteristics. Those are UVA, low-pressure fluorescent tubes; UVA, filtered high-intensity discharge lamps; UVB, low-pressure fluorescent tubes; UVB, filtered high-intensity discharge lamps.

The emission characteristics and the health risks associated with the use of each type of lamp are different. The last two lamp types are associated with high levels of UVB and are now little used. They have been almost universally replaced by the predominantly UVA emitting lamp types.

4. HUMAN EXPOSURE

4.1 Sunlight

Outdoors, exposure to UV constantly changes during the day. People are largely unaware of the degree of these changes. At noon, when the sun is overhead, the level of UV at a wavelength of 300 nm is ten times greater than at either three hours before (9 am) or three hours after noon (3 pm). An untanned person with fair skin may receive a mild sunburn in as little as 25 minutes at noon (depending on the time of year and the latitude) but would have to lie in the sun for at least two hours to receive the same dose after 3 pm. The global biologically effective UV falling on a horizontal surface occurs primarily during the midday hours, about 50% during the four hours centred on noon-time zenith (Sliney, 1987).

Scattering of sunlight by air molecules (due to Raleigh scattering) favours UV and blue light (hence the blue sky). For longer pathlengths through the atmosphere when the sun is low in the sky, more UV and sunlight is scattered. The sun which is white at noonday becomes yellow and then orange as less UV and blue light are present in the direct rays. When the sun is overhead staring at the sun for 90 seconds would cause solar retinitis. A few hours later, with the sun much lower in the sky, it would take many minutes to reach a hazardous retinal dose, and it is virtually impossible to cause any eye damage at sunset. Thus, the geometry of exposure as well as the spectrum (hue) plays a major role in determining the hazards from direct exposure from the sun (Sliney, 1983, 1986).

Estimation of an individual's lifetime UV exposure requires knowledge of the ambient solar UV levels, history of outdoor exposure and the relative exposures at the different anatomical sites. Studies on the anatomical distribution of solar UV have been reported (Diffey et al 1979; Rosenthal et al., 1985; Holman et al., 1983; Gies et al 1992a; Roy et al., 1988). The relative doses at various body sites have been determined using UV sensitive polysulphone film on rotating manikins and headforms. It was found that even though the relative doses to the face and eyes are higher in winter, due to the lower solar elevation, the absolute doses are higher in summer. The presence of a brimmed hat reduced the face exposure by a factor of at least two and the eye exposure was reduced by a factor of 4 to 5 (Diffey et al., 1979, Roy et al 1988).

Polysulphone film badges have also been used to quantify the solar UV exposure received by different subjects and results compared to those calculated from personal diaries and measured ambient solar UVB (Gies et al., 1992a). In general, when UV exposure activities took place under close supervision, good correlations were obtained between the polysulphone badges and the ambient/diaries approach. Results from a recent study (Roy and Gies, 1993), of indoor, outdoor and retired workers indicated that exposures to badge locations of up to 30% of ambient were recorded. Through studies of this type, knowledge is gained on the amount and pattern of exposure from routine activities and this can then be applied in the design of educational campaigns to modify outdoor behaviour and reduce UV exposure. The use of polysulphone or CR39 plastics (Wong et al., 1989; Sydenham et al., 1991) as contact-lens dosimeters have been proposed, but lack of sensitivity and personal comfort has discouraged their use in field studies.

4.2 Skin Exposure Geometry

UV incident on human skin can follow one of three courses, it can undergo absorption, reflection, or scattering. Thus, the actual radiant exposure received by the various layers of the skin will be lower than the incident exposure. Reflection not only occurs at the surface of the stratum corneum, but at all interfaces changing in refractive index. Scattering occurs because of the different structural elements, such as hair follicles and sebaceous glands, and also by cellular components, such as mitochondria and ribosomes. The remaining UV can penetrate into deeper skin layers.

UV penetrates into the dermis exposing a variety of cells and structures, depending in part on the thickness of the human stratum corneum and epidermis. The depth of penetration is wavelength dependent the longer the wavelength the deeper the penetration (Bruls et al., 1984). From figure 4.1 it is seen that the same incident exposure of UVA or UVB radiation will result in a higher actual exposure of UVA than UVB at a given depth. For example, if the incident UV exposure was 100 kJ m^{-2} then 50 kJ m^{-2} of 365 nm radiation would be present at a depth of 30 μm and only 19 kJ m^{-2} at a depth of 70 μm. For 313 nm radiation only 33 kJ m^{-2} would be present at 30 μm and 9.5 kJ m^{-2} at 70 μm. While less than 1% of the UVC wavelengths can barely penetrate the epidermal layer (Bruls et al., 1984), about 1% of the incident UVA dose can penetrate into the subcutaneous tissue (Parrish et al., 1978). The distribution and size of melanin particles also plays an important role in protecting epidermal cells. Melanin particles have a distribution within the stratum corneum and epidermal cells depending upon skin type. In dark skin types (5 and 6) these particles are positioned within cells to provide optimum optical protection for the cell nuclei and in adequate size in the stratum corneum (Kollias et al., 1991).

Figure 4.1 Schematic of human skin depicting the layers, cell types, structural components and percent transmittance of UVA, UVB and UVC radiation at different depths (Bruls et al., 1984).

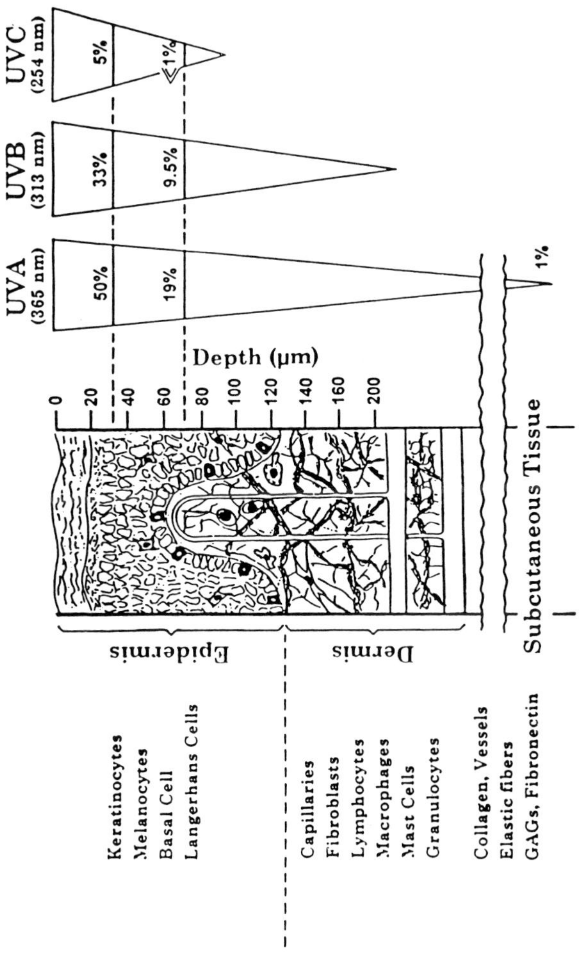

4.3 Ocular Exposure Geometry

People seldom look directly at the sun when it is overhead and very hazardous to view. It is not very hazardous to view when the sun is low in the sky and falls within the normal field-of-view. When the sun is more than 10° above the horizon, the natural tendency is to partially close the eyelids or squint (called squint reflex), thus shielding the retina from direct exposure. These factors reduce the exposure to the cornea to a maximum of about 5% of that falling upon the exposed top of head (Sliney, 1986). If the squint and other behavioural factors are not considered, the dose to the eyelid would be approximately 20% of the dose falling on a horizontal surface.

Although the cornea is more sensitive to UV injury than the skin, people seldom experiences a corneal burn when in sunlight. Using the action spectrum for human photokeratitis and mathematically weighting this with the midday solar spectrum, the time to achieve the threshold for photokeratitis is about 100 seconds (Sliney, 1987, Rosenthal et al., 1988). Again, the geometry of exposure precludes photokeratitis except when ground reflectance exceeds approximately 10%. When the sun is overhead and UV exposure is most severe, the brow ridge and upper lid shield the cornea, and if the eye is turned away from the sun, the more intense scattered UV from overhead strikes the cornea at a grazing angle of incidence where most is reflected and little is absorbed (Sliney, 1983). Only when the incident UV rays are parallel to the pupillary axis are most rays (approx. 98%) absorbed.

When looking at snow, UV is reflected directly into the eye; hence, the traditional eye protector of the Inuit or Eskimo, the slit, in whalebone or in a seal-skin mask, provided geometrical rather than spectral protection against UV exposure (Hedblom, 1961). The lack of protection above and to the sides of sunglasses is a serious shortcoming. However, to obtain a quantitative idea of this component of exposure to the eye, measurements were made using a simulated ocular geometry in sunlight (Sliney, 1986). The human eye received 10 to 25 % of the UV dose when wearing glasses with lenses opaque to UV compared to no lens in the glasses. Therefore, unless goggles with side-shields are used, UV transmission factors in lenses much less than 2-5 % do not provide the eye protection suggested by the transmission factor (Sliney, 1986).

The strong dependence of reflectance with angle of incidence is termed Fresnel's Law of Reflection. This law not only explains the survival of the cornea exposed overhead to UV, but also the glare experienced over water. When the sun is overhead, water reflects about

2% of the UV upward (Sliney, 1986). When low in the sky, much of the sunlight is reflected while the UV and blue light are filtered by the atmosphere. Nevertheless, the strong reflections from water at these low sun angles create discomfort glare and UV exposure of the cornea is further reduced because of the squint.

If dark lenses are placed over the eyes, the natural aversion to bright light, which leads to the squint reflex (that greatly lowers retinal UV or exposure to the eye), would be disabled. This may appear to be an unusual way to consider the comfort that shaded lenses provide. However, poor sunglasses may actually lead to a higher UV exposure (Sliney, 1983).

However, quantifying the protective value of the upper and lower eye lids when they close to squint is difficult. In terms of UV exposure, at least a twenty-fold reduction is likely. For shielding the retina from the direct image of the sun, the upper lid probably provides a protection factor exceeding a thousand (Sliney - personal communication). If a brimmed hat is worn, the direct image of the sun on the retina is rare and overhead UV exposure is virtually eliminated. However, while using a hat the lid opens further and ground reflection of UV could become important.

On an overcast day, the lids open wider, and although the UVB irradiance is reduced by cloud cover, the actual UVB dose rate to the eye from atmospheric scattering near the horizon may be reduced by a factor of only two (Sliney, 1983). Hence, on a cloudy day the eye may receive a greater UVB dose than on a bright sunny day. However, a heavy overcast may attenuate the UVB sufficiently, that this observation may not be true. As sunglasses are not typically worn on an overcast day, one could argue that the concern over sunglasses increasing total ocular exposure is unimportant. However, sunglasses should have sufficient UV filtration so that ocular exposure does not actually increase when they are worn on a sunny day.

Eye and head movements can further reduce UV exposure. Most humans in bright sunlight squint or avoid looking into the sun sector of the sky. These behavioural and physiological factors are not taken into account by simple UV measurements. There is an obvious need to determine accurately the corneal and lenticular exposure to ambient UV. Indeed, the results of previous epidemiological studies of cataract may be questioned because of inadequate dosimetry. Some epidemiological studies may have reached incorrect conclusions regarding risk from UV or sunlight exposure by assigning inaccurate exposure levels to population groups, because they assumed that overhead UV exposure accurately predicts corneal exposure.

4.4 Workplace

4.4.1 *Outdoor work*

Although humans have adapted and acclimatized to solar UV it nevertheless represents the most hazardous source of optical radiation likely to be encountered by the average person and with a few exceptions by the worker. People who work outdoors will be subjected to involuntary UV exposure. The highest exposure will occur during the two hours period either side of noon. Workers must be made aware of this and take appropriate precautions as discussed in chapter 13.

In a study of various work and recreational situations (Challoner et al., 1976; Diffey et al., 1982), it was found that outdoor workers had the highest exposure, receiving approximately 10% of the ambient level, similar to that received during sailing and sightseeing. Higher exposures were found for skiing (20%) and the largest during sunbathing on a beach (80%). Office workers received about 3% of the total ambient radiation with about half that figure from weekend exposure (Leach et al., 1978). The actual exposures vary depending on the time of day and year, duration and frequency of exposure.

4.4.2 *Indoor work*

Examples of indoor workplace exposures to UV are given below.

Photoprocesses

Many industrial processes involve a photochemical component. The large-scale nature of these processes often necessitates the use of high-power (several kilowatts) lamps such as high pressure metal halide lamps which emit significant amounts of UV (Diffey, 1990a). The principal industrial applications of photopolymerisation include the curing of protective coatings and inks and photoresists for printed circuit boards. The curing of printing inks by exposure to UV takes only a fraction of a second. UV drying units can be installed between printing stations on a multicolour line, so that each colour is dried before the next is applied. Another major use of UV curing has been for metal decorating in the packaging industry (Phillips, 1983). UVA is also used to inspect printed circuit boards and integrated circuits in the electronics industry.

Sterilization

UV with wavelengths in the range 260-265 nm is the most effective for sterilization and disinfection since it corresponds to a maximum in the DNA absorption spectrum. Low-pressure mercury discharge tubes are often used as the UV source as more than 90% of the radiated energy lies in the 254 nm line, figure 3.2. These lamps are often referred to as "germicidal lamps", "bactericidal lamps" or simply "UVC lamps" (Diffey, 1990a).

UVC radiation has been used to disinfect sewage effluent, drinking-water, water for the cosmetics industry and swimming pools. Germicidal lamps are sometimes used inside microbiological safety cabinets to inactivate airborne and surface microorganisms (Diffey, 1990a). The combination of UV and ozone has a very powerful oxidizing action and can reduce the organic content of water to extremely low levels (Phillips, 1983).

Welding

Welding equipment falls into two broad categories: gas welding and electric arc welding. Only the latter process produces significant levels of UV, the quality and quantity of which depend primarily on the arc current, shielding gas and metals being welded (Sliney & Wolbarsht, 1980). The levels of UV irradiance around electric arc welding equipment are high; effective irradiance at 1 m at an arc current of 400 A ranged from 1 to 50 W m^{-2} and the unweighted UVA irradiance ranged from 3 to 70 W m^{-2}, depending on the type of welding and the metal being welded (Mariutti & Matzeu, 1987; Cox, 1987). It is not surprising therefore that most welders at some time or another experience "arc eye" or "welder's flash" (photokeratitis) and skin erythema. The effective irradiance at 0.3 m from many types of electric welding arcs operating at 150 A is such that the maximum permissible exposure time for an 8-h working period on unprotected eyes and skin varies from a few tenths of a second to about 10 s, depending on the type of welding process and the material used (Cox, 1987).

4.4.3 Research

Sources of UV are used by most experimental scientists engaged in photobiology and photochemistry and in molecular biology. These applications, in which the effect of UV irradiation on biological and chemical species is of primary interest to the researcher, can be differentiated from UV fluorescence by absorption techniques where the effect is of secondary importance (Diffey, 1990a).

4.4.4 Commerce

Sunlamps emitting UV have been used for tanning, particularly in northern Europe and North America. Prior to the mid-1970s, the source of UV in sunlamps was usually an unfiltered mercury arc lamp which emitted a broad spectrum of radiation, including large quantities of UVB and UVC. There are four distinctly different types of ultraviolet tanning lamps in use, each with different UV emission characteristics viz.; low pressure UVA fluorescent lamps; filtered high intensity discharge UVA lamps; low pressure UVB fluorescent lamps and; filtered high intensity discharge UVB lamps (IRPA/INIRC 1991). The emission characteristics and the health risks associated with each type of lamp are different (Diffey and McKinlay 1983, Gies et al 1986, Diffey 1987). Tanning systems incorporating lamps that emit predominantly UVB are now little used and have been almost universally replaced by the low pressure UVA fluorescent and filtered high intensity discharge UVA types. Tanning requires deliberate exposure of the skin to UV; however, the eyes must be protected. Similarly, staff working in tanning salons must ensure their exposure is kept to a minimum.

Many contaminants of food products can be detected by UV fluorescence techniques. For example, the bacterium Pseudomonas aeruginosa, which causes rot in eggs, meat and fish, can be detected by its yellow-green fluorescence under UVA irradiation. One of the longest established uses of UVA fluorescence in public health is to demonstrate contamination with rodent urine, which is highly fluorescent.

Many flying insects are attracted by UVA radiation, particularly in the region around 350 nm. This phenomenon is the principle of electronic insect traps, in which a UVA fluorescent lamp is mounted in a unit containing a high-voltage grid. The insect, attracted by the UVA lamp, flies into the unit and is electrocuted in the air gap between the high-voltage grid and a grounded metal screen. Such units are commonly found in areas where food is prepared and sold to the public (Diffey, 1990a).

UVA blacklight lamps are sometimes used in discotheques to induce fluorescence in the skin and clothing of dancers. The levels of UVA emitted are usually low (< 10 W m^{-2}) (Diffey, 1990a).

Signatures, banknotes and other documents can be authenticated by exposing them to UVA, under which they fluoresce. UVA exposure of the user is normally to hands and irradiance is low (< 10 W m^{-2}) (Diffey, 1990a).

4.4.5 Medicine and dentistry

In both medical and dental applications of UV, the patient is deliberately exposed to either treat or diagnose a disease or disorder. While non-target areas of the patient must be covered, care must also be taken to ensure staff are fully protected from UV exposure (see chapter 13).

The diagnostic uses of UV are confined largely to fluorescing of the skin and teeth. UV exposure is limited to small areas (< 15 cm in diameter) and the UVA radiation dose per examination is probably no more than 5 x 10^4J m^{-2}. Diagnostic techniques are limited to the use of fluorescence to identify the presence of various fungal and bacterial infectious agents on the skin or in wounds. The source of UV most commonly used for this purpose is the Woods lamp which emits predominantly UVA radiation (365 nm). Exposure of the patient's skin to potentially carcinogenically-effective UV is insignificant (Diffey, 1990a).

UV phototherapy is a well established method for the treatment of a number of skin conditions and in particular for psoriasis (Green et al., 1992). Two general types of UVB emitting lamps are used in phototherapy, high intensity discharge (HID) mercury vapour and mercury/metal halide vapour lamps and low pressure mercury vapour fluorescent lamps. The spectral emissions of these different types of lamps vary greatly and this, with other factors such as the number and power of the lamps, the lamp to skin distance and the individual sensitivity of the patient, determines the treatment time. A treatment dose is chosen to cause erythema in a particular patient. As treatment progresses and the skin becomes increasingly acclimatised, individual treatment doses are increased accordingly. Treatments may be given several times per week. Phototherapy has also been used for the treatment of other skin conditions including severe itching, acne, eczema, polymorphic light eruption (PLE), pityriasis rosea and urticaria, and for renal failure (Green et al., 1992).

Seasonal affective disorder (SAD) is frequently treated by exposure to sources of high illumination. Most treatment regimes have employed sources incorporating so-called "full spectrum lighting" whose emissions contain small amounts of UVA and UVB radiations (Terman et al., 1990).

PUVA

UV photochemotherapy is UV phototherapy used in conjunction with the oral or topical application of a chemical (photosensitising) agent to the patient. The most widely used treatment is PUVA which involves the use of the photosensitising agent 8-methoxypsoralen (8-MOP) in conjunction with UVA irradiation for the treatment of psoriasis. The irradiation sources used for such treatment incorporate either low pressure mercury vapour UVA fluorescent lamps, or HID mercury vapour or mercury/metal halide vapour lamps with an added filter to effectively attenuate the UVB. The UVA irradiance on the skin from sources incorporating fluorescent lamps is generally of the order of 60 W m^{-2} and for the HID mercury systems, around 250 W m^{-2}. Treatments consist of a starting dose of between 500 and 40,000 J m^{-2}, depending on skin type, followed by further incremental doses two to three times weekly. Total treatment radiant exposures of between 10^6 and 2.5 10^6 J m^{-2} have been reported for successful results. However, studies have shown large uncertainties in the dosimetry associated with PUVA treatment and point to equally large consequential uncertainties about the actual treatment doses delivered (Diffey et al 1980).

Hyperbilirubinaemia

Phototherapy is sometimes used in the treatment of neonatal jaundice or hyperbilirubinaemia. The preferred method of treatment is to irradiate the baby for several hours a day for up to one week with visible light, particularly blue light. The lamps used for phototherapy, although intended to emit only visible light, may also have a UV component (Gies & Roy, 1990; Sliney & Wolbarsht, 1980).

Dentistry

Irradiation of the oral cavity with a Woods lamp can produce fluorescence under certain conditions. This has been used in the diagnosis of various dental disorders, such as early dental cavities, the incorporation of tetracycline into bone and teeth, dental plaque and calculus (Hefferren et al., 1971).

Pits and fissures in teeth have been treated using an adhesive resin polymerized with UVA. The resin is applied with a fine brush to the surfaces to be treated and hardened by exposure to UVA radiation at a minimal irradiance of 100 W m^{-2} for about 30 s (Eriksen, 1987; Diffey, 1990a).

4.5 Elective Exposure

By comparison to occupational exposure to UV, where control measures are generally instituted to protect the eye and skin, elective exposures can be much greater. Elective exposure results from outdoor recreational activity, from intentional exposure to sun-tanning equipment and to sunlight at the beach and elsewhere. Actual dose estimates of elective exposure experienced by those who attempt to maintain a tan may exceed 100 MED per year (Challoner et al., 1976; Diffey, 1993a; Diffey et al., 1982).

5. DOSIMETRIC CONCEPTS

5.1 Interaction of UV with Matter

Attenuation of UV occurs due to absorption and scattering. Reflection, refraction and diffraction are phenomena related to boundaries between media. All of these interactions may change the direction, intensity and the wavelength of UV. The quantities describing interactions of UV with matter are dependent on the wavelength.

The total energy absorbed in a material is influenced by reflections from its surfaces. The attenuation coefficient describes the attenuation of UV within tissue and is the sum of the absorption and scattering coefficients. Penetration depth in a tissue is inversely proportional to the exponential attenuation coefficient.

Absorption requires transfer of radiative energy to matter. Apart from possible photomechanical effects, UV is absorbed as a result of electron transitions at the atomic and molecular level. Such molecular absorption can lead to photochemical reactions.

In most molecules the ground state or the singlet state (S_0) consists of two paired electrons. On absorption of radiant energy one of the electrons can make a transition to an excited state (S_1), provided that the incident photon energy corresponds to an existing level in the absorbing molecule. As shown in figure 5.1, the molecule can release this absorbed energy from the excited state by (a) transition directly back to the ground state, S_0, or (b) transition to the generally long-lived excited triplet state, T_1, and then discharging the remaining energy to return to S_0. In either case, transition back to S_0 may be radiative (a photon emitted) or non-radiative (energy dispersed by vibrational-rotational relaxation). The radiative $S_1 \rightarrow S_0$ transition is called "fluorescence" while radiative $T_1 \rightarrow S_0$ is called "phosphorescence". In addition, molecules in the S_1 or T_1 states can return to the ground state either by forming photoproducts or by transferring the energy to an acceptor molecule. The effectiveness of the photochemical process can be amplified by "photosensitizers" or impeded by "quenchers".

Figure 5.1 Three-level electronic energy level diagram. Dashed lines represent non-radiative transitions while solid lines correspond to radiative transitions

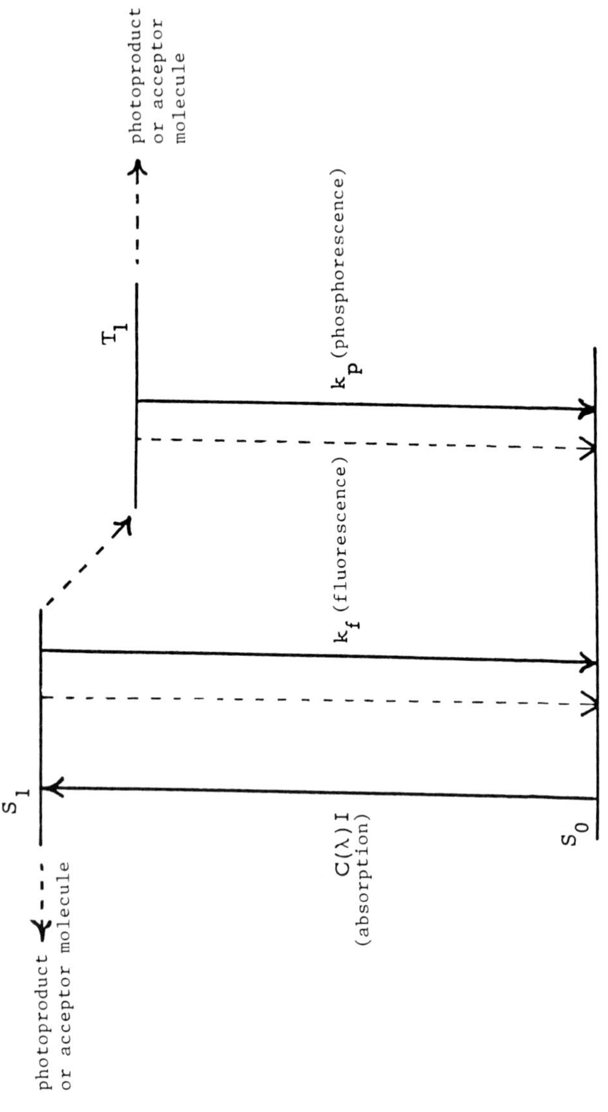

5.2 Biological Weighting Factors and Spectrally Weighted Quantities

Both radiant exposure H and irradiance E are quantities integrated over the total spectrum of interest. To describe the irradiance or radiant exposure in a very narrow spectral (wavelength) interval ($\Delta\lambda$), the quantities of *spectral irradiance* E_λ and *spectral radiant exposure* H_λ are employed. These have the units of: W m^{-2} nm and J m^{-2} nm, respectively. If $E_\lambda \Delta\lambda$ is the irradiance in a narrow interval $\Delta\lambda$ around the wavelength λ, then the integrated irradiance E over the wavelength interval λ_1 to λ_2 can be written as:

$$E = \sum_{\lambda_1}^{\lambda_2} E_\lambda \, \Delta\lambda$$

E_λ and H_λ are spectral functions. Other spectroradiometric quantities exist with analogous definitions, e.g., spectral radiant power, spectral radiant energy, etc, as shown in table 2.2. The spectroradiometric quantities are important in photobiology, and are critical in any discussion of the biological effects of UV. The biological effects of UV are strongly wavelength dependent. As a measure of these effects, "effective" or "biologically active" quantities have been introduced (CIE, 1987). The effective irradiance E_{eff} is defined as:

$$E_{eff} = \Sigma \, E_\lambda \, S_\lambda \, \Delta\lambda$$

and similarly, the effective radiant exposure is

$$H_{eff} = \Sigma \, H_\lambda \, S_\lambda \, \Delta\lambda$$

where S_λ is called the relative spectral effectiveness function or *action spectrum.*

The ***action spectrum*** gives the relative biological response of a tissue to irradiation at different wavelengths, and ideally will correspond to the absorption spectrum of critical absorbing molecules, or "chromophores." In biological systems, however, the action spectrum function is modulated by the shielding (i.e. thickness) of overlying tissue (e.g., stratum corneum of the skin), energy transfer, and the action of sensitizers and quenchers. The action spectrum is therefore specific for a certain effect arising in a certain tissue layer. For example, the action spectrum for erythema (skin) and photokeratitis (cornea) differ.

Based on a statistical analysis of the results of minimum erythema dose studies carried out over the past 20 years or so, and including data by Parrish et al. (1982) on the erythemal efficacy of UVA, the CIE has promulgated a reference action curve (McKinlay and Diffey, 1987), as shown in figure 5.2. This function consists of three straight lines when plotted on a semi-logarithmic scale, and although individual action spectra would not have the two inflection points, the function can be readily expressed by three mathematical functions. The function has been adopted internationally by the CIE and the IEC and is being used by national organizations and authorities for the determination of the erythemal potential of an exposure to a given source of UV. A slightly different action spectrum, which cannot be so readily expressed mathematically, has been recommended by IRPA (1991) for risk assessment in occupational health (see figure 5.2).

The erythemal response of the skin to UV is usually inferred from the minimal erythema dose (MED). This value is determined by exposing adjacent areas of skin to increasing doses of UV, and recording the lowest dose to achieve erythema at a specified time, usually 24 h after irradiation.

The visual detection of erythema is subjective and is affected by unrelated factors such as viewing geometry, intensity and spectral composition of ambient illumination, colour of unexposed surrounding skin, (Chamberlain and Chamberlain 1980, Diffey and Robson, 1992), and the experience and visual acuity of the observer. The difficulty in judging accurately a minimal erythema response is reflected by the varying definitions proposed for this value: these range from the dose required to achieve a just perceptible erythema (Everett et al., 1965, Kelfkens and van der Leun, 1989); to that dose which will just produce a uniform redness with sharp borders (Wucherpfenning, 1931).

The MED will vary according to the wavelength range over which the effective UV is summed and for radiation protection purposes is generally taken to lie in the range 200 to 300 J m^{-2} effective.

5.3 Measurement Techniques

There are three distinct types of measurement systems employed in the detection of UV: radiometers, spectroradiometers and dosimeters. Radiometers and spectroradiometers are direct-reading instruments that use electro-optical (physical) detectors to convert the incident radiation into an electrical signal. Radiometers measure all incident radiant power over a wide spectral range; whereas, spectroradiometers measure the radiant

Figure 5.2 UV-induced action spectrum and the IRPA/INIRC relative spectral effectiveness factor (McKinlay & Diffey, 1987 and IRPA/INIRC, 1991).

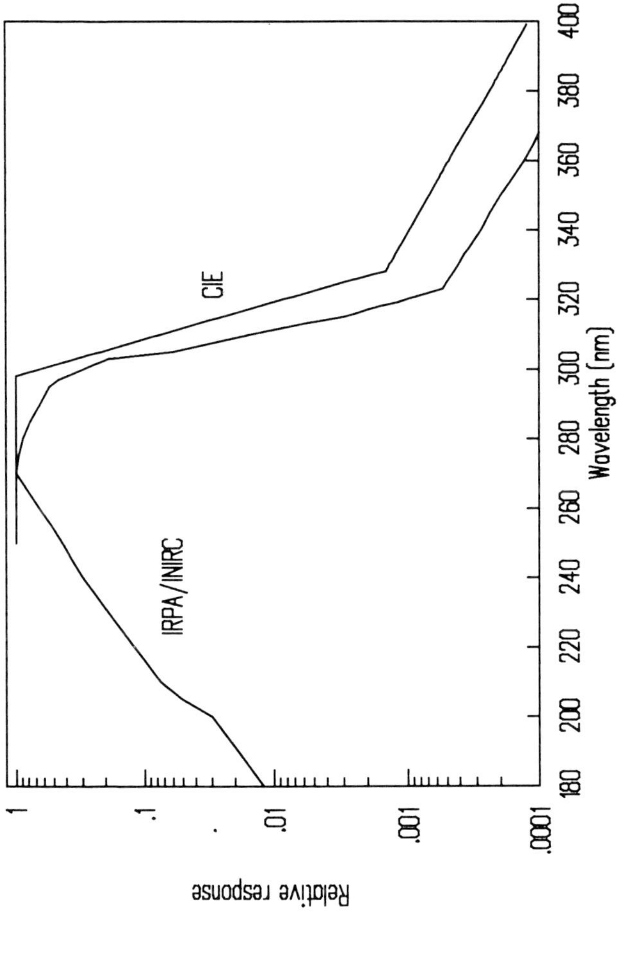

power distribution over a wide spectral range. Either by electronic means or by computer control, radiometers or spectroradiometers may be modified and calibrated to operate as "dosimeters" by time-integration of the output signal from the detector. However, by dosimeters, one usually means devices that by nature respond directly to incident dose, i.e. radiant exposure. Dosimeters may be further optically modified and calibrated to respond according to an action spectrum, thereby serving as a direct-reading instrument for dose to a particular organ.

5.3.1 *Detectors*

The term detector normally refers to an electro-optical device which converts an optical signal (e.g UV or light) into an electronic signal which can be recorded. An important characteristic of any detector is the responsivity, defined as the quotient of the detector output (e.g amperes, A) and the radiant power incident upon the detector (e.g. watts, W). Thus units for responsivity may vary. The unit for irradiance-responsivity is often ampere-per-watt-per-square-metre ($A\ W^{-1}\ m^{-2}$). The spectral responsivity is the responsivity as a function of wavelength. The term detectivity is used to compare the detection capability (the smallest quantity of radiation that can be detected) of different types of detectors, the higher the detectivity the more sensitive the detector. Thermal detectors, such as thermopiles and pyroelectric detectors, have a much lower detectivity (less sensitive) than photodiodes, phototubes and photomultipliers.

The most common types of detectors for UV are semiconductor (junction) photodiodes, vacuum photodiodes (phototubes) and photomultipliers. Junction photodiodes are usually silicon (Si) photodiodes that may be enhanced to improve their UV responsivity and with a spectral responsivity between 190 and 1100 nm. Gallium-arsenide-phosphide (GaAsP) photodiodes have a spectral responsivity between 190 and 670 nm, and gallium-phosphide (GaP) photodiodes have a spectral responsivity between 190 and 520 nm.

Chemical detectors, such as photographic film emulsions or polymer films of polysulphone or CR-39 resins, respond to incident radiant exposure ($J\ m^{-2}$). Their responsivity is generally strongly wavelength dependant, and attempts are made to simulate a photobiological action spectrum directly.

The choice of an optimum detector for a specific instrument or measurement situation depends upon the requirements for ease of data collection, portability, electrical power requirements, size and accuracy.

Each detector type has advantages and disadvantages. Important parameters to consider for instrument requirements are: spectral responsivity, noise-equivalent-power (NEP), linearity, time/frequency response, stability over time, environmental operating conditions, maintenance, ease of operation, the requirements upon additional electronics, and cost.

Biological detectors are also used. For example, biofilms using dried spores of *bacillus subtilis*, immobilized on transparent polyester plastic sheets. After irradiation the biofilm is incubated in a growth medium and the proteins synthesized after spore germination, stained and evaluated by photometry. The biologically effective dose is calculated using a calibration curve. The UV response of this biofilm is additive and follows the reciprocity law in the normal range of fluence rates investigated. The response is independent of temperature (-20°C to 70°C) and humidity. The biofilm can be stored for up to 9 months at room temperature without significant influence on the viability of spores. These detectors have been used in Antarctica and in space to measure the biological consequences of ozone variations (Quintern et al., 1992).

5.3.2 *Radiometers*

A radiometer is a detection system that measures incident radiation. A UV-radiometer usually measures irradiance in watts per square metre (W m^{-2}). The basic layout of a radiometer is shown in figure 5.3.

The diffuser shown in figure 5.3 may not always be present. When used, its purpose is to make the angular responsivity of the radiometer proportional to the cosine of the angle of incidence (measured from the normal to the diffuser surface). This arrangement is often called a *cosine-corrected* radiometer. The diffuser may be made from a flat or slightly curved piece of ground quartz or teflon, or it may be an integrating sphere. The purpose of the optical filter is to limit the spectral responsivity to a certain band, having a lower and upper wavelength cutoff. The band-width can vary upward from about 5 nm, but is often several tens or even hundreds of nanometres wide. Hence, radiometers are called broad-band meters as opposed to spectroradiometers. Ideally the spectral responsivity is constant within the band and zero outside, but in practice this is not possible. If the detector is sensitive to radiation outside the passband of the filter, which is normally the case, there will always be a non-zero responsivity outside the band. Signals which are produced by radiation from outside the band are called "out-of-band signals," "out-of-band leakage," or just "stray light." This limitation of radiometers can often be a serious problem, and is particularly troublesome in UV radiometers based

Figure 5.3 General schematic of a radiometer system. Solid lines indicate the essential elements. Other features (dashed lines) are added to operate in certain environments or to provide spectroradiometric information (i.e., the monochromator). (From Sliney & Wolbarsht, 1980)

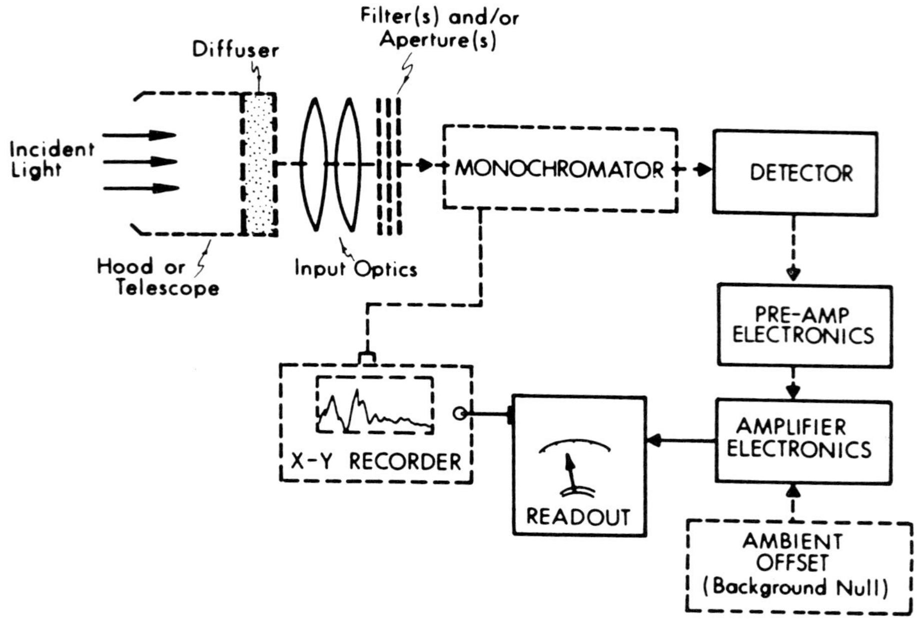

on Si photodiode detectors, because the spectral responsivities of Si photodiodes extend to 1100 nm in the infrared. If one attempts to use such radiometers to measure small quantities of in-band radiation in the presence of large quantities of out-of-band radiation, the results will be prone to large errors. This is frequently encountered when attempting to measure the very small component of biologically active UV present in a light source spectrum.

For many purposes it is desirable to have a UV radiometer which has a spectral responsivity equal to or closely resembling a certain action spectrum. If this is achieved, the radiometer signal is directly proportional to the "effective" or "biologically active" irradiance, because the radiometer will spectrally "weight" the different wavelengths according to the action spectrum S_λ. A well known example of such a radiometer is a photometer (lux-meter or luminance-meter) which has a spectral responsiveness that closely matches the photopic (visual) response of the human eye. Radiometers are commercially available which have spectral responsivities that match, for example, the UV erythema action spectrum (McKinlay and Diffey, 1987) and UV hazard action spectrum adopted by the IRPA/INIRC (1991) and ACGIH.

5.3.3 *Spectroradiometers*

A *spectroradiometer* is a radiometer that is capable of measuring spectral radiometric quantities directly, such as spectral irradiance or spectral radiance. The major difference between the layout of a spectroradiometer and the layout of a radiometer is the waveband selecting device which in a radiometer is usually a broadband filter (see figure 5.3), whereas in a spectroradiometer it is a monochromator or a spectrograph. Radiation entering a monochromator or a spectrograph is dispersed by a grating or a prism and only a small band of radiation is passed to the detector, the so-called bandwidth. The spectroradiometer bandwidth can be selected according to the application, but it is typically 1 - 5 nm. The waveband passed to the detector can be changed manually or automatically by rotating the grating or prism; the instrument is scanned over the spectral range of interest. This type of instrument is called a scanning spectroradiometer.

In a spectrograph, a portion of the spectrum is incident upon a photographic film, or a linear photodiode array which can be read diode by diode. This can occur very rapidly and a spectrum displayed almost instantly. This type of spectroradiometer is therefore useful for studies where time resolution is important. Another advantage is that there are no moving parts compared to a scanning spectroradiometer. However, spectrographs have disadvantages over scanning systems, such as spectral resolution and detectivity.

Spectroradiometers are more complex to operate and maintain than radiometers; they are considerably more expensive; and there are many pitfalls for the inexperienced user. Spectroradiometers generally employ the same kind of input optics as radiometers.

In an ideal spectroradiometer, the monochromator passes a small band of wavelengths to the detector, and passes no radiation outside this band. In practice the out-of-band radiation (leakage or stray-light) that is passed to the detector is of the order of 0.1 percent of the amount of in-band radiation depending upon the quality and size of the monochromator. In certain measurement situations this may give rise to errors (just as in radiometers): the signal caused by out-of-band radiation may be of the same order of magnitude as the signal caused by in-band radiation. For example, if one attempts to measure the solar UV spectrum in the 290-310 nm region, this error occurs because the solar spectrum decreases about five orders of magnitude from 310 nm to 290 nm. To overcome this error, a double monochromator may be used. A double monochromator is essentially two identical monochromators coupled in tandem, the output of the first becomes the input of the second monochromator. The stray light of a double monochromator is typically 0.01 percent.

5.3.4 *Personal dosimetry*

For personal monitoring of UV doses, radiometers are too bulky. A thin-film polymer (eg polysulphone) dosimeter overcomes this problem. It is a thin (0.04 mm) clear plastic film that may be worn as a small badge comparable to those used to monitor ionizing radiation. This allows monitoring of UVB doses on mobile subjects. Polysulphone changes its absorbance (or transmittance) when irradiated with UV (mainly by UVB). The received dose (radiant exposure) is determined by measuring the change in absorbance of the film before and after exposure (Diffey, 1989a). CR-39 plastic resins have also been explored as UVB dosimeters; however, the low sensitivity requires longer exposure periods (Wong et al., 1989).

5.4 Calibration

Improper or inadequate calibration of UV radiometers, spectroradiometers and dosimeters is a serious and common source of error. It is important to maintain a good calibration record for the instruments, but only experience on instrument stability will determine how often calibration is needed. The error caused by calibration provides the minimum uncertainty that can be obtained in measurement situations. Other sources of uncertainty include geometry and spectrum of source emission, detector-source geometry (angular errors), environmental influences and time factors.

Radiometers can be calibrated by using a source of known irradiance. This may either be a line source, such as a mercury lamp or a laser, or by a broadband source, such as a tungsten halogen lamp. It must be realized that the irradiance-responsivity will depend upon the source used for calibration. For example, a radiometer which has been calibrated against a line source will give erratic readings if used to measure a broadband source. In practice it is advisable to have radiometers calibrated against a source which emits a spectrum similar to those of the sources to be measured.

Complete calibration of radiometers and spectral radiometers include analysis of the cosine response of the instrument, the azimuthal response and the temperature sensitivity of the instrument. Recent work on instrument calibration and intercomparison has shown that instruments can vary greatly in these quantities even when the instruments agree on a simple spectral calibration. In the field, instruments will measure different quantities depending on the temperature and angle of incident radiation.

Spectroradiometers are calibrated against standard lamps of known spectral irradiance (or radiance). Such lamps can be obtained from the standards institutes in various countries. Intercomparison of lamp calibration from institute to institute can vary by as much as eight percent in the UV region, while better agreement is common in the visible region of standard lamps. This discrepancy should be noted when comparing results based on instruments calibrated from different lamp standards.

A tungsten halogen lamp is used as the standard lamp for wavelengths between 250 and 2500 nm, whereas a deuterium lamp is used in the region between 180 and 300-400 nm. It is good practice to operate the standard lamp only when calibrating a working-standard lamp and then use the working-standard for routine calibration of a spectroradiometer. For very accurate work it is recommended to maintain three calibrated lamps in order to find out whether a change in response/calibration, at least of a spectroradiometer, is caused by changes in the standard lamp used for calibration or by changes in the spectroradiometer.

Dosimeters are calibrated in the same way as radiometers except that exposure time is an integral part of the calibration process. To obtain a reliable calibration for radiometers and dosimeters, it is advisable to calibrate them against a source which emits a spectrum similar to the one that is to be measured.

6. CELLULAR AND MOLECULAR STUDIES

6.1 Introduction

This chapter provides an overview of the evidence for cellular and molecular effects of UV exposure on biological systems. Since UV exposure has been associated with skin and eye cancers in humans, emphasis will be given to the process of carcinogenesis. It is known that UV exposure results in photochemical modification of the genetic material (DNA), but most of this damage is accurately and efficiently repaired by the cell. However if the amount of damage is too great some of the alterations to the DNA may remain as permanent mutations. It has been proposed that if unrepaired damage occurs to regulatory genes this may be involved in the process of carcinogenesis. In this context mutations to and activation of genes may be important.

Other responses likely to result from UV exposure of cells include increased cellular proliferation, which could have a tumour promoting effect on genetically altered cells, as well as changes in components of the immune system present in the skin. There is evidence to suggest that UV exposure could elicit an immunosuppressive effect which may compromise the body's ability to identify and destroy tumour cells of the skin.

This review includes summary descriptions of UV action and repair of damage to biomolecules, particularly in DNA, cellular chromophores and other target molecules, as well as damage to the cell membrane and proteins. Consequences of damage to the cell, its membranes and activation of genes are also reviewed.

6.2 Interactions with Biomolecules

UV must be absorbed to produce a chemical change. At solar UV intensities normally encountered, the first step in a photochemical reaction is the absorption of a single photon by a molecule and the production of an excited state in which one electron of the absorbing molecule is raised to a higher energy level. Such radiative transition can only occur efficiently when the photon energy of the radiation is close to the energy difference of the atom in the initial and final state (energy level). The photochemistry that may then occur will therefore depend upon the molecular structure and the wavelength of UV as well as the specific reaction conditions. The primary products generated by UV absorption are generally reactive species in a metastable excited state or free radicals both of which form extremely fast. Dark chemical reactions then occur often within microseconds but they may last for hours, as is the case for the lipid peroxidation chain reaction. Finally these relatively rapid processes are translated into photobiological responses which may occur within seconds but can take years or even decades to be manifested.

6.2.1 *Cellular chromophores*

Since chromophores (see chapter 5 for definition) are characterized by the wavelengths at which they absorb, the nature of the critical chromophores will change as a function of wavelength throughout the UV range. The peak absorption of DNA is dictated by its component nucleic acids and occurs at around 260 nm. There is a sharp drop in absorption through the UVB range and absorption is undetectable by conventional means at wavelengths longer than 320 nm. Using special detectors Sutherland and Griffin, (1981) have measured DNA absorption at wavelengths as long as 360 nm. Although overall protein absorption peaks in the UVC range, the aromatic amino acids such as tryptophan (λ max = 280 nm at pH7) and tyrosine (λ max = 275 nm at pH7) exhibit absorptions that extend into the UVA range so that direct damage to proteins can occur at much longer wavelengths than direct damage to DNA.

Several cellular components such as quinones, flavins, steroids and porphyrins are important UVA chromophores. Porphyrins, which exhibit an absorption with a peak around 405 nm, have been implicated in the lethal action of UVA and near-visible light in certain bacteria. Mutants in the bacterium *Escherichia coli* (*E coli*) which are deficient in the synthesis of L-amino levulinic acid, the first step in heme synthesis, are resistant to UVA radiation (Tuveson and Sammartano, 1986) strongly suggesting that porphyrin intermediates can be phototoxic. Porphyrin intermediates evidently also arise during heme synthesis in humans. Indeed, supplementation of human cells with amino levulinate (ALA) bypasses the synthase step and leads to accumulation of protoporphyrin IX (PPIX), the immediate precursor to heme and a strong photosensitiser. ALA appears to be preferentially taken up by skin cancer cells and the selective photosensitisation of such cells by PPIX is the basis of a new type of phototherapy based on endogenous sensitisers (Kennedy et al., 1990). Iron chelators can enhance the sensitising effect by preventing the insertion of iron into the PPIX macrocycle thus preventing the formation of the relatively non-photoactive heme product. Accumulation of iron-free porphyrins is the basis of the acute photosensitivity of skin in patients with a variety of porphyrins. However, it is not clear to what extent PPIX, for example, leads to UVA-mediated cytoxicity in normal human skin cells.

Aside from DNA and proteins, the main chromophores in human skin are urocanic acid and melanins (for review see Anderson & Parrish, 1981).

Trans-urocanic acid (4-amidazoleacrylic acid) is the deamination product of histidine generated by histidase and because of its broad absorption in the UV region has been considered as contributing to a modest extent to the natural sunscreen properties of skin. However, most notable is that the trans form can be photoisomerised to the cis form and it has been proposed that this conversion is a key factor in UV-induced immunosuppression (DeFabo and Noonan, 1983). However, considerable controversy now surrounds this original suggestion (eg. see Gibbs 1993).

Melanins are the major UV absorbing chromophores in skin, exhibiting an extremely broad spectrum of absorption over the UVB, UVA and visible ranges. Melanins are complex polymeric proteins that are produced by melanocytes and transferred to keratinocytes. Although often considered to be neutral density filters, this is not strictly correct since melanins usually degrade upon UV exposure. There is some evidence that melanin may function as a photosensitizer of DNA damage.

In addition to iron-free porphyrins which generate singlet oxygen upon exposure to UVA radiation, other small molecules also have the potential to generate active oxygen intermediates upon UVA exposure (Tyrell, 1992). For example, the photochemical degradation of tryptophan by wavelengths which include the more energetic portion of the UVA spectrum is able to generate hydrogen peroxide and N-formyl kynurenin (McCormick et al., 1976). Although the level of hydrogen peroxide generated *in vivo* by such a pathway would appear to be in the low micromolar range it could nevertheless be crucial to biological processes since iron complexes (such as citrate) that are present in the cytoplasm will react with hydrogen peroxide to generate the highly reactive hydroxyl radical in a superoxide driven Fenton reaction (see Gutteridge, 1985; Imlay et al., 1988). Since the reaction is driven by the continual reduction of ferric iron to the ferrous state by superoxide anions, a cellular source of superoxide anions is also required. In this context it should be noted that both hydrogen peroxide and hydroxyl radical are generated by UVA irradiation of NADH and NADPH (Czochralska et al., 1984; Cunningham et al., 1985). However, it is not at all clear whether this is really the key source of superoxide anions or whether the main source is as a consequence of normal cellular metabolism.

6.2.2 *Cellular targets*

The chromophores for UV effects are not necessarily the critical targets which mediate the effects. The most important cellular target for UV is considered to be DNA since the crucial genetic material exists in unique and very low copy numbers in cells. Radiation in the UVB range is absorbed by DNA and leads to photochemical damage, so that DNA would certainly appear to be the primary chromophore and site of damage for most of the biological effects of short wavelength UV. DNA damage induced by UVB radiation is the key factor leading to sunlight-induced mutations in cancer-related genes and therefore in initiating the carcinogenic process. At longer wavelengths, targets may change. For example, the destruction of mitochondria may be a key factor in the breakdown of cellular integrity following certain types of photosensitisation. Membrane damage clearly takes on added significance when the UV radiation employed (e.g.from sunlight) includes a strong component of longer wavelengths. Breakdown of membranes can lead to aberrant signal transduction as well as dramatic alterations in transport pathways. Leakage of essential components or an influx of extracellular molecules such as calcium can have severe cytostatic and even lethal consequences for the cell and will clearly have an influence on overall tissue/organ function.

6.3 Action Spectra

An action spectrum is a measure of the relative effectiveness of different wavelengths, within the spectral region of study, to produce a given response (see chapter 5 for definition). Clearly the number of photochemical and photobiological endpoints that can be measured is as large as the number of effects themselves and before undertaking action spectroscopy for a given end-point, there should exist a good *a priori* reason for the study. Numerous types of UV induced DNA damage have now been recognized that include stand breaks (single and double), cyclobutane-type pyrimidine dimers, 6-4 pyo photoproducts and the corresponding Dewar isomer, thymine glycols, 8-hydroxy guanine, and many more. In addition, DNA-protein cross-links are produced during UV exposure. Larger scale genetic alterations include chromosome breakage, sister chromatid exchanges and chromatid aberrations. Although partial UV action spectra are now available for many of these lesions, the most studied have been the different types of pyrimidine dimers. Since the indirect oxidising component of radiation damage increases with increasing wavelength, there is a dramatic shift in the type of lesion induced as the wavelength increases. Pyrimidine dimers are characteristic of the direct absorption that occurs at shorter UV wavelengths whereas strand breaks and 8-hydroxy guanine type lesions become increasingly important at longer wavelengths. At a higher level of complexity, action spectra for cell death, mutation, *in vitro* transformation, growth delays, cell permeability, etc, may also be measured.

One goal of determining action spectra has been to correlate end-points with a specific type of initial damage. However, such evaluations are complex partly because the absorbing chromophores and crucial lesions will often change as a function of wavelength. At the whole organism level, action spectra may be determined for effects on entire organs, for example, various markers of leaf damage in plants, erythema induction in skin and even tumour induction.

Studies in cultured cells may be of value in predicting responses in whole organs such as skin but various parameters must be evaluated. In particular, the penetration of UV to the critical chromophores as a function of wavelength must be taken into account by considering the transmission through overlying tissue. As an example, we may wish to calculate the relative cytotoxic action of the different wavelengths in sunlight to cells at the basal layer of the epidermis. In order to do this, an action spectrum must be available for the cytotoxic action of individual wavelengths on cultured epidermal keratinocytes. In addition, data is needed for transmission through human skin to the target cells since this will change as a function of wavelength. Finally if the effect of a particular UV source is required (such as terrestrial sunlight under defined conditions) then this must be determined by spectroradiometry or from available data. The relative biological effectiveness of individual wavelengths of sunlight in killing cells at the basal level of the epidermis may then be predicted by convoluting these three spectra. In practice, interactions (synergistic, additive or antagonistic) exist between different UV wavelength regions and these must also be taken into account in the evaluation of the biological effects of broad spectrum sources. Although action spectra may be of value for predictive evaluations, the primary aim of studies with cultured cells is often to determine chromophores. For this purpose, action spectra must be corrected in order to express results as action per photon before comparison with absorption spectra of critical biological molecules. Thus, DNA is known to be an important chromophore in the UVB region. The results are far more difficult to interpret in the longer wavelength UVA region but at least for simpler organisms such as bacteria, porphyrins have often been implicated. Action spectra, particularly in plants, are often modified by protective absorbing molecules such as carotenoids.

In response to questions posed by the threat to the ozone layer, fairly detailed action spectra have now been determined for squamous cell carcinoma in hairless mice and transmission corrections made to estimate the spectrum in humans. DNA is clearly the primary chromophore in the UVB region but a significant second peak occurs in the long UVA wavelength region.

6.4 Biomolecular Damage

UV radiation can damage many cellular targets including the nucleic acids, proteins and lipids. For the non-solar UVC wavelengths, DNA is clearly the most important target and many photochemical changes can occur as a result of direct absorption. The genotoxic action of solar UVB radiation is also of critical importance, although the spectrum of DNA damage begins to change as oxidative events become more important. At longer UVA wavelengths, indirect effects mediated by active oxygen intermediates are common and except for events directly related to DNA modification (e.g. mutation), it is difficult to discern the crucial targets.

6.4.1 *Nucleic acids*

Cyclobutane type pyrimidine dimers

Cyclobutane type pyrimidine dimers were the first type of UV-induced base damage to be identified (Beukers & Berends, 1960) and being the most frequent lesion induced by either UVC or UVB radiation, they have been the most studied.

Cyclobutane-type pyrimidine dimer formation arises from the production of reactive excited states (normally the forbidden but long-lived triplet state) following absorption of UV radiation. The action spectrum for dimer formation as shown in figure 6.1, closely resembles that for the extinction coefficients of the appropriate monomers, cytosine(C) or thymine(T) for wavelengths as long as 313 nm (Ellison & Childs, 1981) so that the mechanism of formation is probably similar. Although pyrimidine dimer formation (e.g. thymine ◊ thymine or T ◊ T) has been measured in the UVA range, six orders of magnitude more energy is required at 365 nm as compared to 254 nm (Tyrrell, 1973) and the mechanism of formation is unclear. Most of the original observations concerning dimer induction were made in isolated DNA, bacteriophage systems or in *E coli* but essential results have since been confirmed in mammalian cells including human skin fibroblasts. Action spectra determined in human and mouse skin are sharply attenuated at shorter wavelengths, but are otherwise basically similar to those obtained *in vitro*. The action spectra for cyclobutane pyrimidine dimer formation in naked DNA, cell cultures and epidermal DNA is given in figures 6.2 and 6.3. Based on studies with *E coli*, the ratio of T ◊ T, C ◊ T to C ◊ C changes appreciably with wavelength. For example, the ratio of T ◊ T to C ◊ T dimers is 0.63:1 at 313 nm (Ellison & Childs, 1981) but increases to 6:1 at 365 nm (Tyrrell, 1973).

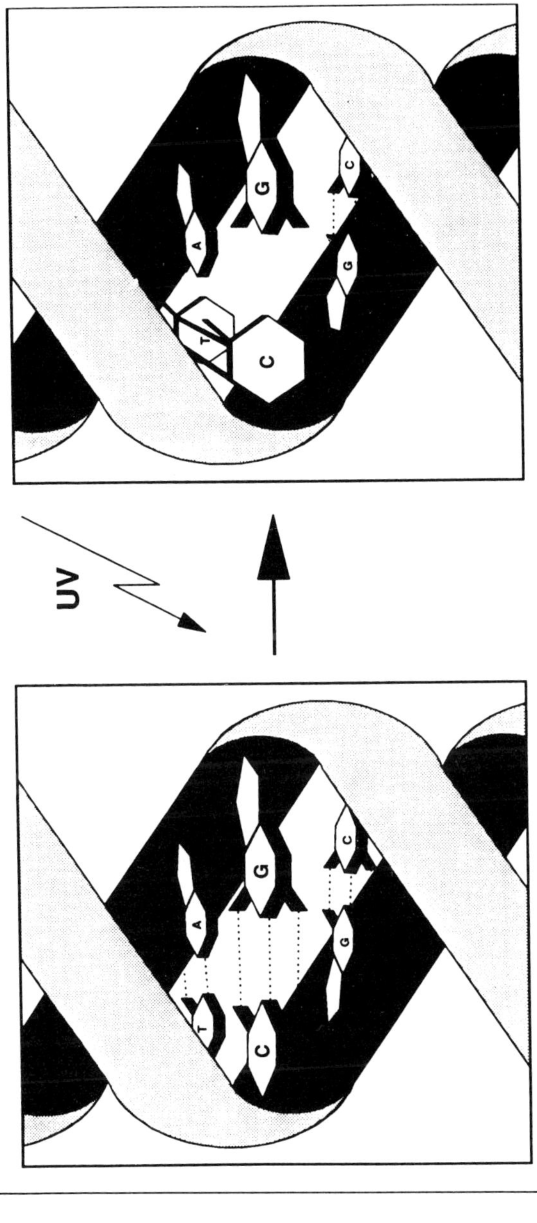

Figure 6.1 Formation of pyrimidine dimers within DNA (courtesy of National Radiological Protection Board, UK)

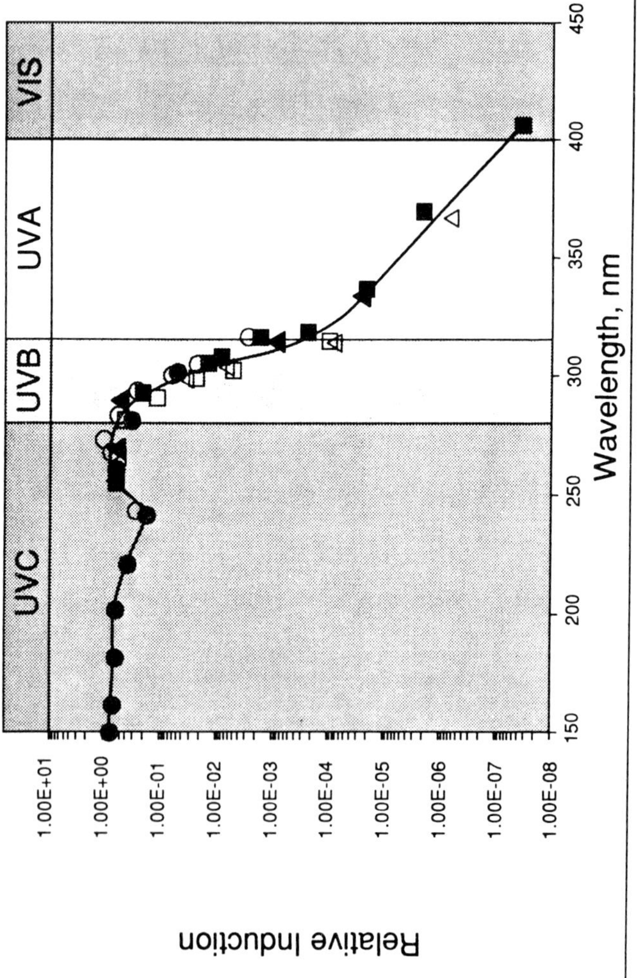

Figure 6.2 Action spectra for cyclobutane pyrimidine dimer formation in naked DNA and cultured cells. ■ Peak et al., 1984; ▲ Chan et al., 1986; ● Matsunaga et al., 1991; □ Enninga et al., 1986; O Doniger et al., 1981 (courtesy of National Radiological Protection Board, UK).

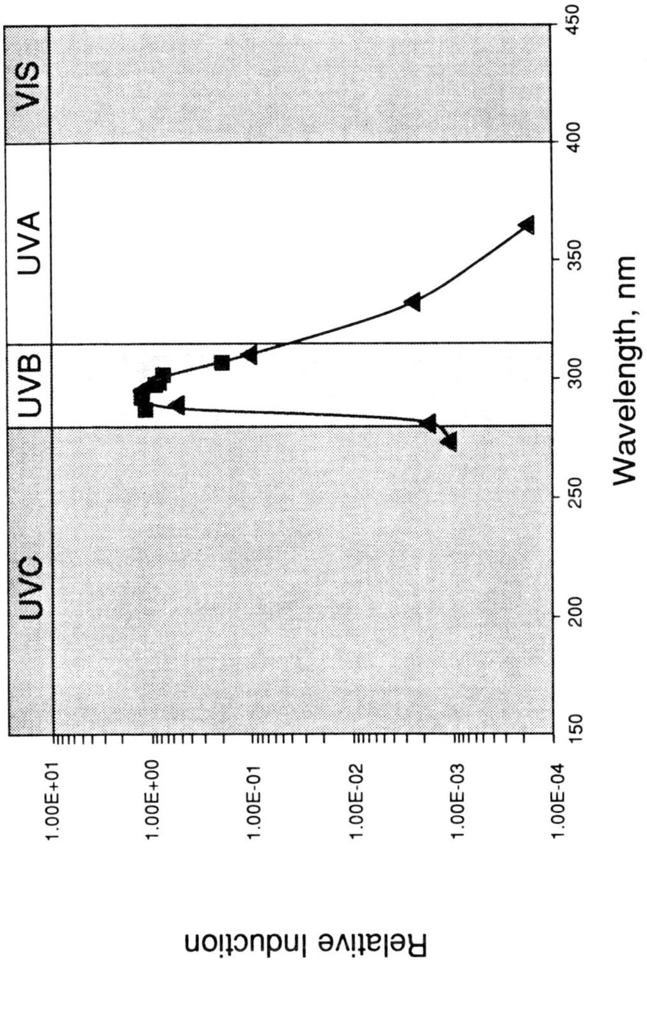

Figure 6.3 Action spectra for cyclobutane pyrimidine dimer formation in epidermal DNA. ■ Ley et al., 1983; ▲ Freeman et al., 1989 (courtesy of National Radiological Protection Board, UK)

Although repair of DNA damage is dealt with separately below, it is worth noting at this point that an extremely specific light-dependant repair process, photoreactivation, exists for repair of pyrimidine dimers *in situ*. Repair proceeds via photolyase which has been shown to be present almost ubiquitously throughout the animal world from *E coli* to non-placental mammals. Recent evidence suggests that photoreactivation may be less important in human cells (Li et al., 1993). Nevertheless, the photoenzymatic splitting of pyrimidine dimers has provided a powerful technique since it has provided a way of linking a specific type of DNA damage (the pyrimidine dimer) with defined biological effects (e.g. cell death, tumour formation).

Thy (6-4) pyo photoproducts

A second type of pyrimidine dimer can be formed by UV (Varghese & Wang, 1967) which was originally termed a pyrimidine adduct and is now more commonly referred to as the thy (6-4) pyo photoproduct. More recently a pyrimidine nucleoside-cytidine lesion was recognized in highly reiterated sequences of human DNA (Lippke et al., 1981) which is almost certainly the precursor of the thy (6-4) pyo photoproduct (Brash & Haseltine, 1982; Franklin, et al., 1982). The (6-4) photoproduct is formed with much greater frequency between cytosines located 5' of adjacent pyrimidines. Action spectra that compare induction of cyclobutane-type pyrimidine dimers are all similar between 265 nm and 302 nm (Patrick, 1977; Chan et al., 1986; Matsunaga, et al., 1991; Rosenstein & Mitchell, 1987) as shown in figure 6.4. However, at longer wavelengths not all the spectra agree. At least for human skin fibroblasts the relative level of (6-4) photoproduct induction is only half that for cyclobutane-type dimers. The reason for this appears to be that the (6-4) photoproducts are converted to a Dewar pyrimidine isomer by UV radiation at wavelengths peaking in the UVB range. This has been confirmed in studies by Mitchell & Rosenstein (1987) using radio-immuno assays for the (6-4) photoproduct and its Dewar isomer.

Although (6-4) photoproducts form with 5-10 fold lower efficiency than cyclobutane type dimers, they may be formed with equal efficiency at certain sites (Kraemer et al., 1988). Furthermore, in the UVB region, a significant level of Dewar pyrimidine isomers will be formed and the precise ratio and level of these three major types of base damage will depend on the wavelength(s) of radiation employed, as well as irradiation conditions.

Other types of dimeric base damage which include purines have been isolated from DNA heavily irradiated with UVC. These include the

Figure 6.4 Action spectra for pyrimidine (6-4) pyrimidone adduct formation in naked DNA and cultured cells. ▲ Chan et al., 1986; □ Rosenstein & Mitchell, 1987; ● Matsunaga et al., 1991 (courtesy of National Radiological Protection Board, UK).

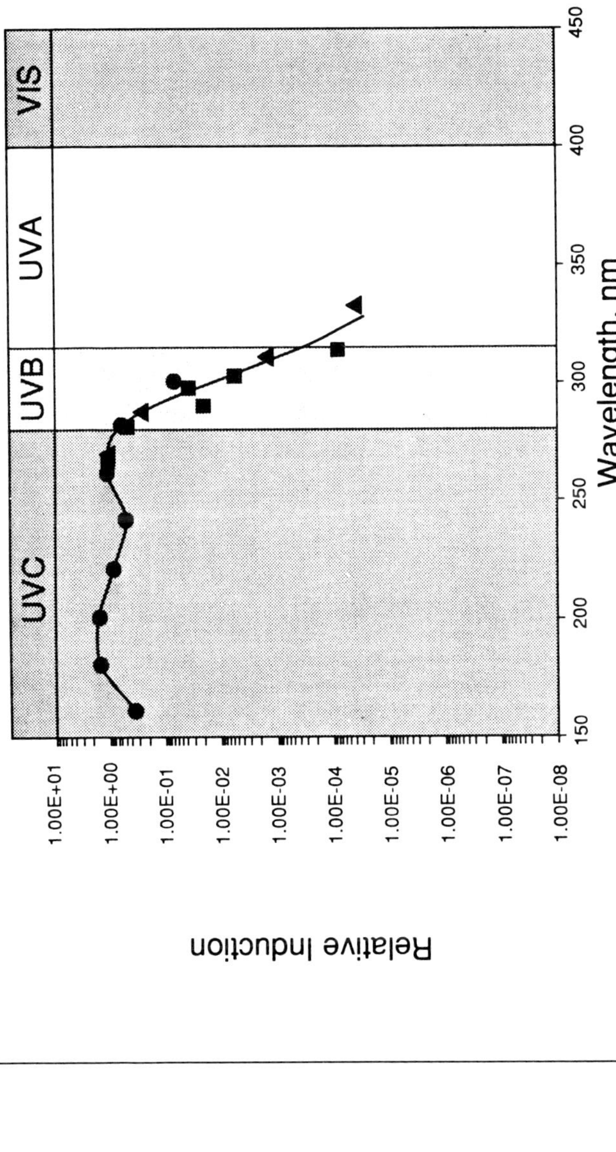

thymine-adenine dimer (Bose & Davies, 1984) and adenine dehydrodimer (Gasparro & Fresco, 1986). Such photoproducts occur at fairly low frequency (approximately 1 percent of that of pyrimidine-type dimers. The relative levels and significance of these photoproducts in the UVB or longer wavelength regions has not yet been determined.

Monobasic DNA damage

Damage to a single base is a relatively low frequency event in UV damaged DNA. Simple hydrates of cytosine and thymine can certainly be formed (Fisher & Johns, 1976) but these low frequency events are unreliable and therefore extremely difficult to study from a biological viewpoint. They may be related to the low frequency cytosine photoproduct identified by sequencing techniques by Gallagher et al. (1989). Sequencing techniques in combination with endonuclease V treatment have also led to the detection of a class of rare and unidentified purine or purine-pyrimidine sites after broad spectrum UV irradiation (Gallagher & Duker, 1986).

A group of lesions induced by both UV and ionizing radiation are ring-saturated thymines of the 5, 6-dihyroxydihydrothymine type (thymine glycols). Although original measurements indicated that they were induced almost as frequently as pyrimidine dimers at 313 nm as against 21:1 at 254 nm (Cerutti & Netrawali, 1979), it has been concluded from more recent data using sequencing analysis (Mitchell et al., 1993) that they do not occur at a significant rate in UVC or UVB irradiated DNA.

Increasingly sophisticated chemical methods are now becoming available to measure oxidative DNA damage (Cadet et al., Methods in Enzymology, in press). Since the proportion of this type of damage will increase with increasing wavelength, such techniques will soon be applied to consolidate the picture of UV-induced based damage throughout the entire solar UV spectrum. Furthermore, an interesting enzyme has been isolated (Boiteux et al., 1987) termed the Fapy glycosylase because of its ability to excise the ring-opened form of N7-methylguanine from DNA. The enzyme will also recognize DNA products generated in photosensitisation reactions involving singlet oxygen (Epe et al., in press) and 8-hydroxyguanine may be a major component. Since the longer UV wavelength in sunlight clearly generate biologically relevant levels of singlet oxygen and other active intermediates (Tyrrell, 1991; Basu-Modak & Tyrrell, 1993), this type of analysis may also be usefully applied to the solar UV spectrum. Certainly, near-visible light alone is able to generate Fapy glycosylase-sensitive lesions in the DNA of cultured mammalian cells and these, at least in part, are probably 8-hydroxyguanine (Epe et al., 1993).

DNA strand breaks

Few DNA strand breaks are induced by UVC radiation but they constitute an increasing proportion of the total lesions as wavelength is increased. For example, in *E. coli* the ratio of DNA strand breaks to pyrimidine dimers is 1:44 at 313 nm (Miguel & Tyrrell, 1983) whereas at 365 nm one strand break is formed for every two pyrimidine dimers (Tyrrell et al., 1974). Action spectra have now been determined for the induction of DNA single strand breaks in human skin cells which show that breaks occur throughout the UVA and into the near-visible range (Peak et al., 1987). Since break measurements involve alkaline denaturation, 10-20 percent of the so-called breaks are due to the fragility of chemical bonds at apurinic and apyrimidinic sites. It is important to note that unlike most of the common forms of base damage, induction of strand breaks is strongly dependent on oxygen throughout the UVB and UVA ranges (Tyrrell, et al., 1974; Peak & Peak, 1982; Miguel and Tyrrell, 1983) and at the longest wavelengths may involve generation of singlet oxygen (Peak et al., 1987). Figure 6.5 gives the action spectra for single strand breaks and figure 6.6 for double strand breaks in cultured cells.

DNA-protein cross links

Photochemically induced DNA-protein cross links, mostly involving cysteine are clearly formed *in vitro* (Smith, 1976; Shetlar, 1980) and appear to be formed *in vivo*, particularly in the UVA range (Bradley, et al., 1979; Peak & Peak, 1991). Despite the obvious importance of this type of damage, there is little known at the molecular level concerning the nature of the damage formed *in vivo*. Action spectra for DNA-protein cross links in cultured cells is given in figure 6.7 (from Peak et al., 1985a, b).

Ribonucleic acid

Messenger RNA is readily susceptible to modification by UV radiation. However, given the fairly rapid turnover of most molecules of this type (half-lives generally of the order of minutes and hours) and the capacity for *de novo* synthesis in the absence of DNA damage, mRNA is not generally considered a critical target of radiation damage in mammalian cells. Bacterial transfer RNA is often extremely photosensitive because of the presence of an unusual nucleoside 4-thiouridine and this leads to some fascinating photobiological phenomena of ecological significance (Jagger,

Figure 6.5 Action spectra for single strand break formation in cultured cells. ▲ Peak et al., 1987; ■ Rosenstein & Ducore, 1983; ● Peak & Peak, 1991 (courtesy of National Radiological Protection Board, UK).

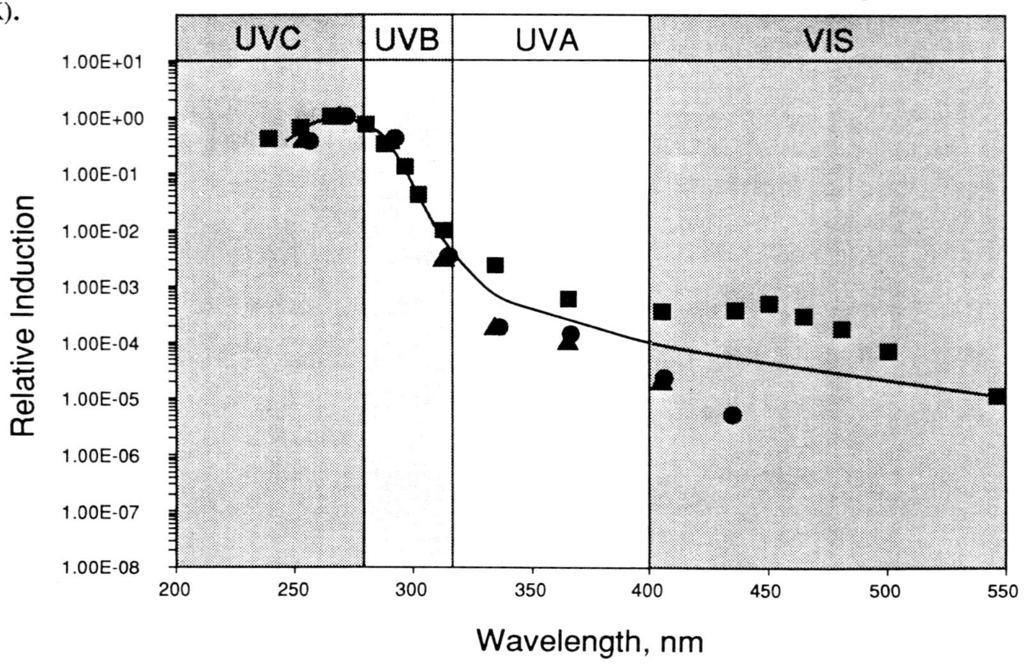

Figure 6.6 Action spectrum for double strand break formation in cultured cells. Peak & Peak, 1990 (courtesy of National Radiological Protection Board, UK).

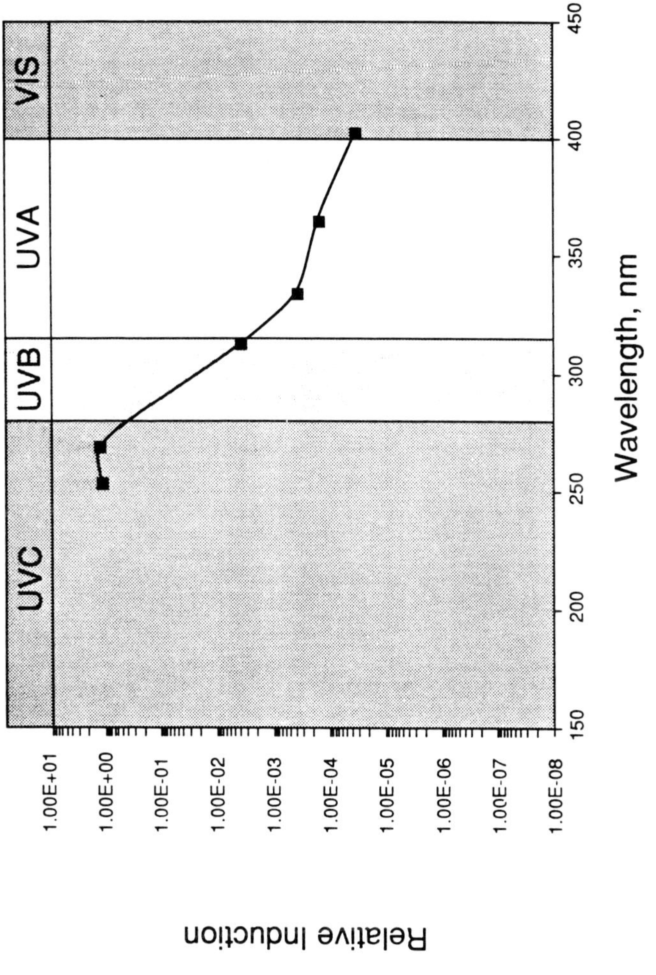

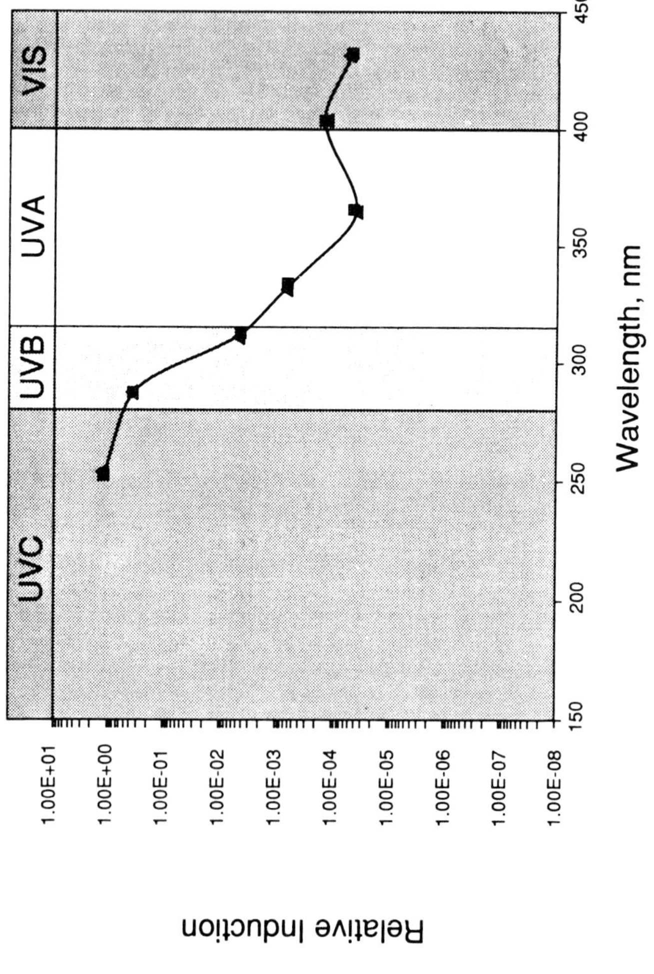

Figure 6.7 Action spectra for DNA-protein cross links formation in cultured cells. ▲ Peak et al., 1985a; ■ Peak et al., 1985b (courtesy of National Radiological Protection Board).

1985). However, such findings are of little significance to eukaryotic cells.

6.4.2 *Membranes*

UV-induced changes in membrane permeability and membrane transport systems would be expected to have fairly dramatic consequences for human skin and eyes. Unsaturated fatty acids are readily oxidised to hydroperoxides. Several reports have now shown that UV radiation can peroxidise membrane lipids (Desai, et al., 1964; Roshchupkin et al., 1975; Putvinsky et al., 1979; Azizova, et al., 1980). Using liposomal models (Mandal & Chatterjee, 1980; Bose et al., 1989), it has been shown that UVA radiation causes a dose-dependent increase in lipid peroxidation as measured by various techniques and that this can be largely inhibited by membrane antioxidants such as butylated hydroxytoluene. In *E coli*, sensitivity to UVA correlates with the levels of unsaturated fat in membranes (Klamen & Tuveson, 1982; Chamberlain & Moss, 1987). An agent which enhances singlet oxygen lifetime, deuterium oxide, enhances the level of membrane damage, sensitivity to UVA and lipid peroxidation. There are now reports that both UVB and UVA (Morlière et al., 1991; Punnonen et al., 1991; Vile et al., 1994) radiation can cause lipid peroxidation at biologically relevant fluences in the membranes of human fibroblasts and keratinocytes.

Cell leakage experiments have been used to assess membrane damage in yeast (Ito and Ito, 1983) and a similar technique has now been used to show UVA-mediated enhancement of membrane leakage in human skin fibroblasts (Gaboriau et al., 1993; Vile et al., 1994). UVA also causes changes in membrane fluidity as assessed using a lipophilic fluorescent probe. UVA-induced alteration of membrane transport systems received considerable attention in prokaryotes (see Jagger, 1985) but little information is available in mammalian cells. A recent study has demonstrated that UVA radiation inhibits both receptor-mediated (low density lipoprotein) and nonspecific (sucrose) uptake of exogenous molecules (Djavuheri-Mergny et al., 1993). These findings may be related to other studies in human fibroblasts which have shown that broad spectrum UV sources cause cytoskeletal damage as manifested by dose-dependent microtubule disassembly (Zamansky & Chou, 1987).

6.4.3 *Proteins*

As the wavelength is increased through the UVB and UVA regions damage to proteins becomes increasingly important because of the absorption properties of the aromatic amino acids relative to nucleic acids. In addition, many proteins that include the antioxidant enzymes catalases and peroxidases contain heme groups thus making them UVA chromophores and potentially photosensitisers. Indeed, catalase is sensitive to sunlight (Mitchell & Anderson, 1965), probably as a result of UVA absorption (Kramer & Ames, 1987). In bacteria there is evidence that endogenous catalase and possibly alkyl hydroperoxide reductase are actually photosensitisers (Eisenstark & Perrot, 1987; Kramer & Ames, 1987) but no similar experiments to have been carried out in mammalian cells. Repair enzymes are also sensitive to UVA radiation and there is evidence that UV-induced repair disruption plays a role in cell death and mutagenesis (Haynes, 1966; Webb, 1977; Tyrrell, 1982). Considerable attention has been given recently to metal ion catalysed oxidation of protein since this is clearly a physiologically relevant process (for review see Stadtman, 1990). Numerous proteins have been shown to be modified by a free radical generating, system modelling those that cells are exposed to during normal metabolism or exogenous insult. It appears that active oxygen/free radical species are generated at specific metal binding sites on proteins and that this leads to reactions with amino acid residues at specific steric locations.

6.5 Cellular Defences

6.5.1 *DNA*

Even one or two pyrimidine dimers in the entire genome of a bacterium such as *E coli* may be lethal if DNA repair processes are defective. However, DNA repair processes are not only crucial for cell survival but also for the maintenance of genetic stability since DNA damage is continuously generated as a by-product of metabolism even in the absence of exogenous insults. Because of the availability of mutants, most of the original studies concerning removal of DNA damage employed bacteria and bacteriophage. The first process to be identified was photoreactivation later known as photoenzymatic repair. In this process, a DNA photolyase forms a specific complex with a pyrimidine dimer which can be split in the presence of UVA and/or visible light to leave the original pyrimidines in the DNA. The process has been widely used to correlate a specific type of DNA damage (the pyrimidine dimer) with a given biological effect (from cell death in bacteria to cancer in fish), although recent evidence for an enzyme which recognizes (6-4) photoproducts may cast doubt on the validity of this approach. Photoenzymatic repair is entirely error free (i.e. it does not lead to mutations) and occurs in a wide variety of single and multiple-celled organisms. Although photoenzymatic repair and associated photolyases occur in non-placental mammals such as the marsupials, evidence for photoreactivation in placental mammals, including humans, has been fragmentary and controversial. Recent evidence suggesting that photoreactivation of UV damage may not be a significant process in human skin (Li et al., 1993) could be of crucial importance when considering potential interactions between wavelengths.

Evidence for two broad categories of DNA repair, originally denoted as dark repair processes, were revealed by bacterial studies (see Friedberg, 1984 for review). Post-replicational repair, as the name implies, can occur only after DNA synthesis and includes many of the complex pathways of genetic recombination. Humans with the genetic disease Xeroderma pigmentosum (XP) of the variant complementation group are deficient in this type of repair. However, the SOS repair process in bacteria which involves the inducible activation of a post-replication error-prone (mutagenic) repair pathway, has no equivalent in humans. On the other hand, excision repair is the most widespread of DNA repair processes and occurs from bacteria to man. In excision repair, damaged or incorrect bases are excised from the genome and replaced by the correct nucleotides. The first step in the process involves recognition of the damage and incision at or close to the damaged site. This can occur by two distinct mechanisms. Damaged bases may be recognised by a series of specific glycosylases. In this case, incision occurs by a two-step reaction which involves the sequential activities of the DNA glycosylase and an apyrimidinic/apurinic endonuclease. However, a second mechanism of incision involves the direct action of a damage-specific DNA incising activity without the need for glycosylase action. At least in *E Coli*, incisions are made at either side of the damaged base so that exonucleolytic removal of bases is unnecessary in this case. Repolymerization of the gap created by endonuclease/exonuclease activity is an essential step and can take place using the undamaged strand as a template. The action of DNA ligase restores the original integrity of the double-stranded DNA.

DNA excision repair in humans is also an extremely complex process as evidenced by the considerable genetic heterogeneity in XP which is a rare but extensively studied disease whose cellular basis involves a defect in DNA repair. Genomic clones of several human DNA repair genes have now been derived by transfecting DNA from repair proficient human cells into a series of UV-sensitive mutant rodent cell lines (Westerveld et al., 1984). A considerable amount of information is now available concerning the molecular genetics of eukaryotic DNA excision repair (Hoeijmakers & Bootsma, 1990). The repair genes isolated to date often have DNA binding and/or nucleic acid helicase domains. Most recently, a repair gene product has been identified as one of the components of a transcription factor complex involved in the transcription of polymerase II genes (Schaeffer et al., 1993). This is currently an extremely active area of research and further genes are expected to be isolated.

In vitro repair systems are now available (Wood et al., 1988). In addition, animal models are now being developed using homologous recombination techniques and genetic manipulation of embryonic stem cells.

6.5.2 *Human excision repair disorders*

Several human diseases involve defects in DNA repair. The most studied example is the genetic disorder XP which actually involves several types of excision repair defect as well as the variant form which is defective in post-replication repair. These cell lines are crucial to basic studies of DNA repair in humans. Cell lines derived from the excision-defective individuals are many times more sensitive to inactivation and mutation by UVC and UVB radiation (Arlett et al., 1992). This appears to be directly correlated with the fact that individuals with this disease are extremely prone to tumours of the skin, eye and lips (Kraemer et al., 1987). Indeed, it is the study of cancer incidence in these individuals which provides the strongest evidence that the induction of photoproducts in skin by UV is the first event in a sequence which eventually leads to basal cell carcinoma, squamous cell carcinoma and melanomas in man.

The above conclusion is now complicated by studies with cells from patients with the rare disease, Trichothiodystrophy. Although, cells from most of the patients studied so far have a marked defect in DNA excision repair, the patients do not show elevated evidence of skin tumours. They are, nevertheless, sun-sensitive in terms of their erythemal response (Bridges 1990). A partial explanation may be that XP patients but not Trichothiodystrophy patients have defects in both DNA repair and oxidative metabolism and both these processes are involved in carcinogenesis (Vuillaume et al., 1992).

Fibroblasts from patients with Cockayne's syndrome are specifically defective in excision of dimers from DNA undergoing active transcription (Mayne et al., 1988) and are sensitive to killing and mutation by UVC radiation. (Arlett & Harcourt 1983). However, these individuals are not exceptionally cancer-prone (Barret et al., 1991).

6.5.3 *Antioxidant pathways*

Small antioxidant molecules

Recent reviews have evaluated the nature and importance of small antioxidant molecules in human blood plasma (Stocker & Frei, 1991), the eye (Spector, 1991) and human skin (Fuchs & Packer 1991; Tyrrell 1991).

Glutathione is a major constituent of lens epithelial cells (Rathbun 1989) and these cells have a high capacity for maintaining glutathione in the reduced state because of extremely active hexose monophosphate shunt activity. This compound may be involved in a number of antioxidant reactions that are relevant to UV-mediated oxidative stress including detoxification of hydrogen peroxide (as a cofactor of GSH peroxidase), detoxification of free radicals, reduction of protein disulphides, and competition with protein thiols for oxidising species. The role of ascorbate as an effective antioxidant in lens is less clear because of the potential of ascorbate to be involved in the generation of deleterious components (Spector, 1991). Vitamin E is also a potentially useful antioxidant but there is no general agreement as to the usefulness of vitamin E therapy for cataract.

Free radical intermediates have been implicated in UV-induced carcinogenesis in investigations originally stimulated by the isolation of the putative carcinogen cholesterol epoxide from human skin (Black 1987). Various components present in skin are potent antioxidants including ascorbate, uric acid, carotenoids and sulphydrils. Carotenoids have been shown to inhibit UV-induced epidermal damage and tumour formation in mouse models (Mathews-Roth & Krinsky, 1987). In cell culture models using human skin cells, it has been clearly shown that glutathione depletion leads to a large sensitization to UVA (334 nm, 365 nm) and near-visible (405 nm) wavelengths as well as to radiation in the UVB (302 nm, 313 nm) (Tyrrell & Pidoux, 1986,1988). There is a direct correlation between the levels of sensitisation and cellular glutathione content. Additional evidence that glutathione is a photoprotective agent in skin cells is derived from experiments which have demonstrated that glutathione levels in both dermis and epidermis are depleted by UVA treatment (Connor & Wheeler, 1987).

Water-soluble antioxidants in plasma include glucose, pyruvate, uric acid, ascorbic acid, bilirubin and glutathione. Lipid soluble anti-oxidants include α-tocopherol, ubiquinol-10, lycopene, ß-carotene, lutein, zeaxanthin and α-carotene. Since, the long wavelengths in sunlight can penetrate through tissue and into blood at the longer wavelengths, these defenses may be critical under certain circumstances.

Antioxidant proteins including enzymes

The major classes of antioxidant enzymes characterized to date in eukaryotic cells are superoxide dismutase (which converts superoxide anion to hydrogen peroxide), catalase (which destroys hydrogen peroxide) and glutathione peroxide and associated enzymes (which in addition to metabolizing hydrogen peroxide can also reduce hydroperoxides such as those that result from lipid peroxidation). Both glutathione peroxide and catalase are present in the lens, although the latter is present at low levels and concentrated in the epithelial cells (Bhuyan & Bhuyan 1983). Spector (1991) claims that these enzymes are present at sufficient concentrations to handle the normal levels of hydrogen peroxide generated in the lens. This author suggests that the thioredoxin/thioredoxin-reductase system may also be involved in the defense of lens against oxidative stress. This system can quench free radicals and also reduce some protein disulphides.

All the major antioxidant enzymes are present in skin but their role in protecting cells against oxidative damage generated by UV radiation has not been elucidated. Acute UV exposures lead to changes in glutathione reductase and catalase activity in mouse skin but insignificant changes in superoxide dismutase and glutathione peroxidase (Fuchs et al., 1989). Consistent with original studies in bacteria, neither endogenous catalase nor superoxide dismutase play a major role in protecting cells against the lethal effects of UVA irradiation (Tyrrell & Pidoux 1989). Iron plays a critical role in oxidative reactions as a catalyst in the Fenton reaction so that cellular levels of free iron need to be kept low. The intracellular storage protein, ferritin may therefore play a critical role in cellular antioxidant defense. UVA radiation (and other oxidant stress) leads to high levels of expression of the heme oxygenase 1 gene (HO1) (Keyse & Tyrrell 1989) which in turn leads to the catabolism of heme and release of free iron. The increased ferritin levels that result appear to be directly responsible for a UVA-mediated adaptive response involving the protection of human fibroblast membranes against subsequent UVA radiation damage (Vile et al., 1994).

6.5.4 *Summary*

Repair of UV-induced DNA damage is crucial in removing potentially mutagenic damage from cells although errors in repair can themselves lead to mutations. The repair capacity of human skin cells therefore directly relates to the probability of initiation of the carcinogenesis process and eventually tumour formation. At longer UV wavelengths, an increasing component of oxidative damage to DNA, membranes and proteins influences the biological effects. Both endogenous and exogenous photosensitisers normally generate active oxygen intermediates. Cellular antioxidant defense mechanisms are therefore crucial for the prevention or removal of the damage caused by the oxidising component of UV radiation.

6.6 Cellular Consequences of Damage

6.6.1 *Membrane disruption*

Lipid and protein damage by UV associated with cytoskeletal damage may lead to severe disruption of plasma membrane functions including a breakdown in the permeability barrier and interruptions in active transport functions. Crucial signalling molecules such as cytokines may be inappropriately released leading to aberrant cell to cell communication and toxins present in the external cellular environment may gain free access to the interior of the cell. Critical ion pumps may be damaged, thereby influencing a wide range of processes that rely on ion homeostasis. Breakdown of internal lipid membranes in eukaryotic cells will also be highly disruptive leading to many pathological consequences including mitochondrial damage, leakage of proteases from disrupted lysosomes and breakdown of the nuclear membrane permeability barrier. Details in this important area of UV effects are sparse but it is clear that consequences of UV damage to membrane components need to be better understood and incorporated into current models for cellular and organ damage.

6.6.2 *Activation of genes*

UV inducible defense pathways in bacteria and human cells

In bacteria, UVC radiation induces a large set of genes under the regulatory control of the *rec A* gene which lead to enhanced DNA repair, mutagenesis, prophage induction and inhibition of cell division (for review see Walker, 1987). Many groups have sought a similar SOS response in eukaryotic cells. Reactivation of several different UVC damaged viruses (human cytomegalovirus or Herpes Simplex virus) has been observed upon infection into UVC treated cultured human skin fibroblasts. The effects are not generally large (Dion & Hammelin, 1987; Abrahams et al., 1984). In one study, a parallel phenomenon has been observed using split doses of UV in arrested cultures of human fibroblasts (Tyrrell, 1984). Cell populations irradiated with low doses of UV developed enhanced resistance to a second UV challenge dose with a maximum response occurring between 2-4 days. The level of reactivation was much higher in a repair deficient (XP variant cell line). As for viral reactivation, protein synthesis is necessary. No mutation studies have been carried out under similar conditions. Furthermore, these phenomena have not been investigated in the solar UVB region although it is likely that the response will be similar. Although these adaptation responses appear to reflect enhanced gene expression, there are few clues as to the molecular mechanism underlying these observations.

Bacteria also respond strongly to oxidative stress by either the oxyR pathway (Christman et al., 1985) or the soxRS pathway (Greenberg et al., 1990) which is induced by superoxide-generating redox cycling agents such as menadione and paraquat. The oxyR pathway is induced by agents such as hydrogen peroxide and the regulatory protein encoded by this gene controls expression of at least 9 proteins including the antioxidant enzymes, catalase, glutathione reductase and alkyl hydroperoxide reductase. This pathway is emphasised here because it also appears to be involved in protection of bacterial cells against the cytotoxic action of UVA radiation (Kramer & Ames 1987). However, although several eukaryotic genes are induced by both UVA radiation and hydrogen peroxide (see below), none of them involves such a clear-cut direct activation of antioxidant enzymes.

Gene activation in mammalian cells by UVC and UVB radiations

A large number of genes have been shown to be activated by UVC radiation (listed in Table 1 of a review by Keyse 1993). However, in many cases the doses required are very high, so that by the criterion of colony-forming ability, the majority of the population is dead. Although it is a reasonable assumption that the same genes will be induced by UVB radiation, this has only been shown in certain cases. Damage to DNA may be a critical intermediate in triggering the response since induction of certain genes has been shown to occur at much lower doses in mutant cell strains lacking DNA repair. (Stein et al., 1989, Miskin & Ben-Ishai, 1981). Furthermore, crude action spectra for induction of several genes by UV radiation correspond to the action spectra for DNA damage induction (Stein et al., 1989). However, at least for the induction of the *fos* gene (see action spectrum in figure 6.8), events at the membrane also appear to be involved (Devary et al., 1992). There is still a controversy as to whether or not the initial signal occurs in the nucleus and is then transduced to the membrane or whether the crucial initiating events occur at the membrane itself. UVC activation of the HIV-1 promoter also appears to involve membrane events (Devary et al., 1993).

Metallothioneins are also induced by both UVC and UVB radiation (Angel et al., 1986). However, in general, the relationship between

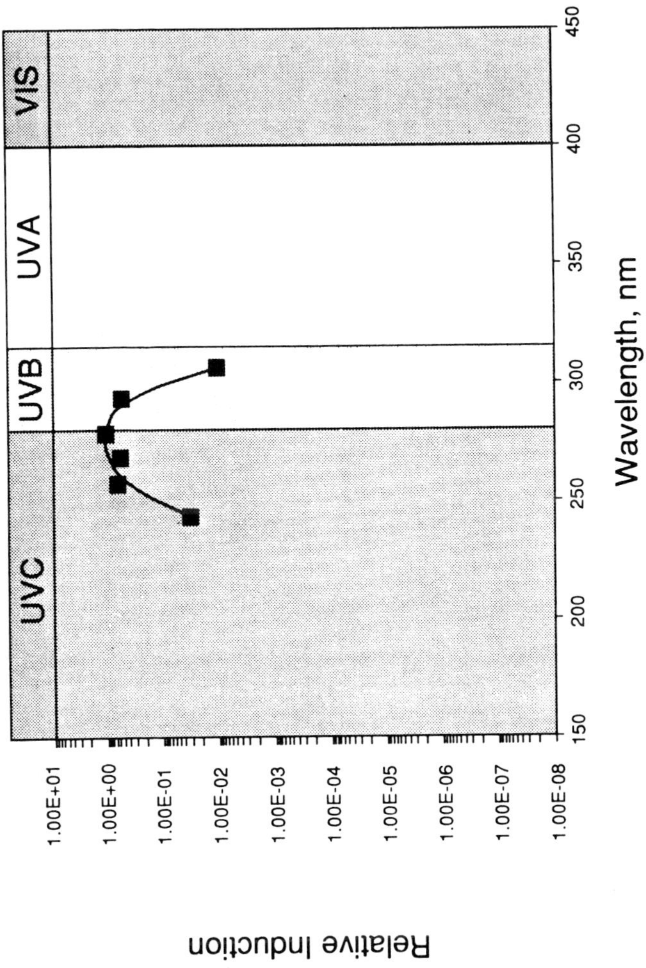

Figure 6.8 Action spectrum for early phase of *c-fos* induction in cells. Stein et al., 1989a (courtesy of National Radiological Protection Board, UK).

UVC/UVB activation of genes and cellular defense against short wavelength UV radiations remains obscure. The synthesis of a constitutive damage specific DNA-binding protein has been shown to be stimulated by UV radiation in both monkey and human cells (Hirschfield et al., 1990). Although the binding activity was shown to be absent in certain strains of XP (group E) (Chu & Chang 1988), subsequent studies showed that not all strains from this group lacked the damage specific protein (Kataoka & Fujiwara 1991).

Gene activation in mammalian cells by UVA radiation

The eukaryotic genes induced by UVA radiation are, for the most part, distinct from those induced by the shorter wavelengths. This appears to be largely due to the fact that UVA radiation acts indirectly by generating active oxygen intermediates rather than being directly absorbed by biomolecules. Although UVA radiation can activate antioxidant enzymes such as catalase in prokaryotic cells, there is no evidence that UVA radiation can activate any of the common antioxidant pathways in mammalian cells. In contrast to the studies with UVB/UVC radiations, UVA radiation can activate genes at doses which kill only a small percentage of the total population in cultured cell models. This is crucial since it indicates that gene activation by UVA radiation may actually relate to events in living tissue and could reasonably be expected to be involved in protective pathways.

For simplicity, we can distinguish three groups of genes that are activated in cultured mammalian cells by UVA radiation. These may involve secreted molecules in cell to cell interactions: collagenase (Scharffetter et al., 1991) and intracellular adhesion molecule 1; proteins involved in early cellular events and signal transduction (protein kinase C, phospholipase A2, and a phosphatase, see Keyse, 1993) or catabolic enzymes (currently only represented by heme oxygenase 1). To date only heme oxygenase 1 has been implicated in a cellular defense pathway in which human fibroblasts adapt to oxidative damage to membranes (Vile et al., 1994).

UV activation of viruses

UV radiation has long been known to activate Herpes Simplex virus. Experimental evidence now indicates that UVC and UVB radiation can activate the promoter of the human immune deficiency virus (see figure 6.9) as well as complete HIV (Valerie et al., 1988). This activation may contribute to the faster development of AIDS in seropositive individuals. Current evidence in both cell systems and transgenic animal models have

Figure 6.9 Action spectrum for HIV-1 activation in cells. Stein et al., 1989b (courtesy of National Radiological Protection Board, UK).

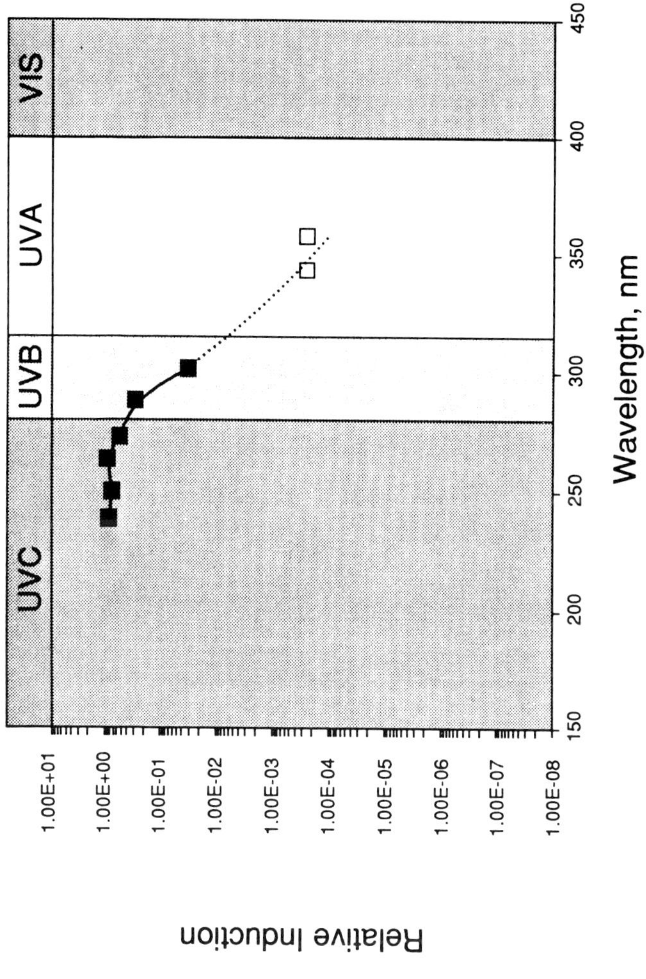

led to the conclusion that UVA radiation cannot activate the virus (see Beer & Smudzka, 1991). However UVA at solar radiation levels can clearly activate binding of the NFKB transcription factors to the corresponding DNA binding site which is present in several promoters including the long terminal repeat of the HIV promoter (Tyrrell, R.M Personal communication). This issue clearly merits further study in view of the importance to human health.

6.6.3 *Cell death*

Cells irradiated with UV may show changes in permeability, inhibition of macromolecular synthesis, loss of ability to divide and total metabolic disruption eventually leading to cellular disruption. A discussion of how to define and measure cell death is beyond the scope of this overview, but the most commonly accepted parameter employed is the loss of the ability of a cell to divide and form colonies. Many classical studies of UV effects were based on these parameters and survival curves and their interpretation have been extensively discussed (Jagger, 1985). Inactivation rates can be derived from survival curves and used to construct action spectra for inactivation of cultured organisms ranging from viruses to human cells. Such survival curves are particularly useful for defining sensitive and resistant cell populations, often an indication of genetic defects in repair processes. Action spectra for inactivation of cell populations generally follow DNA absorption at wavelengths as long as 320 nm. However cells are killed more efficiently than predicted by DNA damage at longer wavelengths as a result of multiple effects of the longer wavelength including disruption of DNA repair and the increasing importance of targets such as the membrane.

At solar UV levels that lead to erythema and acute skin burn in human beings, extensive cell death may occur. This may be particularly important to the eventual appearance of melanomas which have been linked to severe sunburn early on in life in epidemiological studies. It should also be noted that action spectra data taken together with solar spectroradiometric measurements and the known transmission of human skin have led to the conclusion that the UVA component of sunlight is a major factor in the cytotoxic action of sunlight at the basal layer of the epidermis (Tyrrell and Pidoux 1987).

6.6.4 *Mutation, chromosomal damage and transformation*

Studies in microorganisms have unambiguously shown that damage induced by UV throughout the whole range is mutagenic (Webb, 1977). Until the present decade, UVB and UVA studies in mammalian cells were much less conclusive because most of them employed broad spectrum lamps and mutagenic effects could be partially or entirely attributed to wavelengths at the short end of the emitted spectrum. Nevertheless, a large body of work now supports the conclusion that both UVC and UVB radiations are mutagenic to cultured human cells. Studies using predominently UVA sources or monochromatic radiations in three different cultured human cell systems have reported positive (Enninga et al., 1986), ambiguous (Jones et al., 1987) or negative (Tyrrell 1984) results. These results are clearly a function of the system employed and merely underline the fact that although pre-mutagenic lesions are induced by wavelengths longer than 320 nm in human cells, the efficiency of mutation induction is several orders of magnitude lower than that induced by the short wavelengths. It should be stressed at this point that UVA radiation is clearly carcinogenic in animal models (De Gruijl et al., 1993).

Most DNA photoproducts are likely to be pre-mutagenic lesions because of the potential for error occurring during repair. Recent attention has focused on the relative mutagenicity of the cyclobutane type pyrimidine dimers compared with the second most common DNA lesion formed by UVB and UVC radiation, the (6-4) pyo photoproduct (reviewed by Mitchell et al., 1993). Most of the conclusions are based on the specific type of sequence changes (transitions, tandem transitions) that occur in a variety of test systems. In certain cases, clear evidence has emerged that the minor (6-4) pyo photoproduct may be highly mutagenic relative to the pyrimidine dimer (Leclerc et al., 1991). Much additional study will be required to resolve the mutagenic potential of each photoproduct, especially considering the rapid expansion in numbers of additional photoproducts that are now being recognised.

Except for UVC radiation, most of the studies of the chromosomal effects of UV radiation have been carried out with broad spectrum sources. The data has been extensively tabulated in a recent evaluation of UV effects (IARC 1992). A similar comment applies to the studies on morphological transformation.

6.7 Conclusions

DNA is the most critical chromophore and target for damage by UVB and UVC radiation. The fraction of oxidative type damage involving other chromophores and additional targets increases with increasing wavelength. The determination of accurate action spectra in cultured cells and animal models is critical to obtaining clues as to the nature of these chromophores and for predictive evaluation in the many cases in which human data is lacking.

A considerable amount of knowledge is available concerning the interaction of UV radiation with nucleic acids. Controversy still exists as to which type of lesion constitutes the most important type of pre-mutagenic damage, although (6-4) pyo photoproducts and cyclobutane type pyrimidine dimers may both be relevant. Damage to membranes and other organelles is also being given increasing attention since non-DNA events may also be involved in UV mediated biological effects.

Studies of DNA repair defective disorders in humans have clearly established a link between UV induced DNA damage in skin and various types of cancer. A clear understanding of endogenous defense pathways including antioxidant defense is essential for understanding the origins of UV-related human disease and to the elaboration of adequate protective measures.

Cell death, chromosome changes, mutation and morphological transformations are observed after irradiation of prokaryotic and eukaryotic cells with UV. Many different genes and several viruses (including HIV) are activated by UV radiation. However, the genes activated by UVC and UVB are different from those activated by UVA radiation.

7. ANIMAL STUDIES

7.1 Skin Carcinogenesis

7.1.1 *Domestic animals*

Skin tumours have been reported in some domestic and food animals including cats, dogs, cows, sheep and goats (Dorn et al., 1971; Emmett, 1973; Madewell et al., 1981). That the tumours observed often develop in sparsely haired, light-coloured skin suggests that sunlight was involved. Cancers of the external membranes of the eye are also observed, particularly in cattle, and are thought to be related to sun exposure (Russell et al., 1956).

7.1.2 *Experimental animals*

The experimental induction of skin cancers in mice following exposure to a mercury arc lamp was first reported by Findlay (1928). Since then, carcinogenicity of UV has been investigated in many experiments, mostly in mice, less often in rats, and infrequently in other species (Blum et al, 1959; Urbach et al., 1974; Kripke & Sass, 1978; WHO, 1979; van der Leun, 1984; Epstein, 1985). Spontaneous skin tumours are rare in rodents but have been consistently observed following experimental UV exposure with a clear dose-response relationship in well-conducted studies. A recent review concluded that there was sufficient evidence that UV caused skin cancer in experimental animals (IARC, 1992).

Broad Spectrum UV

The carcinogenicity of sunlight was tested in two studies in mice and rats (Roffo, 1934; 1939). In the first study of 600 rats, 165 (70%) of 235 which survived the acute heat load of exposure to sunlight for 5 hours a day developed tumours of the skin (mainly squamous cell carcinomas on the ears) or conjunctiva (spindle cell sarcomas). No tumours developed when sunlight was filtered through glass. Similar results were obtained in a second study in 2 000 rats and mice.

"Solar-simulated radiation" has been studied in a number of experiments (Forbes et al., 1982; Staberg et al., 1983; Young et al., 1990; Menzies et al., 1991). In the study by Forbes et al. (1982), 1 000 hairless mice were exposed for up to 80 weeks to radiation from a xenon arc lamp passed through various filters to simulate sunlight. More than 90% of the mice developed tumours, particularly squamous cell carcinomas.

UVB

Many studies have been conducted with sources emitting mainly UVB radiation. A few of the more informative studies in different species are summarised below.

Mouse: Freeman (1975) exposed one ear of each haired albino mouse in groups of 30, three times a week, to one of four wavelengths of narrow band UVB (290, 300, 310 and 320 nm), produced by a high-intensity diffraction grating monochromator with a half-power band-width of 5 nm, at doses proportional to the MED of each wavelength for untanned human skin. Tumours were produced in about 50% of surviving animals at each wavelength except 290 nm where no tumours were produced although all animals survived. Most tumours were squamous cell carcinomas (SCC).

De Gruijl et al. (1983) exposed six groups of 22 to 44 (total 199) male and female Skh-hr 1 hairless albino mice to daily doses of from 57 to 1 900 J m^{-2} of mainly UVB from Westinghouse FS40TL12 sunlamps. Most of the mice developed skin tumours, mainly squamous cell carcinomas, even though the highest daily dose was sub-erythemal. A power relationship (linear on log-log scales) was observed between the daily dose and the time required for 50% of the animals to develop tumours (figure 7.1). SCC developed in 71% of mice in the lowest dose group and two skin tumours of different types were observed late in the lives of 24 control mice (received no UVB radiation).

Other Species: Stenbäck (1975a) exposed groups of shaven NMR rats, Syrian golden hamsters and guinea pigs to mainly UVB from Westinghouse FS40T12 sunlamps for 60 weeks at weekly doses of 5.4 to 10.8 J m^{-2}. Tumours developed in 16 of 40 rats (mainly papillomas on the ears), 14 of 40 hamsters (mainly papillomas of skin not on the ears) and 2 of 25 guinea pigs.

A number of experiments were carried out in which groups of a South American opossum, *Monodelphis domestica*, were exposed to mainly UVB from Westinghouse FS40 sunlamps. *M domestica* is unusual in showing photoreactivation of cyclobutylpyrimidine dimers (Ley, 1985). Regular exposures of 250 mJ m^{-2} produced melanomas in 5 of 13 surviving animals by 100 weeks from commencement of the experiment. No melanomas were seen in a much larger colony not exposed to artificial UV (Ley et al., 1989). In other experiments, nonmelanocytic skin tumours (mainly fibrosarcomas and squamous cell carcinomas) and fibrosarcomas of the corneal stroma were produced (Ley et al., 1987, 1989). The latter were delayed in appearance and reduced in number when UV exposure was

Figure 7.1 Relationship of the logarithm of relative UVB dose to the logarithm of median time (t_m) to first detectable skin tumours (threshold < 1mm diameter) in albino hairless mice irradiated with Westinghouse FS40TL12 sunlamps. The maximum daily dose was measured at 190 mJ m^{-2} (From De Gruijl et al., 1983).

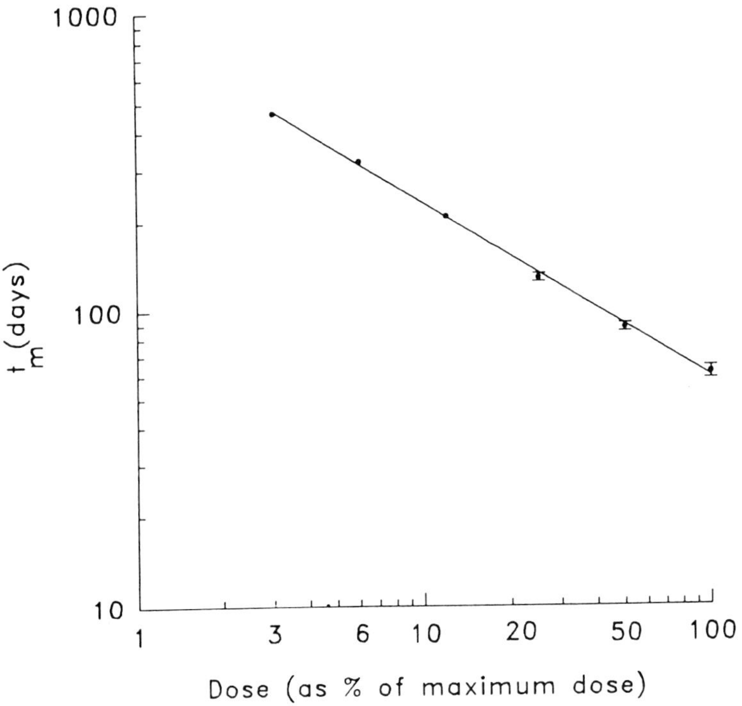

followed immediately by photoreactivating light.

A group of 460 hybrid fish of two strains developed by crossing platyfish (*Xiphophorus maculatus*) and swordtails (*Xiphophorus helleri*) were exposed for 5 to 20 days to mainly UVB from Westinghouse FS40 sunlamps filtered through acetate sheets transmitting > 290 nm (150 or 300 mJ m^{-2}) and >340 nm (850 and 1700 J m^{-2}). Between 19% and 40% of exposed fish developed melanocytic tumours compared with 12% and 2% in control fish (Setlow et al., 1989).

In an attempt to confirm a suspected association between sunlight and cancer of the eye in cattle, four Hereford cattle were exposed to mainly UVB from Westinghouse FS40 sunlamps. Visible tumours developed in the eyes of three of them and one was confirmed histopathologically as a preneoplastic growth (Kopecky et al., 1979).

UVC

Experiments have been carried out in which animals have been exposed to low-pressure mercury discharge germicidal lamps which emit most of their radiation at 254 nm with weaker spectral lines in the UVB, UVA and visible spectra (IARC, 1992). Examples are given below.

A group of 40 mice was irradiated with germicidal lamps at weekly doses of 3×10^4 J m^{-2}. By 52 weeks, 97% of mice had developed skin tumours, the majority of which were squamous cell carcinomas (Lill, 1983). In another study, groups of 24 hairless albino mice were irradiated daily at 230, 1460 or 7000 J m^{-2}. The prevalence of tumour-bearing mice (with mainly squamous cell carcinomas) increased with time to over 75% in each exposure group (Sterenborg et al., 1988). A comparison with other studies showing response to exposure to UVB led the authors to conclude that the small amounts of UVB emitted by the germicidal lamps could not explain the response observed. Interaction between UVC and UVB could not be excluded. Yields of keratoacanthoma like skin tumours, proportional to dose, were observed in small groups of rats exposed to radiation from Westinghouse G36T6L germicidal lamps (Strickland et al., 1979).

UVA

A number of studies have been conducted in which skin tumours have been produced in hairless mice by UVA under conditions in which the exclusion of UVB from the exposure was adequately documented (IARC, 1992). For example, groups of 24 albino hairless mice were exposed to UVA from Philips TL40W/09 fluorescent tubes filtered through 10mm of glass, highly absorbent for UVB, for 12 h/day, seven days a week, for one year. The daily dose was 220 kJ m^{-2}. Skin tumours appeared in all animals and histopathological examination of the larger lesions showed the majority to be SCC. On the basis of the known dose-response to UVB, it was estimated that 100,000 times more UVB than was residually present in the exposure would have been necessary to produce the incidence of tumours observed (van Weelden et al., 1986, 1988). Similar findings were obtained in a study in which UVA at > 340 nm was produced by passing radiation from Philips HPA 400 W lamps through liquid filters (Sterenborg and van der Leun, 1990).

7.1.3 *Interactions between radiations of different wavelengths*

Simple photoaddition is commonly assumed for the interaction of different wavelengths of UV in producing cancer. That is, exposure at each wavelength contributes to the effective dose in an additive way. Several studies, however, suggest that the true position is more complex and the subject has been reviewed in detail by van der Leun (1987, 1992).

For exposures to UV at different wavelength ranges administered simultaneously, or in close temporal proximity, both reductions and increases in the carcinogenic effect have been reported by comparison with what would have been expected on the basis of simple addition. Following detailed review, these effects were described as "nonexistent, unproven or small" (IARC, 1992) and this conclusion is consistent with the results of a recent study (Berg et al., 1993). Such interactions play only a small role in the evaluation of risks of UV (Health Council of the Netherlands, 1986).

There is a well-established protective effect of visible light against UV carcinogenesis (and other effects) in *M. domestica* (Ley, 1993) and lower animals (see, for example, Setlow et al., 1993) which possesses the photoreactivating enzyme, photolyase. Whether or not humans possess a DNA photolyase or show photoreactivation is controversial (Ley, 1993, Li et al., 1993).

Several experiments, with somewhat conflicting results, have been carried out in which exposures to UV to one wavelength range have been separated in time from exposures to another (Forbes et al., 1978; Staberg et al., 1983; Bech-Thomsen et al., 1988a, b; Slaper, 1987). On review of these studies, it was concluded that the combined effects tend to be slightly less than what would be expected from simple photoaddition (IARC, 1992).

7.1.4 *Dose-response*

The accurate and quantitative description of the relationship between UV and the occurrence of skin tumours, usually SCC, has been based on experiments in which mice have been exposed regularly, usually daily, to UV from standard sources. In most relevant experiments, a UV dose, usually much lower than that of the outdoors environment, was delivered daily or several times per week until skin tumours developed. The UVB dose which induces tumours in mice is lower than for acute reactions such as erythema or oedema and up to 33 times lower in one experiment which produced an abundance of skin cancers (De Gruijl et al., 1983). The higher the dose given, the less time it takes for tumours to appear. In most experiments, the time taken for 50% of mice to develop tumours has ranged between a few months and one year but can be brought down to as low as 18 days (IARC, 1992; Willis et al., 1981).

Quantitative dose-effect relationships have been derived for mice exposed regularly (usually daily) to UV. The median time to first tumour (t_m) has been used as the measure of effect. Dose-effect relationships of the following form have been proposed (IARC, 1992):

$$t_m = k_1 D^{-r}$$

or, equivalently,

$$log\ t_m = -r\ \ log\ D + log\ k_1\ .$$

In these expressions, k_1 is a constant representing both the susceptibility of the mouse strain and the effectiveness of the radiation spectrum administered, *D* is the daily dose of radiation and *r* is a numerical exponent giving the slope of the dose response curve. Estimates of *r* vary between 0.5 and 0.6 in most experiments, with broad-spectrum UV and broadband UVB; the value of 0.5 is typical for large tumours, and 0.6 for small tumours (Blum et al., 1959; de Gruiji, 1983). In one experiment with UVC a value r=0.2 was found (Sterenborg, 1988). The relationship found by de Gruijl et al. (1983) for the induction of skin tumours less than 1 mm in diameter by UVB in albino hairless mice is shown in figure 7.1; the value of *r* in this relationship is 0.6.

A corresponding expression for the dose-response relationship in albino hairless mice is given by:

$$Y = k_2\ D^c\ t^d$$

where Y is the average number of tumours per mouse (the yield), k_2 is a constant, D is the daily dose of UV radiation, t is the number of days of exposure to UV and c and d are numerical exponents describing the dose response relationship (van der Leun & der Gruijl, 1993). By describing the response in terms of a measure of incidence of tumours rather than time to tumour development, this expression may be more useful for risk assessment in humans.

7.1.5 *Effect of pattern of exposure*

Tumours can be induced by a single dose of UV (Hsu et al., 1975; Strickland et al., 1979). In mice, this has required a dose that caused ulceration of the skin which is known to be a tumour promoter.

Two experiments have reported on the effects of pattern of UV (mainly UVB) exposure in albino hairless mice. At constant instantaneous intensity and constant weekly dose of UV, increasing fractionation of the dose from once weekly to three times weekly to five times weekly increased the incidence of tumours (Forbes et al., 1981). Similarly, with a constant daily dose of UV, incidence of tumours increased with extension of the period of delivery (and corresponding reduction in instantaneous intensity) from 1.25 to 4 or 12 hours (Kelfkens et al., 1991); there was no appreciable difference between exposures of 4 and 12 hours. Similar results had been obtained by Forbes and Davies (cited in Kelfkens et al., 1991).

7.1.6 *Action spectrum*

Ideally, to determine the action spectrum of UV carcinogenesis, experiments would be carried out with monochromatic radiation to determine the relationship between dose and median time to first tumour for each wavelength. However, narrow-band monochromatic sources suitable for experiments of these types are difficult to achieve. An alternative approach is to conduct experiments with a number of overlapping broad band sources and to derive an action spectrum by appropriate mathematical analysis of the results.

Recently two large collections of data on carcinogenicity of UV in albino hairless mice following exposure to multiple overlapping sources in the UVC, UVB and UVA ranges, supplemented with results of experiments using highly filtered UVA sources, have been combined to produce what is probably the best estimate to date of the action spectrum for skin carcinogenesis in any strain of animals (de Gruijl et al., 1993). As far as possible, the end point in the experimental results used was the appearance of SCC.

The action spectrum produced is shown in figure 7.2. The upper and lower dashed (- -) curves result from a sensitivity analysis showing the boundaries of the effects of displacements of 5 nm segments of the action spectrum that do not increase the χ^2 for the fit of the spectrum to the data by more than 1.0. Effectiveness rises as wavelength increases to a peak at about 295 nm, falls steeply to an initial minimum at about 350 nm, rises again to 380 nm and then appears to fall away sharply. The definition of this action spectrum is very good in the UVB range, there is substantial uncertainty in the UVA range and essentially no information below 280 nm except at 254 nm. Even with the uncertainty, if there is not actually a second peak in the UVA range, there is at least a plateau from about 340 to 380 nm. This action spectrum is very similar to the action spectra for erythema in humans (McKinlay and Diffey, 1987) and the induction of oedema in the skin of mice (Cole et al., 1986).

Recently, results have been reported on the action spectrum for the production of melanomas in hybrid fish (Setlow et al., 1993). Groups of between 20 and 124 fish were exposed to single doses, at two to six exposure levels, of UV or visible light at wavelengths of 302 nm, 313 nm, 365 nm, 405 nm and 436 nm. Narrow band radiation was produced by use of a grating monochromator and, for the higher wavelengths, various filters to eliminate any radiation at substantially lower wavelengths. The experiment was terminated after four months and all fish examined for melanomas which occurred in 5% to 24% of control fish and 24% to 45% of irradiated fish. The estimated action spectrum obtained is shown in figure 7.3 superimposed on published action spectra for mammalian cell mutagenicity and cytotoxicity. Relative to an effectiveness in producing melanomas of 1.0 for UV at 302 nm, the effectiveness at 313 nm was 0.16 and that at 365 nm, 0.32; for visible light, the relative effectiveness were 0.017 at 405 nm and 0.023 at 436 nm. The effectiveness of UVA in producing melanoma in this model relative to the effectiveness of 300 nm radiation was some 3 orders of magnitude greater than the effectiveness of UVA, relative to the same baseline, in producing SCC in hairless albino mice (figure 7.2; de Gruijl et al., 1993). An action spectrum has not yet been determined for production of melanoma in *M. domestica.*

Figure 7.2 Estimated action spectrum (called the SCUP action spectrum) for induction by UV of SCC in the skin of albino hairless mice (Skh-hr 1). The dashed lines (--) show the upper and lower limits for 5 nm displacements of the action spectrum that do not increase the χ^2 for fit of the spectrum to the data by more than 1.0 (Reprinted with permission from de Gruijl et al., 1993).

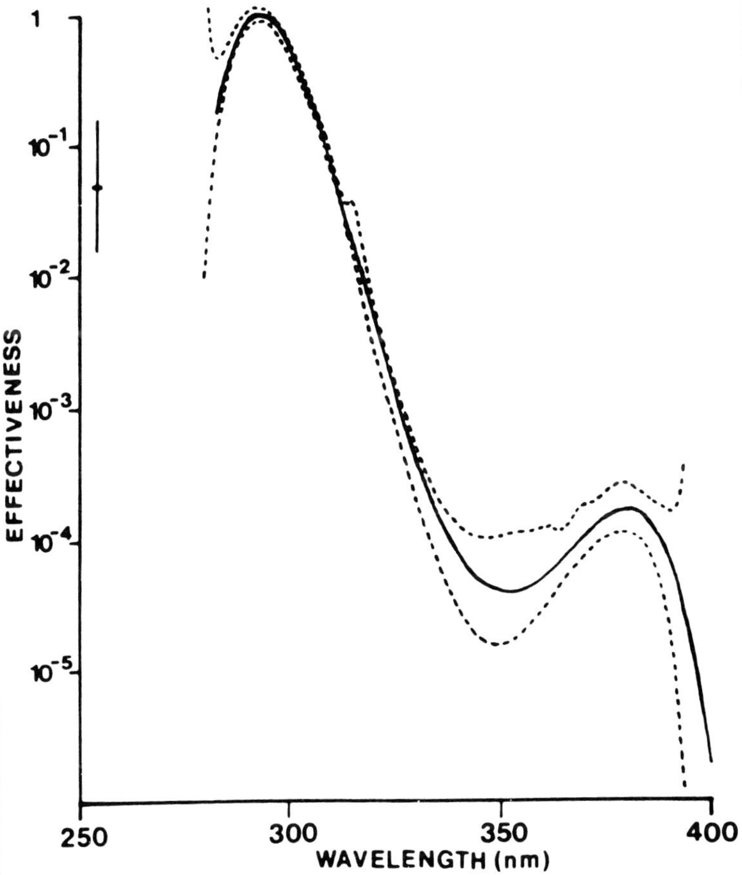

Figure 7.3 Estimated action spectrum for induction by UV and visible light of melanocytic tumours in hybrid fish of the genus *Xiphophorus* compare with published action spectra for mammalian cell mutagenicity and cytotoxicity. o, cytotoxicity; ●, mutagenicity; ■, induction of melanocytic tumours (Reprinted with permission from Setlow et al., 1993).

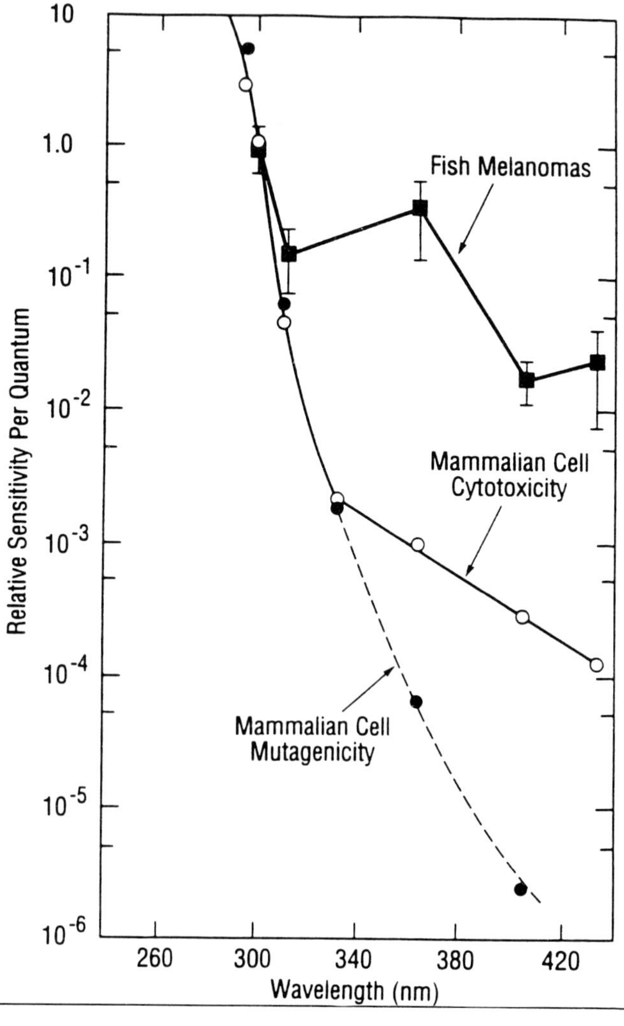

7.1.7 *Interaction between UV and chemicals*

Interaction with chemical carcinogens

A number of studies have been carried out in which UV has been administered before or after administration of a known chemical carcinogen. A period of irradiation with UVB before application of 3,4-Benzo[a]pyrene to the skin of mice increased the carcinogenic response to high-dose 3,4-Benzo[a]pyrene (Gensler & Bowden, 1987; Gensler, 1988). A number of studies in which mice were irradiated with UV after application of 7,12-Dimethylbenz[a]anthracene (DMBA) to the skin showed an increase in tumour production over that produced by DMBA alone (Epstein & Epstein, 1962; Epstein, 1965; Reeve et al., 1990; Husain et al., 1991). Of particular interest in this regard is the production of melanoma-like lesions in mice by the combination of DMBA and UV. In a number of experiments, DMBA alone has produced benign pigmented naevi. Subsequent administration of UVB, UVB + UVA, and UVA alone caused these naevi to grow into lesions that had the appearance of malignant melanoma; these lesions did not develop in mice treated with DMBA alone (Epstein, 1965; Epstein et al., 1967; Husain et al., 1991). Irradiation with UVB from Westinghouse FS40 sunlamps before application of DMBA and the promoter 12-O-tetradecanoylphorbol 13-acetate (TPA) reduced the incidence and number of tumours produced in CDF1 mice both when the site of subsequent application of the chemicals was irradiated and when a distant site was irradiated (Gensler and Welch, 1992). This effect, therefore, appeared to be mediated systemically.

Both croton oil and TPA, applied to skin after irradiation with UV, have been shown to increase the carcinogenic response to UV (Epstein & Roth, 1968; Pound, 1970; Stenbäck, 1975b; Strickland et al., 1985). Of two other, suspected cancer promoters, one, methyl ethyl ketone peroxide increased tumour production (Logani et al., 1984) and the other, benzoyl peroxide, did not (Epstein, 1988; Iversen, 1988).

Interaction with other chemicals

In several experiments, mice exposed to either solar-simulated radiation or UVA and topical application of 5-methoxypsoralen showed higher incidences of skin papillomas or SCC than did mice exposed to UV or 5-methoxypsoralen alone (Zadjela & Bisagni, 1981; Cartwright & Walter, 1983; Young et al., 1983). Methoxsalen (8-methoxypsoralen) shows the same effects when given with UV (IARC, 1980).

7.1.8 *Mechanisms of UV carcinogenesis*

DNA damage

There is abundant evidence that UV causes DNA damage, both by direct photochemical effects (for example, the production of cyclobutylpyrimidine dimers and 6-4 photoproduct) and by oxidative effects leading to DNA strand breakage and DNA-protein cross-linkage (see Chapter 6).

There is evidence that UV-induced DNA damage, and particularly the formation of pyrimidine dimers, is one step in the mechanism whereby UV can cause cancer in experimental animals. First, Hart et al. (1977) showed, in the clonal fish, *Poecilia formosa*, that the transplantation of UVC irradiated thyroid cells from one fish to another induced thyroid tumours in the host fish. If irradiation of the thyroid of the donor fish was followed immediately by application of photoreactivating light (which monomerizes the pyrimidine dimers), the development of thyroid tumours was almost completely prevented. Second, and similarly, Ley et al. (1991) showed that exposure to photoreactivating light, after exposure to UV, delayed and reduced the yield of skin tumours produced in *M. domestica* by irradiation with Westinghouse FS40 sunlamps. The same result was obtained for corneal tumours but, unexpectedly, exposure to photoreactivating light was as effective in reducing carcinogenesis when given immediately before UV as when given after. There is evidence that photoreactivating light may also inhibit the production by UV of melanocytic lesions in the skin of *M. domestica* (Ley et al., 1989). Third, Yarosh et al. (1992) applied liposomes containing T4 endonuclease V, an enzyme that specifically repairs cyclobutyl pyrimidine dimers, to the skin of albino hairless mice, three times a week, after they had been irradiated with Westinghouse FS20 sunlamps. The incidence of skin tumours observed in the mice fell in proportion to the quantity of active liposomes applied.

There is also evidence that activated oncogenes and a mutated tumour-suppressor gene are present in some skin cancers induced experimentally by UV. Husain et al. (1990) reported studies of expression of the cHa-*ras* oncogene in three papillomas and three carcinomas from among lesions that developed in 17 of 90 Sencar mice following a single exposure, at 7 x 10^4 J m^{-2}, to UVB from Westinghouse FS20 sunlamps. RNA preparations from all six tumours showed elevated levels of Cha-*ras*-specific messenger RNA sequences, suggesting overexpression of this oncogene. DNA from the carcinomas, but not the papillomas, was able to induce transformation of NIH-3T3 cells which demonstrated overexpression and amplification of the Cha-*ras* oncogene. Subsequently, in their studies of melanocytic tumours produced by DMBA and UV in hairless mice (Skh-hr 2), Husain et al. (1991) found mutations in codon 61 of the N-*ras* oncogene in three of eight precursor naevi and one melanoma. The base transitions, however, were not of a type to suggest that they had been caused by UV. Kress et al. (1992) screened exons 5 to 8 of the p53 tumour-suppressor gene for mutation in 35 epidermal tumours induced in four strains of mice by UV from Westinghouse FS40 sunlamps. Mutations were found in seven tumours. All mutations occurred at dipyrimidine sequences. C → T and CC → TT transitions were present in five of the seven tumours with mutations, strongly suggesting that these mutations were due to UV.

Oxidative processes

Oxidative processes in the skin may also mediate the carcinogenicity of UV, particularly UVA (Morlière et al., 1992), in skin, either by direct oxidative damage to DNA or by way of potentially carcinogenic intermediates, such as cholesterol-5,6-epoxide (Black, 1987; Morin et al., 1991). A number of studies have shown that relative increases in dietary polyunsaturated fatty acids, which may lead to lipid peroxidation, can increase the tumour response to exposure to UV in experimental animals and that this effect can be inhibited by the simultaneous feeding of antioxidants (Reeve et al., 1988; Black et al., 1992). In addition, the feeding of antioxidants, such as tocopherol, can reduce the tumour response to UV in the absence of any manipulation of dietary fat (Black & Chan, 1975; Gerrish & Gensler, 1993).

Immune-suppression

UV-induced immune-suppression appears to play a major role in UV carcinogenesis in mice. A review of the literature on the association between UV-induced immune suppression and increased susceptibility to tumours may be found in section 7.3.2.

There is evidence also that administration of immunosuppressive drugs will increase the carcinogenic response to UV in experimental animals (IARC, 1992). Experiments have been carried out with anti-lymphocyte serum, azathioprine, cyclophosphamide, cyclosporine and 6-mercaptopurine. Consistent increases in the carcinogenic response to UV over two or more experiments were seen with azathioprine and cyclosporine (Reeve et al., 1985; Nelson et al., 1987; Servilla et al., 1987; Kelly et al., 1987, 1989).

7.1.9 *Conclusions*

From a review of the animal studies one can conclude the following about UV exposure of the skin:

Carcinogenesis by sunlight is a widespread phenomenon among domestic and food animals. Most tumours found are squamous cell carcinomas (SCC). In experimental animals skin cancer is mainly caused by UV radiation. Again, most tumours induced are SCC. For the induction of SCC in albino hairless mice, the effectiveness is a function of wavelength:

- the effectiveness is found to peak in the UVB range;
- UVA is also carcinogenic, but at a much lower level of effectiveness-similar to what is found for erythema and tanning;
- the effectiveness in the UVC range is unknown, except for one wavelength, 254 nm; at that wavelength the effectiveness is lower than that in the UVB peak
- it is still unknown if there is any effectiveness of visible light.

For the induction of SCC in hairless mice by daily exposures to UVB the dose effect relationship was found to be a power function. It showed no indication of a threshold dose, even at doses as low as 3% of that required for an acute reaction, such as oedema. Radiations of different wavelengths can cooperate in the induction of SCC.

Melanomas are much less common among animals. Only two animal models have been found where exposure to UV induced melanomas:

- the South American opossum *M. domestica*, and

- a hybrid fish, derived from the swordtail and platyfish.

An initial action spectrum was determined for the hybrid fish. It peaks in the UVB range but also shows a high effectiveness in the UVA. An action spectrum for the induction of melanoma in *M. domestica* has not been determined.

Basal cell carcinomas are uncommon in animals. Suitable animal models for the induction of BCC are not available.

7.2 Immune Responses

7.2.1 *Immune function assays*

The immune system depicted in figure 7.4 is composed of primary lymphoid organs (bone marrow and thymus), secondary lymphoid organs including spleen and lymph nodes, and several cell types. In addition a number of mediators including cytokines, antibodies and complement regulate and/or are produced by the immune system. A number of studies have shown that exposure to UV suppresses contact hypersensitivity (CHS) and other delayed-type hypersensitivity (DTH) responses of the immune system. Both of these responses provide a measure the competence of T lymphocytes, suppression of which would be expected to compromise host resistance to infectious agents such as viruses and mycobacterium. Unless otherwise indicated animal studies have utilized FS sunlamps (see Chapter 3 for spectral characterization) and exposed shaved skin.

Two types of experiments have been described in the literature. In experiments designed to investigate local immune suppression, mice were exposed to UV and a hapten chemical such as dinitrofluorobenzene (DNFB) was applied to the site of irradiation. After an incubation period of several days, animals were challenged by painting the chemical on the ear, and the immune response was assessed by measuring ear thickness, which is an expression of CHS. Mice exposed (usually for 4 successive days prior to chemical application) to doses of UV, which might cause a minimal erythemal response in an untanned human, failed to show ear swelling (Toews et al., 1980; Noonan & De Fabo, 1990; Jeevan et al., 1992a). The failure to respond appeared to be due to the development of suppressor T cells which rendered the mouse tolerant to the particular antigen. This concept was supported by the observation that the same mice could not be sensitized with the same chemical through unirradiated skin 14 days later. Moreover, antigen-specific unresponsiveness could be adoptively transferred to naive mice by spleen and lymph node cells obtained from mice skin-painted with DNFB through UV-irradiated skin (Elmets et al., 1983). It should be noted that the precise nature of the activity of these suppressor cells remains the subject of some debate.

In a second type of experiment the effects of UV on systemic immune responses were demonstrated by irradiating mice at one site and subsequently (3-5 days later) exposing them to a contact allergen (CHS) or injecting a protein antigen (DTH) at an unirradiated site. These mice failed to respond when subsequently challenged on the ear (CHS) or in the footpad (DTH) with the same antigen (Noonan et al., 1981a, Kim et al., 1990; Ullrich et al., 1986a; Ullrich, 1986; Jeevan & Kripke, 1990;

Howie et al., 1986; Denkins et al., 1989; Giannini, 1986a,b). Again unresponsiveness was attributed to the development of antigen specific "suppressor T cells" (Noonan et al., 1981b; Ullrich 1985). These experiments suggest that immune suppression could occur even when the site of entry for the antigen was not the same as the site of UV exposure.

Noonan et al. (1981a) reported a 50% suppression of CHS in BALB/c mice after a single dose of 2 KJ m^{-2} UV. She also reported that there was no difference in the dose response curves for UV-induced local and systemic immunosuppression of CHS responses; however, the dose of UV required to suppress CHS in C57BL/6 mice was 6.4 times less than that required to produce similar immune suppression in BALB/c mice (Noonan & De Fabo, 1990). Also, while local suppression could be demonstrated in mice sensitized immediately after irradiation, systemic suppression occurred only if the sensitizer was applied 3 or more days after radiation (Noonan & De Fabo, 1990).

Fifty percent suppression of CHS and DTH has been reported at doses ranging from 2.3 kJ m^{-2} to 20 kJ m^{-2}, (Kim et al., 1990; Jeevan & Kripke, 1990; Jeevan et al., 1992b) levels which produce minimal or no edema. The dose needed to produce 50% suppression varies depending on the strain of mouse and type of antigen used, and on the laboratory producing the data. Suppression of virus-specific DTH was observed in mice exposed to a suberythemal dose of UVB 3-7 days prior to infection with Herpes simplex virus (HSV) but not 14 days and persisted for at least 3 months after irradiation (Howie et al., 1986). Elimination of wavelengths below 315 nm with a mylar filter either eliminated or greatly reduced the suppression of CHS following exposure to UV indicating that most if not all the suppression is due to UVB (Noonan et al., 1981b; Noonan and De Fabo, 1990). Using narrow bands of UV at 10 wavelengths from 250 to 320 nm, it was reported that maximum suppression of CHS occurred between 260 and 270nm, there was a shoulder in the action spectrum from 280-290 nm and then a steady decline to 3% of maximum at 320 nm (De Fabo and Noonan, 1983).

There are two subpopulations of T helper cells, designated Th1 and Th2 which appear to be differentially affected by UV exposure. These two populations are thought to regulate different sets of immune responses. Th1 cells produce interleukin (IL) 2 and γ interferon (γIFN) as well as other cytokines, promote delayed-type hypersensitivity (cell mediated, type IV) responses such as CHS, provide help for certain antibody subtype responses including complement-fixing antibodies, activate macrophages, and may be particularly important for dealing with antigens expressed on cell surfaces, such as viral and tumour antigens (Coffman et al., 1988).

Figure 7.4 Schematic of the immune system. The immune system is composed of primary lymphoid organs (bone marrow and thymus), secondary lymphoid organs (not shown) and several cell types. A number of mediators including cytokins, antobodies, and complement regulate and/or are produced by the immune system. The above schematic depicts some of the interactions that occur when the immune system responds to an antigen.

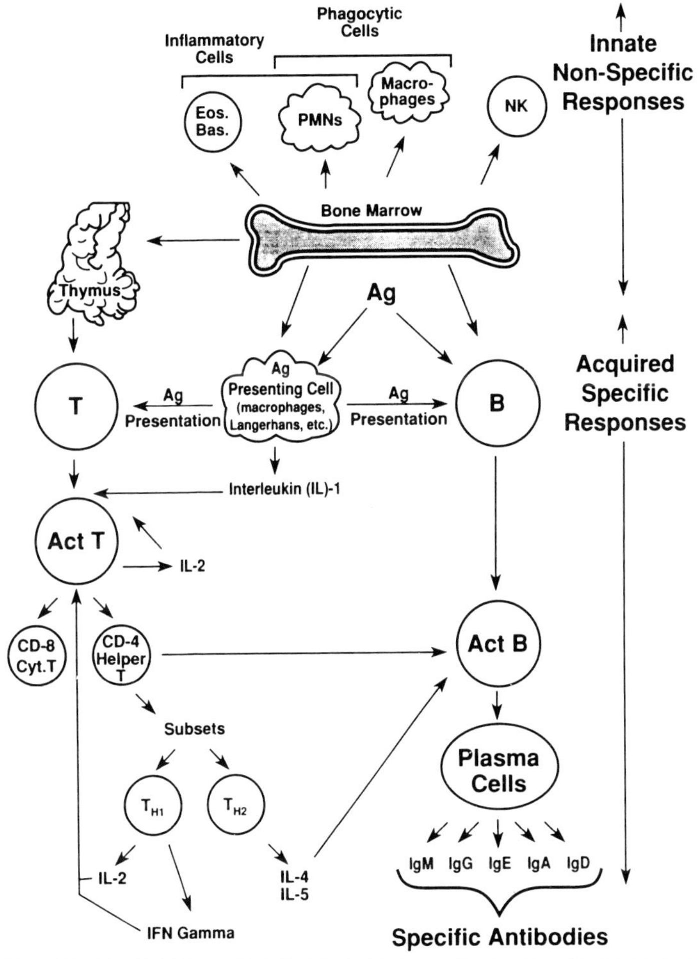

Th2 cells produce a different array of cytokines including IL-4 and IL-5 which promotes antibody responses. Only Th2 cells can stimulate a primary IgE response which is mediated by IL-4 and inhibited by γIFN (Coffman et al., 1988). Thus, Th2 cells may be particularly important in responding to certain parasitic infections, and also play an important role in immediate-type hypersensitivity including reactions to common allergens such as pollen and dust mite.

Recent studies have suggested that both local and systemic immune suppression induced by UV may be the result of an inability to present antigen to and hence activate Th1 cells (Simon et al., 1990, 1991; Araneo et al., 1989).

Suppression of systemic CHS and DTH responses similar to that observed following UV exposure have been obtained by injecting mice with supernatant from UV-irradiated keratinocytes (Kim et al., 1990; Rivas & Ullrich, 1992; Jeevan et al., 1992c). Among factors derived from keratinocytes, the cytokines tumour necrosis factor α (TNFα) (Yoshikawa & Streilein, 1990; Vincek et al., 1993) and IL-10 (Rivas & Ullrich, 1992) are thought to be important in UV-induced immunosuppression. Also, cis-urocanic acid, the product of UV isomerization of urocanic acid located in the stratum corneum, when injected subcutaneously or painted on the epidermis, produces immunosuppressive effects which mimic UVB-induced immunosuppression (Ross et al., 1986), and the action spectrum of UV-induced immune suppression closely follows the absorption spectrum of urocanic acid (De Fabo and Noonan, 1983). In all three cases it is thought that these mediators act by modifying antigen presentation (Vermeer & Streilein, 1990; Rivas & Ullrich, 1992; Noonan et al., 1988).

In summary, it appears that UVB causes the release of mediators from the skin which alter the antigen presenting capability of Langerhans cells as well as antigen presenting cells at other sites, resulting in the development of "suppressor T-cells". It may be that these suppressor T cells are Th2 cells. The net result is the failure to activate Th1 cells and suppression of DTH responses thought to play an important role in host defences against certain types of tumours and microbial infections. The immune suppression is antigen specific, (i.e. only responses to antigens administered within 7 days after irradiation are affected) and is long lasting (at least 3 months).

In addition to DTH and CHS responses, UV affects several other immune functions frequently included in the standard protocols for immunotoxicity testing. Spleen cells taken from UV-exposed mice (single exposure, 54 kJ m^{-2}) failed to respond in a mixed lymphocyte response assay *in vitro* (Ullrich, 1985), and spleen cells from tumour-implanted UV-treated (10 kJ m^{-2}, 3 times/wk, for 3 months) mice were not cytotoxic *in vitro* against UV-induced tumours (Fisher & Kripke, 1977). In contrast, exposure to approximately 2-3 kJ m^{-2} day^{-1}, for 23 days did not affect responses of spleen or inguinal lymph node cells to the mitogens, phytohaemagglutinin, concanavalin A or bacterial lipopolysaccharide. Similarly, lymphocyte responses to these mitogens and peritoneal macrophage phagocytic and tumouricidal activities were unaffected by exposure to 10 kJ m^{-2}, 3 times per week, for up to 6 months (Funnell & Keast 1985; Norbury et al., 1977).

Kripke et al., (1977) reported no effect of UV (in mice exposed to 10 kJ m^{-2}, 3 times per week for up to 6 months) on the primary haemagglutonin antibody response to sheep red blood cells; however in another study, the IgM and IgG plaque forming cell responses of lymph node cells to sheep red blood cells given intradermally (through irradiated skin) were suppressed (Funnell & Keast, 1985). Also, suppressor cells generated by irradiating mice with a single exposure of 30-40 kJ m^{-2}, 5 days prior to sensitization with trinitrochlorobenzene prevented the development of hapten specific antibody-forming cells when injected intravenously along with hapten conjugated sheep red blood cells into syngeneic recipients (Ullrich et al., 1986b).

UV exposure enhanced poly I.C augmented natural killer cell (NK) activity in mice (Lynch & Daynes, 1983); however, suppression of NK activity in rats has been reported following exposure to suberythemal doses of UV (Garssen et al., 1993). Hence, in laboratory animals UV exposure appears to affect mixed lymphocyte responses, cytotoxic T cell activity, possibly NK activity, and in some circumstances antibody responses. With the exception of NK activity all of these responses are antigen specific responses. In contrast UV does not appear to alter several non-specific responses including macrophage phagocytic or tumouricidal activities, or T or B cell responses to mitogens. However, unlike CHS and DTH, none of these responses has been studied in detail in rodents, and dose response information is not available.

7.2.2 *Susceptibility to tumours*

Interest in the immunosuppressive properties of UVB was first sparked by the observations of Kripke and associates that UV exposure induced highly antigenic tumours which did not grow when transplanted into syngeneic, immunocompetent mice but did grow when transplanted into immunosuppressed or UV treated mice (Kripke 1974; Kripke & Fisher, 1976). The precise nature of the tumour antigens has not been defined.

Mice treated with 1.8 kJ m^{-2}, 3 times per week, for 3 months were unable to reject UV-induced syngeneic tumours when challenged subcutaneously at any time from 2 weeks into the irradiation exposure regimen to as late as 5 months after the end of UV treatment (Kripke & Fisher, 1976). Hence susceptibility to tumour challenge was detectable well before the appearance of primary skin cancers induced by the UV and persisted long after exposure ended. Similarly, more UV-induced fibrosarcoma tumour colonies were detected in the lungs following i.v injection of tumour cells in mice treated with 7 kJ m^{-2}, 3 times per week, for 5 weeks (Kripke & Fidler 1980) as compared to unirradiated controls. Susceptibility to tumour challenge was directly proportional to dose of UV and a dose fractionated over time was no more effective than the same total dose given as a single treatment (Kripke & Fidler 1980; De Fabo and Kripke 1979).

In BALB/cAnN mice 50% tumour incidence following subcutaneous tumour challenge at an unirradiated site occurred at a dose of approximately 40 kJ m^{-2}. Enhanced tumour incidence was observed in mice exposed to 21.6 kJ m^{-2} as much as 32 weeks before tumour challenge. A number of studies (Fisher & Kripke, 1977; Daynes & Spellman, 1977; Daynes et al., 1977; Spellman & Daynes, 1978; Spellman et al., 1977; Ullrich & Kripke, 1984, de Gruijl and van der Leun 1982, 1983) have demonstrated that susceptibility to challenge with UV-induced tumours following UV exposure, like suppression of CHS and DTH, is mediated by antigen specific "suppressor T cells" which are present in spleen and lymph nodes of UV-irradiated mice. As with suppression of DTH and CHS responses, enhanced susceptibility to UV-induced tumours is antigen specific and long lasting.

While it is very clear that UV increases the susceptibility of mice to UV-induced tumours, much less work has been done on the effects of UV on susceptibility to other types of tumours. UV treated mice that were unable to reject syngeneic UV-induced tumours were able to reject 2 types of non-UV-induced tumours, B16 melanoma tumours and a spontaneous mouse leukaemia tumour (Kripke et al., 1977). Roberts and Daynes (1980) reported that mice irradiated with subcarcinogenic doses of UV for 3 weeks prior to treatment with either benz[a]pyrene or methycholanthrene at an unirradiated site had reduced latency periods for the development of these chemically-induced tumours. Also, chemically induced tumours from these UV-treated mice appeared to be more antigenic than those induced in untreated mice in that they were incapable of progressive growth when transplanted into normal (immunocompetent) syngeneic mice but were capable of progressive growth in UV-treated mice. The authors suggested that decreased selective pressures exerted by the host (due to UV-induced suppressor cells) at the time of tumour induction allowed more immunogenic tumours to emerge and progress.

7.2.3 *Susceptibility to infectious disease*

Several types of infectious disease models have been developed to study the effects of UV exposure: 1) the infectious agent was injected through irradiated skin, 2) exposure to the infectious agent occurred at a site distant from the site of irradiation, or 3) in the case of some herpes simplex virus (HSV) studies, exposure to UV occurred after infection. The first exposure scenario is representative of vector-borne infections and some vaccinations while the second exposure regimen is representative of infections which do not necessarily enter the host via the skin. The third scenario was designed to mimic reactivation of HSV in humans following sun exposure. In all cases the focus has been on microbial agents that are controlled, at least in part, by DTH responses.

An example of the first type of model is that of *Leishmania major* infection in mice (Giannini 1986a, 1986b, 1987, 1992). Mice were irradiated only on the tail with suberythemal doses (0.06-6 kJ m^{-2}), 3 times/week, for 1 month and were infected intradermally through the irradiated surface of the tail 24 hr after the first UV exposure. In UV-treated mice the DTH response to *L. major* antigens 2 and 6 weeks post infection was suppressed, the number of organisms recovered from skin at the injection site was (Giannini, 1986a) and, a larger number of parasites was observed in the draining lymph node (Giannini, 1987, 1992). Finally, mice which were infected through irradiated skin failed to develop protective immunity such that lesions following reinfection at an unirradiated site were significantly larger when compared to lesions of previously infected but unirradiated mice (Giannini, 1986b).

In a similar model mice treated with 13 or 33 kJ m^{-2} for 4 consecutive days and infected intradermally with HSV at the site of irradiation had a higher incidence of zosteriform lesions than unirradiated mice, and at the higher exposure level 100% mortality was observed as opposed to no mortality in unirradiated mice (Yasumoto et al., 1987). A decreased DTH response to viral antigen was observed and appeared to result from the induction of suppressor T cells (Yasumoto et al., 1987, Aurelian et al., 1988). Also, following *in vitro* exposure to UV, a defect in the ability of Langerhans cells to present HSV antigen to lymphocytes was demonstrated (Hayashi & Aurelian, 1986).

In contrast, no effect of UV on either parasite specific DTH responses or recovery of parasite from internal organs was observed following percutaneous injection of *Schistosoma mansoni* through UV-irradiated (0.4 kJ m^{-2}, 4 consecutive days) skin (Jeevan et al., 1992a). In this same study, suppression of microbe specific DTH responses were not observed following intradermal injection of *Mycobacterium bovis* (BCG) or subcutaneous injection of *Candida albicans* at the site of irradiation; however, the number of viable mycobacteria recovered from the lymphoid organs of BCG-infected mice was increased significantly in the UV treated mice for a period of more than 2 months post infection.

BCG has also been used as an infectious disease model to illustrate systemic effects of UV immunosuppression. In this model mice were irradiated on the back and injected with BCG subcutaneously in the footpad. Mice exposed from 1 to 15 times (3 times/week for up to 5 weeks) to one minimal erythemal dose (2.25 kJ m^{-2}) showed significant suppression in their DTH response to tuberculin (PPD) and increased numbers of live bacteria in the spleen and lymph node compared to unirradiated controls (Jeevan & Kripke, 1990). However, when exposures were continued beyond 5 weeks, the DTH response recovered and mice challenged with bacteria at that point did not exhibit increased numbers of organisms in the spleen and lymph node, suggesting that eventually some sort of adaptation to exposure occurs. Significant suppression of DTH was observed in mice which received a single dose as low as 1.4 kJ m^{-2} 3 days prior to infection and significant increases in bacteria in spleen and lymph node were observed in mice which received as little as 0.7 kJ m^{-2}. Similar effects were observed when supernatants from keratinocyte cultures exposed to UV *in vitro* were injected intravenously 3 days prior to infection (Jeevan et al., 1992c).

In a similar model, mice treated with a single high UV dose (45 kJ m^{-2}) 3 days before infection with *Mycobacterium lepraemurium* exhibited significant suppression of DTH responses to mycobacterial antigen 3 and 6 months after infection and had significantly more bacteria in the infected footpad, lymph node, and spleen 3-6 months post infection (Jeevan et al., 1992b). This high dose also reduced the median survival time in mice infected i.v. With a lower exposure dose (2.3 kJ m^{-2}) 50% suppression of the DTH response to mycobacterial antigen was observed 3 months post infection, and increased numbers of bacteria were observed in the footpad, spleen and lymph node of mice exposed to UV doses greater than or equal to 5.6 kJ m^{-2}. When mice were treated with 2.25 kJ m^{-2}, 3 times/week from 3-15 times, the DTH response to *M. lepraemurium* was suppressed, but as with BCG, the DTH response was normal in mice which received more than 15 exposures.

Effects of systemic UV-induced immune suppression have been demonstrated in mice infected with HSV, 3 days after irradiation with 1 kJ m^{-2}, at a site distant from the site of infection. In this model suppression of DTH was mediated by modulation of epidermal antigen presenting cells and the development of suppressor T cells (Howie et al., 1986, 1987). Subcutaneous injection or epidermal application of UV-treated urocanic acid produced similar immune suppression (Ross et al., 1986). Effects of UV on the actual progression of disease in this model have not been reported.

While most of the work to date has been done in mice, recent work in the rat suggests that suberythemal doses of UV also suppress immune responses. In addition rats exposed to suberythemal doses of UV had higher levels of microorganisms in target organs following oral infection with *Trichinella spiralis* or intraperitoneal infection with cytomegalovirus (Garssen et al., 1993).

In summary, exposure to suberythemal doses of UV has been shown to exacerbate a variety of infections in rodent models. Both infections which are initiated at the site of UV exposure and infections initiated at distant sites have been affected. While most of the infections test, have evolved in some manner more recent work indicates that systemic infections without skin involvement may also be affected. Enhanced susceptibility appears to result from suppression of T-helper-1 cell activity. The mechanisms associated with this suppression appear to be the same as those identified in association with suppression to CHS responses.

Reactivation of latent HSV infections can be induced in mouse and guinea pig by exposure of the previously infected site to sub- or minimal erythemal doses of UV. However, the role that immune suppression plays in this reactivation has not been established (Blyth et al., 1976; Norval et al., 1987; Laycock et al., 1991).

7.2.4 *Susceptibility to immunologically-mediated diseases*

Several studies have suggested that stimulation of Th2 cells may remain intact or be enhanced in UV-exposed mice (Simon et al., 1990; 1991; Araneo et al., 1989). Since Th2 cells are the only cells that can stimulate a primary IgE response (Coffman et al., 1988), it is possible that UV exposure may increase the risk of immediate-type hypersensitivity. This possibility has not yet been studied, but deserves attention in light of the increasing incidence of morbidity and mortality due to asthma, which is often triggered by allergic responses (NIH, 1991; Danielle, 1988).

Acceleration of autoimmunity following UV exposure has also been reported in mice. Both acute (2 hr/day, for 7 days) and chronic (3 hr/wk, for 4 wks) exposure to 20 J m^{-2} s^{-1} enhanced mortality in an autoimmune strain of mice (NZB X BZW F1). These exposures also caused increased serum antibodies to single stranded DNA, enhanced polyclonal B-cell activity in the spleen, and caused more severe renal glomerular inflammatory changes (Ansel et al., 1985), all hallmarks of autoimmunity. It is unclear whether there is a relationship between these reactions and the effects of UV on immunological processes described above.

7.2.5 *Conclusions*

Exposure of mice to UV radiation impairs certain immune responses, enhances susceptibility to a variety of infectious agents and UV-induced tumours. While fewer studies have been done in rats, similar effects have been observed. Suppression of contact and delayed type hypersensitivity responses have been studied most extensively; however, several other cell mediated responses are also affected. Suppression of these immune responses appears to be mediated by release of soluble mediators from UB exposed skin which alter antigen presentation by Langerhans (and other) cells such that they fail to activate TH 1 cells. The resulting immune suppression is antigen specific, can occur regardless of whether antigen is applied at the site of exposure or not, and is relatively long lasting.

Enhanced susceptibility to a variety of infections in mice and rats corresponds to suppression of DTH responses to microbe specific antigens. UV exposure also prevents the development of protective immunity to these infections.

7.3 Ocular Studies

7.3.1 *Introduction*

The large number of animal studies enhances our understanding of both acute and delayed ocular effect from UV exposure (Zigman 1993; Andley 1987; Dillon et al., 1990). Studies of the action spectrum of delayed or permanent effects such as cataract or retinopathy and UV damage mechanisms in the cornea, lens and retina are only possible in animal models.

7.3.2 *General effects*

Photokeratitis is an acute reversible radiation-induced injury of the corneal epithelium. It is analogous to acute sunburn of the skin. Animal studies have clearly demonstrated that exposure to an artificial source of UVB can lead to acute photokeratitis, and action spectra have been determined (Cogan & Kinsey, 1946; Pitts et al., 1977; Zuclich and Kurtin, 1977). Pitts (1974; 1978) estimated the mean threshold of UVB (290-315 nm) for photokeratitis was 35 J m^{-2} at 270 nm.

Damage to corneal endothelium has been reported in rabbits (Doughty & Cullen, 1990). The effects on the corneal stroma have also been observed in rabbits, where reversible damage to the stromal keratocytes has followed exposure to UV (Ringvold & Davangar, 1985). This histological study showed that keratocytes disappear following UV exposure and later reappear. More recent animal studies have reported the use of a UVB filtering contact lens or the application of UVB absorbing chromophores to the cornea of rabbit eyes protects against photokeratitis (Bergmanson et al., 1988; Oldenburg et al., 1990).

7.3.3 *Cataractogenesis*

There is substantial evidence that exposure to UV induces discrete opacities in the anterior lens of experimental animals. Several studies have shown that UVB, but not UVA, induces anterior opacities in animals (Bachem, 1956; Pitts et al., 1977; Jose & Pitts, 1985; Söderberg 1990). Supra threshold doses of UVB at 300 nm cause a Na-K shift between the lens and the surrounding (Söderberg (1991). This leads to swelling and disruption of lens cells, probably causing zones of deviating refractive index within the lens observed as opacities (Söderberg 1989). Anterior lens opacities have developed in albino mice after daily exposure for 1-2 months to mixed UVA and UVB source (290-400 nm), but not when the source was filtered to remove radiation <320 nm (Jose & Pitts, 1985). Anterior cataract have also been produced in young albino mice exposed to black light (predominantly UVA, with some UVB) (Zigman et al., 1974). With more prolonged exposure of mice, cortical and posterior subcapsular opacities have been induced (Zigman et al., 1975; Jose, 1986). By contrast, a dose of 2 kJ m^{-2} applied every day produced anterior polar cataract within 8 weeks. Extension of the irradiation to 5 months created an opacity in the deeper cortex (Weager et al., 1989). In testing possible cataractogenic efficacy of UVA and UVB, UVB alone was cataractogenic, whereas, UVA showed the same effect only when other cataractogenic factors were added (e.g. X-ray) (Schmitt et al., 1988).

Ham et al. (1989) irradiated rhesus monkeys to 1 mW cm^{-2} daily for three years to UVA radiation (UVB radiation was carefully excluded) and was unable to detect lenticular opacities.

7.3.4 *Retinal effects*

It is well accepted that short wavelength visible non-coherent and coherent light, as well as UVA, can cause photochemical, mechanical and thermal damage to the retina and the pigment epithelium (review: Ham et al., 1984; Organisciak & Winkler, 1993). Aphakic monkeys revealed retinal lesions after exposure to UVA (Guerry et al., 1985). Exposure of aphakic albino rats to UVA created acute retinal lesions with 50-80% more effectiveness than blue light (Rapp & Smith 1992). Mechanical and thermal lesions are almost entirely limited to exposure to high energy laser light. Photochemical damage can occur through two different light exposure regimes: short term, high irradiance (minutes to hours) and long-term (days to weeks) low irradiance (Kremers & van Norren, 1988; Remé et al., 1991; Rapp & Smith, 1992). Whereas damage thresholds differ depending on the animal species, basic mechanisms at the molecular and structural level are essentially the same (for review: see Organisciak and Winkler, 1993). Photochemical lesions are strongly dependent on wavelength, i.e. the absorbing chromophore and its quantum efficiency, obey, at least within a certain time frame, the reciprocity of intensity and exposure duration (e.g. Kremers & van Norren, 1988).

Action spectra for high irradiance short exposure duration lesions have been obtained in several studies (e.g. Ham et al., 1984). Action spectra for prolonged exposure to relatively low light levels are less clear and were first evaluated by Noell et al. (1966). Prolonged exposure to low light levels may elicit secondary tissue responses that may not be directly related to the initial action spectrum. These tissues responses include acute cellular necrosis and apoptotic cell death, an inflammatory response with oedematous changes and macrophage invasion, and tissue proliferation with scar formation and neovascularization (e.g. Hoppeler et al., 1988; Yoshida et al., 1993). Action spectra, tissue responses, preventive measures as well as enhancing factors, which are all intensively investigated in many laboratories, are likely to be similar to the human.

Studies of photochemical retinal injury in aphakic rhesus monkeys have extended the action spectrum for short-wavelength light damage down to 310 nm (Ham et al., 1984). These studies showed that the retina, if exposed, is up to six times more vulnerable to photochemical damage in the UV than in the visible. These results are therefore of direct relevance to pseudophakic individuals without a UV-protective lens, and may also indicate a contributory role to light damage from the small fraction of UV that reaches the retina of the normal eye.

8. HUMAN STUDIES: THE SKIN

8.1 Characteristics

8.1.1 *Structure and optical properties*

The skin is a large organ with an area of more than 1.5 m^2 in adults. It provides the first stage of protection for chemicals, radiations, xenobiotics and also prevents the evaporation of water and the loss of ions and proteins. The skin has developed specific mechanisms for photoprotection and biological responses to UV as discussed below.

Skin is composed of three very different parts (as shown in figure 4.1): the epidermis, dermis and subcutaneous tissue. The epidermis is the outermost layer of the skin and varies in thickness from 50 μm to 600 μm (palmoplantor skin). The fibrous proteins known as keratin are produced in the keratinocytes of the epidermis. It is keratin that serves as a major protective tough substance in the skin; hair and nails are composed almost entirely of keratin. The daughter cells of the keratinocytes in the basal layer (stratum basale) of the epidermis differentiate and become "prickle cells" of the malpighian layer of the epidermis - the *stratum malpighii.* As these cells migrate outward, changes continue to occur; granules appear in the cytoplasm of each cell; the cells tend to flatten and form the *stratum granulosum.* Still later, the cells lose their nuclei, die, dehydrate and flatten out to form the tough *stratum corneum* (horny layer). It is generally agreed that the entire process of cell migration from the basal layer of the epidermis to final shedding from the surface of the stratum corneum takes 28 days in normal skin. Of this 28-day period, the cell spends about 14 days in the epidermis and 14 days in the stratum corneum.

The skin contains millions of tiny glands, including: apocrine (sweat) glands which discharge sweat into hair follicles, eccrine (sweat) glands which carry saline from the dermis and subcutaneous layer directly to the skin surface, and sebaceous glands which secrete sebum - an oily substance which lubricates hairshafts and maintains a slightly acidic, oily film over the stratum corneum. The collection of eccrine sweat glands plays a major role in the body's thermoregulatory mechanism, since evaporative cooling is the most efficient means the body has for removing excess heat, as long as the humidity is not 100%. More than two litres of sweat can be discharged in one day. On average, the skin contains about as many sebaceous glands as eccrine sweat glands, except that there are few sebaceous glands on the palms of the hands and soles of the feet.

The dermis, or corium, is much thicker than the epidermis, but consists of much larger cells. The dermis is largely connective tissue which gives the skin its elasticity and supportive strength. Nerve cells, blood vessels and lymphatic glands are found in the outermost dermal layer - the papillary dermis. Unlike the epidermis, the thickness of the dermis is not at all uniform throughout the body; it varies from 1 mm to 4 mm.

The basal layer of the epidermis is delineated from the dermis by a complex basement membrane. The keratinocytes are anchored to the basement membrane by semi desmosomes. This is the only layer where cell division takes place. The division of keratinocytes, under normal conditions, occurs every 17 to 38 days. The division rate may vary in different parts of the body.

Melanocytes are formed in the basal layer of the epidermis loosely attached to the neighbouring keratinocytes (ratio 1 melanocyte for 46 keratinocytes). The melanocytes synthesize the pigment melanin which matures into melanosomes. Then the melanosomes are transferred to the keratinocytes where they are digested if their size is below 1 cubic micron. Large melanosomes, as in dark skin, are not digested but transferred intact to the stratum corneum with the normal shedding of the epidermis.

Melanocytes are cells of nervous origin which have migrated during the 10th week of embryonic life in the epidermis and in the hair roots. These cells divide very slowly (one division every 3-5 years). There is a boost of division when new hairs are growing or after exposure to UV light.

Chemically, melanins are bipolymers: red melanins contain sulphurs and are soluble at PH 7.2, black melanins are insoluble. The ratio of red and black melanins within a melanocyte is genetically determined. Mixed types of melanins are deposited on a protein matrix contained in the melanosomes. Both types absorb UV and participate in the screening effect of the whole epidermis. Two major steps in the melanin synthesis take place: the enzymatic (tyrosinase) oxidation of the tyrosine to produce dopa (di-hydroxyphenylalanine) and the spontaneous oxidation of dopa in quinones.

Black melanin absorbs UV. In the presence of oxygen, it produces a free radical which, in sufficient quantities, can be deleterious to the melanocytes and the cellular environment, including keratinocytes or in the dermis, fibroblasts and fibres.

A third type of cell is present in the upper layers of the stratum Malpighi: the Langerhans cell. It is a migrating dendritic cell which is able to recognise foreign or abnormal structures. This cell plays a major role in immunological recognition and its activity is very sensitive to UV. Its function is impaired by a UV dose as low as one half of a minimal erythema dose.

The innermost layer of the skin is generally known as the subcutaneous layer. It is composed largely of fatty tissue that serves a shock-absorbing and insulating role. The thickness of this layer varies considerably from one body region to another and from one person to another.

Skin optics are governed by two basic processes, the absorption and scattering of light. Absorption is the loss of a photon when its energy is reduced within the atom or molecule, and more specifically in a target species called a chromophore. UV absorption occurs in wavelength bands where the molecules have characteristic absorption spectra. The absorbed photon energy is dissipated as heat or reemission of light when the excited molecules return to their ground state, or the energy is spent on photochemical reactions. Scattering is a process where the direction of propagation of UV is altered, especially at boundaries of refractive index. Scattering and absorption of the photons limit the depth of penetration of UV in the skin (see section 4.2 and figure 4.1).

In the white skin, the change in the refractive index causes 5% of the normally incident light to be reflected. The remaining 95% is absorbed or reflected at the dermis. The back-scattered light is reflected again at different interfaces. This phenomenon explains why, in the epidermis and in the upper papillary dermis, the strength of the light becomes several times that of the incident light itself.

The transmission of UV through isolated epidermis is strongly dependent on the chromophores contained in the structure. Aromatic amino acids (tryptophan, tyrosin, phenyl-alanine) absorb strongly near 275 nm, urocanic acid and melanins play the role of endogenous sunscreens. The DNA absorbs 260 nm wavelengths. Melanin is the unique chromophore with an absorption extending into the UVA and visible regions.

8.1.2 *Skin types*

The sensitivity of skin to UV has been defined by six phototypes: types I to IV are characteristics of caucasoid populations; type V represents mongoloid Middle Eastern populations (Fitzpatrick et al., 1974);

and type VI represents African and American negroid populations. The capacities to acquire natural tan or to present naturally a deep pigmentation are keys to the response to UV exposure. Among caucasians, there is a general correlation between skin type and resistance to sunburn and capacity to tan.

8.2 Beneficial Effects

8.2.1 *Vitamin D3*

An established beneficial effect of UV exposure is the synthesis of vitamin D3 (Adams et al., 1982). In adults, the epidermis contains nearly 50% of the total concentration of 7-dihydrocholesterol in the skin. UVB exposure causes the provitamins D3 to be isomerized to pre-vitamin D3. During continual exposure to sunlight, the pre-vitamin D3 forms by photo-isomerization the biologically inert photo-products lumisterol and tachysterol. Once formed, the pre-vitamin D3 spontaneously isomerizes into vitamin D3 (reaction with a maximum efficacy at 37°C), a more stable form. After crossing the basal membrane of the epidermis, vitamin D3 is linked to a circulating α1-globulin: vitamin D-binding protein. The protein linked vitamin D3 is transformed to 25-OH-T3 which can be measured in the blood. Transported to the kidney, it is metabolised to 1,25 dihydroxy vitamin D3 which is the biologically active form.

Vitamin D3 is required for the intestinal absoprtion of calcium (Davies 1985). After a single whole body exposure to one MED the circulating vitamin D3 level increases by an order of magnitude (2 ng/ml to 24 ng/ml within 24 hours) and returns to normal levels within a week (Holick 1985). Since active vitamin D3 is metabolised by the kidney, it was expected that in the circulating blood it does not change dramatically after repeated solar exposures. Chronically reduced vitamin D3 synthesis may lead to a deficit in active vitamin D3, as was found in elderly subjects (Omdahl et al., 1982).

The use of sunscreens was found to suppress cutaneous vitamin D3 synthesis (Matsuoka et al., 1988). This was also found in children, pregnant or lactating women and debilitated patients with poor intestinal absorption. Widespread use of sunscreens could lead to vitamin D deficiency in some groups and inadequate fixation of calcium (Prystowsky 1988). More recently, receptors for the active form for vitamin D3 were found in the keratinocytes of the epidermis. Vitamin D3 inhibits the proliferation of cultured keratinocytes and induces them to terminally differentiate (Smith et al., 1986). The topical or oral administration of 1, 25-OH-D3 has proved to be effective for the treatment of psoriasis, in replacement or in addition to the classical PUVA treatment. This is a new approach for the treatment of this condition and a possible explanation for the success of the heliotherapy (Morimoto and Kunihiko, 1989).

For the entire system of vitamin D3 production the amount of UV radiation reaching the skin is critical. The doses needed are small, and daily exposures of the face and hands to sun and light for 15 minutes is considered sufficient. The minimum dose requirement was estimated to be equivalent to 55 MED per year (Health Council of the Netherlands, 1986). When too little UVB reaches the skin, deficiencies of vitamin D may occur, resulting in a weakening of the bones. Groups at risk are particularly dark-skinned children in high latitude cities and elderly people living entirely indoors. Supplementation of vitamin D3 in the diet is then recommended.

8.2.2 *Skin adaptation*

Another beneficial effect of modest exposure to UVB radiation is the maintenance of the ability of the skin to sustain further UV exposures. Loss of this adaptation forms an important component in photodermatosis, skin diseases where the lesions are caused by light. These patients can be treated by regular exposures to UVB. The doses required are in the same range as that needed for the synthesis of vitamin D3.

8.2.3 *Other benefits*

It has been suggested that beneficial effects of UV exposures may occur such as: improvement of cardiopathy and functions, and better microorganism defense. These effects have not been confirmed in well designed studies. Bright light therapy for winter depression is most likely to be the consequence of visible light stimulating the ocular system. Because of the high illumination needed for this treatment special care is needed to avoid the emission of UV light by these sources (Terman et al., 1990).

Treatment of portwine stains and pigment dyschromia by lasers are applications of selective absorption of some wavelengths by specific chromophores contained in the lesion. Phototherapy by specific dyes absorbed by tumour cells or specific structures, is currently a growing field.

8.3 Acute Effects

8.3.1 *Erythema and sunburn*

In its mildest form, sunburn consists of a reddening of the skin (erythema) that appears up to about 8 h after exposure to UV and gradually fades after a few days. In its most severe form, it results in inflammation, blistering, and peeling of the skin. The degree to which a person will experience sunburn depends critically on skin type. For fair-skinned people, the relative effectiveness of UV for tanning and for erythema are approximately the same over the entire UVB and UVA ranges of wavelengths (Parrish et al., 1982).

The most important factors that define if a dose of UV will induce erythema are the wavelength of the radiation, the skin type, and the pigmentation of the subject. UVA, UVB and UVC are all able to induce the erythema.

The relative effectiveness of the different wavelengths to induce erythema is expressed as an erythema action spectrum (McKinlay and Diffey 1987). For minimal erythema, the most erythemogenic wavelengths are in the 250-290 nm range and a decrease in effectiveness is observed as the wavelengths increase. Erythema occurs 3-5 hours after UV exposure and reaches a maximum intensity between 8 and 24 hours, fading over 3 days. The vasodilatation of capillary vessels within the papillary dermis can be observed before the erythema becomes visible, and occurs in the same way for children, adults and elderly. However, the exposure time required to produce UVB erythema increases after about 60 years of age.

Histologic alterations from erythema are observed in the photodyskeratotic keratinocytes as well as intercellular edema with exocytosis (lymphocytes in the epidermis). Superficial vascular plexus, endothelial cell enlargement, perivenular edema, red blood cells in the capillary are characteristic features observed between 3 hours and 72 hours after UV exposure. Dermal neutrophils appear immediately after irradiation reaching a peak level at 24 hours.

DNA may be the primary chromophore involved in the induction of erythema (Ley, 1985, Wolf et al., 1993). Subsequently, a number of inflammatory mediators are induced. Cutaneous blisters have been used extensively to study these mediators. Prostaglandin (E_2 and F_2) levels were elevated in these blisters within 6 hours, peaked at 24 hours and returned to control levels by 48 hours after UV exposure, although erythema persisted beyond that time. Indomethacin suppressed prostaglandin formation, however, blood flow was only slightly altered by this treatment suggesting that other factors must play an important role in UVB induced inflammation (Greaves et al., 1978). Similarly while elevated histamine levels have been observed, antihistamines have little effect in diminishing UV induced erythema (Gilchrest et al., 1981).

Finally, UV exposure causes keratinocytes, to release the cytokines interleukin-1 (IL-1) and tumour necrosis factor α (TNF α) both of which are potent mediators of inflammation (Oxholm et al., 1988; Rasanen et al., 1989). UVB exposure also causes up-regulation of adhesion molecule such as ELAM-1 which facilitates inflammatory cell infiltration (Murphy et al., 1991).

Irradiation of human skin with 3 MED is associated with increased levels of transforming growth factor, suggesting a role of this molecule in keratinocyte proliferation, epidermal hyperplasia and angiogenesis.

8.3.2 *Skin pigmentation and tanning*

When skin is exposed to UV, two distinct tanning reactions ensue. Immediate pigment darkening (IPD) begins immediately on exposure to UV and is caused by the darkening of the pigment melanin that is already present in the skin; it is normally seen only in people who have at least a moderate constitutive tan. Such pigmentation begins to fade within a few hours after cessation of exposure. UVA is regarded as being most effective for IPD.

Delayed tanning (melanogenesis) takes about three days to develop and is more effectively produced by UVB than by UVA (Parrish et al., 1982; Gange et al., 1985). Delayed tanning is more persistent than IPD and results from an increase in the number, size and pigmentation of melanin granules. Exposure to UVB results also in an increase in the thickness and scattering properties of the epidermis (outer layer of the skin). Because UVA does not produce thickening of the epidermis, the tan obtained from it, while perhaps cosmetically acceptable, is not as effective in protecting against further exposure to UV as the equivalent pigmentation induced by exposure to UVB or solar radiation.

8.3.3 *Photosensitization*

The use of certain medicines may produce a photosensitizing effect on exposure to UVA as may the topical application of certain products, including some perfumes, body lotions, etc. Many medications and other agents contain ingredients that may cause photosensitivity, which is defined as a chemically induced change that makes an individual unusually sensitive to light. An individual who has been photosensitized may develop a rash, sunburn, or other adverse effect from exposure to light of an intensity or duration that would normally not affect that individual.

Reactions to photosensitizing agents involve both photoallergy (allergic reaction of the skin) and phototoxicity (irritation of the skin) after exposure to ultraviolet radiation from natural sunlight or artificial lighting (particularly from tanning booths). This photosensitization of the skin may be caused by creams or ointments applied to the skin, by medications taken orally or by injection, or by the use of prescription inhalers.

In addition to an exaggerated skin burn, itching, scaling, rash, or swelling, exposure to UV in combination with certain medications may result in (FDA 1992); Skin cancer, Premature skin aging, Skin and eye burns, Allergic reactions, Cataracts, Reduced immunity and Blood vessel damage.

This can result in photoallergic or phototoxic reactions that are accelerated by UV exposure. Phototoxic contact dermatitis often occurs clinically as exaggerated sunburn but occasionally blisters may also occur on the erythematous areas. Most phototoxic sensitizers have an action spectrum in the UV from 280-430 nm. Window glass which absorbs UV below 320 nm will protect patients from phototoxic compounds with absorption below 320 nm, but fails to protect against photosensitizers such as tar and psoralens which are efficient at longer wavelengths. Examples of photocontact drugs and substances are given below in table 8.1.

The concentration of drugs needed to elicit a photoallergic reaction is much lower than that needed to cause a phototoxic reaction. On the other hand, photoallergic reactions occur only in a small proportion of exposed individuals while phototoxic reactions may occur in anyone, given sufficient exposure. Generally, no clinical reaction occurs on first exposure to an agent causing subsequent photoallergy. Even sunscreen agents used to protect against photocontact dermatitis may be photoallergenic. A small number of individuals who develop photocontact dermatitis may retain a persistent reactivity to light (including UV) long after exposure to the photosensitizing compound.

8.4 Chronic Effects on the Skin Other than Cancer

UV radiation causes a number of chronic degenerative changes in the skin, mainly in caucasian populations, as a result of its action on keratinocytes, melanocytes and components of the dermal stroma including

Table 8.1 Some photosensitizing substances (CIE, 1990, FDA, 1992)

Sulphonamides
Salicylanilides
Coal-Tar derivatives
- acridine
- anthracene
- phenanthrene

Dyes
- anthraquinone
- eosin
- methylene blue
- rose bengal

Psoralens
Some fragrances
Cyclamate (artificial sweetener)
Non-steroidal anti-inflammatory drugs (pain reliever, antiathritics)
Deodorant and bacteriostatic agents in soaps
Fluorescent brightening agent for cellulose, nylon or wool fibres
Phenothiazines (major tranquilizers, anti-emetics)
Sulfonylureas (oral anti-diabetics, hypoglycemics)
Sunscreen ingredients
- 6-Acetoxy-2,4, - dimethly-m-dioxane (preservative)
- Benzophenones
- Cinnamates
- Oxybenzone
- Para-aminobenzoic acid (PABA)
- Paba esters

Tetracyclines (antibiotics, anti-infectives)
Tricyclic antidepressants

fibrous tissue (collagen and elastin) and blood vessels. These changes include freckles (ephelides), melanocytic naevi, lentigines, telangiectasia, skin wrinkling and atrophy, yellow papules and plaques on the face, colloid milium (firm, small, yellow, translucent papules on the face, forearms and hands), diffuse erythema, diffuse brown pigmentation and ecchymoses (Goldberg & Altman, 1984). These or related changes are sometimes grouped into syndromes such as cutis rhomboidalis nuchae (thick, yellow, furrowed skin, particularly on the back of the neck), Favre-Racouchot syndrome (yellow, thick comedones and follicular cysts of the periorbital, malar and nasal areas) and reticulated poikiloderma (reddish brown reticulated pigmentation with telangiectasia and atrophy and prominent hair follicles on the exposed chest and neck). With the exception of freckles and melanocytic naevi, these changes are also referred to collectively as "photoageing" (Gilchrest, 1990) because of their association with increasing age but presumed correlation with total accumulated exposure to the sun rather than with age per se.

In the US National Health and Nutrition Examination Survey (Engel et al., 1988), age-adjusted prevalence proportions of senile elastosis, actinic (solar) keratosis, fine telangiectasia, localized hypermelanism, senile (solar) lentigines and freckles, in whites 1 to 74 years of age, were associated with lifetime exposure to the sun as estimated by dermatologists.

Freckles and solar lentigines

Freckles and solar (also called senile) lentigines are pigmented macules occurring on the sun exposed skin of caucasians. Their prevalence is increased in those with highly sun-sensitive skin (Azizi et al., 1988). Freckles occur most commonly in children while the frequency of solar lentigines increases with age and is greatest in those over 60 years of age (estimated at 75% in the USA: Rhodes et al., 1991). They show similar histological patterns: their are increased numbers of melanocytes and an increased concentration of melanin in the basal layer of the epidermis (Rhodes et al., 1991). Melanocytic atypia has been observed in both. An increased risk of melanoma has been observed in relation to freckling in childhood and an increased risk of non-melanocytic skin cancer in relation to both freckling and prevalence of solar lentigines (see sections 8.4.1 and 8.4.2).

Melanocytic naevi

Melanocytic naevi are benign proliferations of melanocytes usually beginning in the basal layer of the epidermis and later extending into the dermis. They are common in white populations and rare in black and

Asian populations (Armstrong & English, 1988; Gallagher et al., 1991), are associated, in white populations, with phenotypic indicators of constitutional sensitivity to the sun, particularly fair skin colour (Green et al., 1988b; Gallagher et al., 1990b), occur mainly on body sites that are maximally or intermittently exposed to the sun (Kopf et al., 1978, 1985; Augustsson et al., 1990; Gallagher et al., 1990a), occur more commonly in Australian than British children (Green et al., 1988b) and in persons born in Australia than immigrants who arrived in Australia after about 15 years of age (Armstrong et al., 1986), and somewhat inconsistently with measures of sun exposure, including sunburn in early life (Armstrong et al., 1986; Gallagher et al., 1990c; Coombs et al., 1992). They are associated with an increased risk of cutaneous melanoma (see section 8.4.2).

Solar keratoses

Solar keratoses are benign proliferations of epidermal keratinocytes. They are very common on exposed body sites in older people in caucasian populations living in areas of high ambient solar irradiance (see for example, Marks et al., 1983 and Holman et al., 1984a). Solar keratoses have been reported to be associated with phenotypic indicators of cutaneous sun sensitivity (Vitasa et al., 1990), to be more common in people born in Australia than in migrants to Australia (Goodman et al., 1984), to be associated with estimates of total and occupational sun exposure (Goodman et al., 1985; Vitasa et al., 1990), and to be associated with other benign indicators of cutaneous sun damage (Holman et al., 1984b; Green 1991). Their number on the skin is strongly associated with risk of non-melanocytic skin cancer (see section 8.4.1).

8.5 Cancer

Epidemiological evidence relevant to the effects of UV on risk of cancer in humans derives mainly from study of the effects of sun exposure (presumably solar UV but not separable from other solar radiation) on cancer risk. There are four general lines of evidence available from which it may be inferred that sun exposure causes any particular cancer. They are that: the cancer in question occurs more frequently in people who are sensitive to the sun, occurs mainly at sun-exposed body sites, is increased in residents of areas of high ambient solar irradiance, and is increased in people with high personal sun exposure.These lines of evidence will not apply to all cancers that may be linked to sun exposure. They form nonetheless, a useful framework within which most of the relevant evidence can be described. To this framework will be added a consideration of evidence relating to artificial sources of UV when it is available.

The most direct evidence of the carcinogenicity of UV in humans should come, in principle, from observation of the effects of personal exposure to the sun. In practice, it is very difficult to make measurements of personal sun exposure accurately.Most often they are made by questionnaire and require recall of rather non-salient details of life over 60 or more years. This is a very difficult task (Kricker et al., 1993). A difficulty is presented by the fact that people who have sun sensitive skin and are at higher risk of skin cancer will tend to expose themselves less to the sun. To obtain an accurate measure of the effects of personal sun exposure, this confounding with sun sensitivity should be controlled - this has not always been done. It may not be surprising, therefore, that measures of personal exposure to the sun have not been consistently associated with risk of cancers thought to be related to the sun and that more indirect evidence has proved to be stronger.

8.5.1 *Nonmelanocytic skin cancer*

Introduction

There are two major histopathological types of nonmelanocytic skin cancer: basal cell carcinoma (BCC) and squamous cell carcinoma (SCC). BCC is the commoner type in white populations.

The epidemiology of nonmelanocytic skin cancer is difficult to describe accurately. Its routine recording is often not attempted by cancer registries because of the large numbers of cases involved and, if attempted, is invariably incomplete because of the rarity with which primary nonmelanocytic skin cancers require hospital treatment and the frequency with which probable nonmelanocytic skin cancers are not sent for histopathological verification of the diagnosis (Muir et al., 1987).

These difficulties have influenced the quality of the epidemiological evidence relating nonmelanocytic skin cancer to sun exposure. In addition, most of the earlier cross-sectional and case-control studies of nonmelanocytic skin cancer , and some of the more recent ones, (see, for example, table 11 in IARC, 1992) are deficient in that the control series were rarely population-based, appropriate effect measures or p values were often not estimated, and confounding by age and sex were not controlled in the analysis. In the narrative that follows, little reliance will be placed on these studies which include those reported by Lancaster & Nelson (1957), Gellin et al. (1965), O'Beirn et al. (1970), Urbach et al. (1974), Aubry & MacGibbon (1985), O'Loughlin et al. (1985), Herity et al. (1989), Hogan et al. (1989) and Gafa et al. (1991).

The results of most of the studies referred to below have been described and their results tabulated in detail in other publications (e.g., IARC, 1992) thus only the immediately salient features will be described here.

Sun-sensitivity

Race

Nonmelanocytic skin cancer is much less frequent in populations with dark skins than those with light skins (Fitzpatrick & Sober, 1985; Hoffman, 1987; Urbach, 1987). Data from cancer registries represented in Cancer Incidence in Five Continents Volumes II-VI (Doll et al., 1970; Waterhouse et al., 1976, 1982; Muir et al., 1987; and Parkin et al., 1992) in which direct comparisons of nonmelanocytic skin cancer incidence in different ethnic groups can be made within a single geographical area show that the incidence rates in the light skinned populations are consistently the highest. Similarly, in the 1977-78 US survey of nonmelanocytic skin cancer; rates in whites were 232.6 per 100 000 person years compared with 3.4 in blacks (Scotto et al., 1983).

Available evidence suggests that BCC occurs less frequently than SCC among dark skinned populations. The opposite is the case in light skinned populations. BCC was the most common nonmelanocytic skin cancer reported in South African whites in 1949-1975 but was rare among black Africans, occurring mainly in albinos (Oettlé, 1963; Oluwasanmi et al., 1969; Rippey and Schmaman, 1972; Isaacson et al., 1978). SCC, principally on the lower limb and associated with previous trauma, was the commoner of the two in blacks (Oettlé, 1963; Oluwasanmi et al., 1969; Rippey and Schmaman, 1972; Isaacson et al., 1978; Rose, 1973). Melanesians (Foster & Webb, 1988) and Polynesians (Paksoy et al., 1991) had less BCC than SCC, while no BCCs were reported in the Melanesians of North Samoa, a particularly heavily pigmented people (Foster & Webb, 1988).

Ethnic background is an important determinant of risk of nonmelanocytic skin cancer in Caucasians. In people of southern European ethnic origin born in Australia, relative to other people born in Australia, risk of BCC was 0.56 (95% CI 0.14-1.65) for those with one southern European grandparent, 0.17 (0.00-1.05) for two and 0.00 (0.00-0.86) for three or four (p for trend 0.002; Kricker et al., 1991a). No subject with SCC in this study had any southern European grandparents (RR 0.00, 0.00-1.23).

Individual sun sensitivity

Among recent cross-sectional, case-control and cohort studies several have reported significantly elevated relative risk (RR) estimates for red or light hair colour with BCC (RRs between 1.5 and 2.9; Hunter et al., 1990; Green & Battistutta, 1990; Kricker et al., 1991a) and SCC (RR=2.4; Kricker et al., 1991a). However, a light complexion was significantly associated only with SCC (RR=3.3; Kricker et al., 1991a), and high RRs (of 3.4) for light hair colour with BCC and SCC were reported in only one study (Vitasa et al., 1990).

Sensitivity of the skin to the sun, as measured by ability to tan and susceptibility to sunburn, was more consistently related to risk of BCC and SCC than hair, skin and eye colour. RRs of 2.0 or more for BCC were found with a skin that burns rather than tans (Marks et al., 1989; Vitasa et al., 1990; Hunter et al., 1990; Kricker et al., 1991a). For SCC, the evidence of an increased risk with sun-sensitive skin was somewhat weaker, with RRs around 2.0 and 95% confidence intervals (CI) that were wide and included 1.0, in the two studies that reported RRs adjusted for age, sex, and other relevant confounders (Vitasa et al., 1990; Kricker et al., 1991a).

Xeroderma pigmentosum and albinism

Xeroderma pigmentosum (XP) is a recessively inherited syndrome characterised by clinical and cellular hypersensitivity to solar radiation and a defect in the capacity to repair UV-induced damage in DNA (Fitzpatrick et al., 1963, Cleaver, 1973). Evidence of cutaneous sun damage may appear as early as 1-2 years of age in the absence of specific protection from the sun, and skin cancers are very frequent (Kraemer et al., 1987). In a survey of 830 cases of XP located through published case reports, 45% were reported to have had skin cancers (Kraemer et al., 1987). The median age of diagnosis of the first skin cancer was 8 years. Ninety seven per cent of BCC and SCC were on constantly exposed sites, that is, the face, head, and neck, compared with an estimated 80% in the general US population. In 220 XP patients in whom the number of skin cancers was stated, half had more than two cancers and 5% had more than 30; 79 patients were described as having BCC and 112 SCC (Kraemer et al., 1987).

Albinism is an inherited disorder of melanin metabolism with a decrease in or complete absence of melanin; as a result, the skin of albinos is highly sensitive to the sun. The most common type of albinism occurs in 1 in 15,000 American blacks, 1 in 40,000 European or American Caucasians, and has estimated frequencies as high as 1:3,900 in Soweto, South Africa (Kromberg and Jenkins, 1982), and 1 in 1,000 in Nigeria

(Cervenka et al., 1979). African albinos have been reported to have a high incidence of SCC and a somewhat lower rate of BCC (Cervenka et al., 1979; Luande et al., 1985; Kromberg et al., 1989).

Body-site distribution

It is commonly stated that the site distributions of non-melanocytic skin cancers, particularly SCC, correspond well to what would be expected from the exposure of different body sites to the sun. They do generally conform to this pattern with more than 60% of lesions occurring on the head and neck (Kricker et al., 1993). It is consistently observed, however, that the proportion of SCC on the upper limbs is higher than that of BCC while BCC has the higher proportion (some 10% or more) on the trunk (Scotto et al., 1983; Østerlind et al., 1988a; Giles et al., 1988; Glass & Hoover, 1989; Levi et al., 1988; Karjalainen et al., 1989; Kricker et al., 1990; Gallagher et al., 1990a; Roberts, 1990; Magnus, 1991; Serrano et al., 1991; Kricker et al., 1993). At the sub-site level, BCCs are almost completely absent on the heavily exposed backs of hands, and infrequent on the forearms compared with the upper arms (Brodkin et al., 1969; Scotto et al., 1983; Goodman et al., 1984; Kricker et al., 1990); in addition, this subsite distribution on the face is not highly correlated with the distribution of UV erythema on the face (Diffey et al., 1979).

Residence in areas of high ambient solar irradiance

Geographical variation

Annual incidence rates of nonmelanocytic skin cancer in 29 populations of mainly Western European origin in Cancer Incidence in Five Continents, volume 6 (Parkin et al., 1992) show little evidence of any consistent relationship between incidence and latitude. The highest incidence rates were in the populations of Tasmania, Australia (42°S) (213.2 per 100,000 in men and 113.1 per 100,000 in women) and British Columbia, Canada (49°N) (134.1 in men and 91.2 in women), and were also comparatively high in Switzerland (47°N) (78.7 in men and 50.2 in women) and Southern Ireland (53°N) (71.5 in men and 48.0 in women).

In contrast to these international patterns, incidence rates of nonmelanocytic skin cancer within countries do appear to increase with proximity to the equator as indicated by broad place of residence, latitude, or measures of solar irradiance. Geographical variation in nonmelanocytic skin cancer incidence in the USA has been described in three National Cancer Surveys (Mountin & Dorn, 1939; Dorn, 1944a, 1944b; Auerbach,

1961; Haenszel, 1963; Scotto et al., 1974) and several related studies (Scotto et al., 1982, 1983; Serrano et al., 1991). Incidence of all types increased with increasing proximity to the equator, with similar gradients for men, women and all ages. The same pattern is seen in Australia (Marks et al., 1993)

Migrants

The nonmelanocytic skin cancer experience of light-skinned migrants from areas of low to areas of high ambient solar irradiance has generally been consistent with an effect of sun exposure on skin cancer incidence. In Australia, incidence and mortality were found to be lower in migrants, most of whom had come from the UK, an area of lower sun exposure, than in those born in Australia (Armstrong et al., 1983; Giles et al., 1988). Kricker et al. (1991a) examined in some detail the relationship between BCC and SCC and migration to Australia. Migrants (excluding those from southern Europe who may be at lower constitutional risk for skin cancer) had a lower risk of BCC and SCC (RRs around 0.3) than did those born in Australia. In addition, for BCC (which had sufficient cases to analyze) the RR in those who migrated in the first 10 years of life (1.05) was the same as that in those born in Australia (1.0) but then fell to low levels in those who migrated later in life (RR about 0.2). Hunter et al., (1990) observed an association between risk of BCC and residence in southern parts relative to elsewhere in the USA (RRs of 1.6 for residence in California and 2.1 for Florida).

Personal sun exposure

Total sun exposure

Reported measurements of total current or accumulated sun exposure in studies of nonmelanocytic skin cancer are likely to be subject to substantial error not only because of the difficulties in recalling sun exposure over periods of 60 years or more (Kricker et al., 1993) but also because of the use of broad summary variables such as "estimated average daily outdoor exposure" (Gellin et al., 1965). The two studies which attempted a more quantitative measure found no evidence of a positive association between estimates of total sun exposure and risk of BCC (RRs of 1.0 or less) (Hunter et al., 1990; Vitasa et al., 1990). Only one of these studies included SCC (with only about 50% confirmed histopathologically); for sun exposure above the 75th centile the estimated RR was 2.5 (95% CI 1.2-5.4) (Vitasa et al., 1990).

Occupational sun exposure

Early clinical reports associated skin cancer with outdoor occupation (Molesworth, 1927; Blum, 1948; Emmett, 1973). However, the relationship between occupation and skin cancer has been examined adequately in relatively few studies and the evidence for an association is weak. At the population level, the best conducted studies which attempted to classify occupational sun exposure on the basis of occupational title found only small differences in skin cancer incidence between outdoor and indoor workers. Several population studies reported associations with employment in agriculture (Atkin et al., 1949; Whitaker et al., 1979; Teppo et al., 1980) and outdoor employment generally (Beral & Robinson, 1981; Vågerö et al., 1986) but their interpretation is complicated by incomplete and potentially biased case ascertainment (Vågerö et al., 1986; Teppo et al., 1980), inclusion of other cancers (Atkin et al., 1949), and confounding between occupation and social class (Beral & Robinson, 1981).

There have been few well-conducted studies of occupational sun exposure at the individual level. They show a generally consistent but not strong association between BCC and SCC and various crude measures of outdoor employment, e.g., "indoors", or "outdoors" occupation. The RRs have generally been under 2.0 for BCC (Hogan et al., 1989; Marks et al., 1989; Green and Battistutta, 1990; Gafa et al., 1991). One study reported a high RR for SCC with an "outdoors" occupation but with an extremely wide confidence interval (Green and Battistutta, 1990). Other studies found RRs close to 1.0 (Aubry and MacGibbon, 1985, Hogan et al., 1989; Marks et al., 1989; Gafa et al., 1991) and only one appeared to be statistically significant (Hogan et al., 1989).

Recreational exposure

The relationship of exposure to sunlight in non-working hours (largely recreational sun exposure) with nonmelanocytic skin cancer has been described in only two studies. One study reported an RR below 1.0 for BCC in those with "mainly outdoor leisure" and a positive but not statistically significant association for SCC: RR of 3.9 (95% CI 0.5-30.9) (Green & Battistutta, 1990). In the study of Aubry & MacGibbon (1985), the highest category of a "non-occupational exposure score" showed an elevated risk of SCC (RR 1.6; p-value=0.07).

Sunburn

Risk of BCC was significantly increased in subjects with a history of sunburn in one of two recent studies. Hunter et al. (1990) observed an increasing risk with increasing frequency of painful sunburns (RR 2.91, 95% CI 2.37-3.58, for 6+ occasions). Green and Battistutta (1990), on the other hand, found no discernible association between BCC and number of painful sunburns. The risk of SCC, however, was increased with any history of painful sunburn in this study: RRs 3.3 (95% CI 0.9-12.3) for 1-5 sunburns and 3.0 (0.7-12.2) for 6+.

Other sun-related skin conditions

Cutaneous microtopography (a measure of loss of the fine skin markings on the backs of the hands presumed due to loss of dermal collagen; Holman et al., 1984a), prevalence of solar elastosis of the neck, solar telangiectasia and solar lentigines and a history of solar keratoses have been taken as indicators of a high level of total accumulated exposure to the sun in those who have BCC or SCC. The evidence that sun exposure causes these conditions, however, is no stronger, and may be weaker, than the evidence that it causes BCC, SCC or cutaneous melanoma.

Increasingly severe sun-related skin damage as measured by cutaneous microtopography was associated with increasing risks of both BCC (RR 3.1, 95% CI 1.5-6.4 for the highest grade) and SCC (RR 1.8, 95% CI 0.8-4.2 for the highest grade) (Kricker et al., 1991a). Other indicators of sun damage to the skin (e.g. freckles, telangiectasia, and elastosis) were also strongly related to risk of both BCC and SCC, whether considered separately (Green and Battistutta, 1990; Kricker et al., 1991a) or together (Holman et al., 1984a; Green et al., 1988a), and including when adjusted for cutaneous sun sensitivity (Kricker et al., 1991a). The RRs associated with the presence of 40 or more solar keratoses were 10.4 (95% CI 5.8-18.8) for BCC and 34.3 (95% CI, 14.0-84.0) for SCC (Kricker et al., 1991a).

Exposure to artificial sources of UV

Any use of a sunlamp was associated with a statistically significantly increased risk of SCC in the study of Aubry & McGibbon (1985) but three other studies (O'Loughlin et al., 1985; Herity et al., 1989; Hogan et al., 1989) found no association with "artificial sunlight" or use of sunlamps or sunbeds.

8.5.2 *Cutaneous Melanoma*

Introduction

Cutaneous melanoma began to be studied epidemiologically in 1948 when it was separated from other primary malignancies of the skin in the 6th Revision of the International Statistical Classification of Diseases (WHO, 1948), and Eleanor MacDonald published the first population-based study, covering 272 incident cases of melanoma in Connecticut (MacDonald, 1948). Because of its likely fatality if not treated, melanoma is much more likely to come to medical attention and to be diagnosed histopathologically than nonmelanocytic skin cancer. It has, therefore, been more readily recorded on a population basis than nonmelanocytic skin cancer and better studied epidemiologically. Thus, while generally considered less clearly associated with sun exposure, a series of large and well-conducted studies in different countries over the last 10 years have served to clarify this issue.

Sun-sensitivity

Race

Melanoma is a disease primarily of light-skinned populations and occurs much less frequently in people with darker skins. In the United States, the incidence in whites is ten fold or more higher than in blacks living in the same areas (Parkin et al., 1992). Rates are lowest (less than 0.7 per 100 000 person years) in parts of Asia (eg Japan, Singapore, India, China, Philippines) while in Los Angeles, USA, incidence was less than 1 per 100 000 in Japanese and Chinese people compared with slightly higher rates, around 2.0, in blacks (Parkin et al., 1992).

Among Caucasians, ethnic background is an important determinant of melanoma incidence. The incidence is substantially lower among Hispanics than among other whites in the United States. For example, the incidence among Hispanics in New Mexico is less than 2 per 100,000 person years, but in other whites it is about 11 per 100,000 (Muir et al., 1987). In several case-control studies, subjects with a southern or eastern European background had substantially lower risks than those of northern European or United Kingdom origins (Elwood et al., 1984; Holman and Armstrong, 1984a; Graham et al., 1985).

Individual sun sensitivity

Blue eyes, fair or red hair, and pale complexion in people of European origin are well established risk factors for melanoma. These pigmentary characteristics were documented in most melanoma case-control studies (see table 16 in IARC, 1992 and, as examples, Elwood et al., 1984, Holman & Armstrong, 1984a, and Green et al., 1985). Relative risk for light skin colour ranged from a little more than 1.0 to about 3. Compared with those with dark brown to black hair, those with fair hair generally had a less than two-fold increase in risk, but those with red hair usually had a 2 to 4-fold increase in risk. Eye colour was generally a weak risk factor with relative risks less than 2, and what increased risk there was generally disappeared after adjustment for the other traits.

Increased risks of melanoma in those with a reduced ability to tan and an increased tendency to sunburn were observed in all case-control studies in which these sun-sensitivity measures were examined (see, for example, Elwood et al., 1984, Holman & Armstrong, 1984a, and Green et al., 1985).

Xeroderma pigmentosum and albinism

In a review of reports of 378 patients with XP in which cancer was mentioned, 37 patients had a melanoma (Kraemer et al., 1987).

African albinos have been reported to have a low rate of melanoma (Cervenka et al., 1979; Luande et al., 1985; Kromberg et al., 1989). Levine et al. (1992) state that there have been only 16 documented cases of melanoma in albino patients reported in the English language literature. Since albinos generally have a normal number of melanocytes (Dargent et al., 1992), the rarity of melanoma in them may indicate that melanin plays an important role in the genesis of this cancer.

Body site distribution

The distribution of melanoma appears to favour sites which are less heavily sun exposed, that is the back and face in Caucasian men and the lower limbs in women (Crombie, 1981). However, when whole-population series of cancer cases have been examined and body surface area taken into account, sites that were usually covered by clothing had lower rates than those usually exposed, with the exception of the forearms and hands for which the rates per unit area were low (Elwood & Gallagher, 1983; Green et al., 1993). The anatomic site distribution of melanoma in blacks is quite different from that in Caucasians with the majority of melanomas on the soles of the feet (Higginson and Oettlé, 1959; Lewis, 1967; Fleming et al., 1975).

Residence in areas of high ambient solar irradiance

Geographical variation

Internationally, the incidence of melanoma varies over 100-fold. Among countries included in Cancer Incidence in Five Continents, Volume VI, the lowest rates reported around 1983-87 were 0.1-0.2 per 100 000 person years in China (Qidong), Japan (Osaka), India (Bombay), and in Kuwaitis in Kuwait, while the highest were about 25 per 100 000 person years in parts of Australia (Parkin et al., 1992). In the USA and Australia, which have reasonably homogeneous populations of mainly European origin distributed across a wide latitude range, melanoma incidence increases with increasing proximity to the equator or with increasing measured, annual ambient UV irradiance (Scotto & Fears, 1987; Jones et al., 1992).

A simple latitude gradient for melanoma is not evident in Europe. Armstrong (1984) showed that the incidence of melanoma in Europe decreased from about latitude 35° N to a minimum around 55o N and then rose with increasing latitude because of high rates in Scandinavian and Scottish populations. The gradient of risk for melanoma from north to south in northern Europe matches the increasing natural pigmentation of the skin and may also, in part, be due to differing patterns of sun exposure, particularly recreational and vacation sun exposure.

Migrants

If a person migrates in childhood to a country of high ambient solar radiation such as Australia, Israel, and New Zealand, their risk of melanoma is observed to be similar to that in those born in the country to which they migrate, whereas if they migrate after this age their risk is substantially less than that in the locally-born population (Katz et al., 1982; Cooke and Fraser, 1985; McCredie & Coates 1989; Steinitz et al., 1989; Khlat et al., 1992). Overall, British immigrants to Australia and New Zealand, where the populations are of predominantly British origin, had incidence and mortality rates of melanoma of about a half the levels in those born in these countries (Cooke and Fraser, 1985; Khlat et al., 1992).

Residence history

Studies of individual lifetime ambient solar radiance, based on latitude, location (eg, tropical, near coast), or average sunshine hours of all places of residence are consistent in showing an increased risk of melanoma with increased average radiance (Green & Siskind, 1983; Holman et al., 1984b; Graham et al., 1985; Østerlind et al., 1988b; MacKie et al., 1989; Weinstock et al., 1989; Beitner et al., 1990). RRs for the highest category of ambient solar radiance were 2.8 for mean annual hours of bright sunlight at places of residence in Australia (Holman et al., 1984b), between 1.4 and 2.6 for a southerly latitude in the USA (Graham et al., 1985; Weinstock et al., 1989), or a tropical or Mediterranean residence (MacKie et al., 1989; Beitner et al., 1990). RRs differed greatly for residence near the coast in Denmark (RR=1.7; Østerlind et al., 1988b) and Australia (RR=5.0; Green & Siskind, 1983).

Personal sun exposure

Lifetime total exposure

Inconsistent results have been obtained in studies in which lifetime total sun exposure were assessed by questionnaires. RRs for the highest exposure category were between 0.6 and 5.3 (see table 18 in IARC, 1992). Two of five studies showed a statistically significant positive association with RRs of 3.4 and 5.4 (Grob et al., 1990; Lê et al., 1992) while one study showed a significant negative association (RR 0.6; Graham et al., 1985). The other two RRs were 1.1 (Dubin et al., 1986) and 5.3 (95% CI 0.8-30.8; Green, 1984).

Usual or recent total exposure

In this context, total means exposure from all sources (i.e. occupational and non-occupational) rather than the total over some period of time. This concept has been measured in a variety of ways. For example, it has been common to enquire about present "usual" exposure to the sun or usual exposure in some time period in the fairly recent past. The evidence of any effect of such exposures on risk of melanoma is weak. Of five studies, four had relative risks for the highest categories of exposure ranging from 0.7 to 1.2 (Elwood et al., 1985b; Dubin et al., 1986; Holman et al., 1986; Cristofolini et al., 1987). The remaining study found a relative risk of 2.5 ($p < 0.001$) for the highest category of exposure of average daily sun exposure 10-20 years ago (Rigel et al., 1983).

Occupational exposure

Four studies of melanoma have shown statistically significant positive associations with estimated lifetime occupational exposure to the sun (see table 20 in IARC, 1992) with RRs ranging up to 6.0 (95% CI, 2.1 to 17.4) for outdoor employment (Paffenbarger et al., 1978; Dubin et al., 1986; Garbe et al., 1989; Grob et al., 1990). On the other hand, four studies showed statistically significant results in which the RR for the highest category of exposure was < 1.0 (Elwood et al., 1985b; Holman et al., 1986; Østerlind et al., 1988b; Beitner et al., 1990). The remaining studies have shown RRs around 1.0.

Recreational exposure

Recreational exposure to the sun has generally been measured by either the type of recreational activity or the frequency or duration of outdoor recreation (see table 22: in IARC, 1992). Some studies have also recorded sun exposure during vacations separately from other recreational sun exposure. At least one statistically significant positive association was found in 11 of 16 studies in which recreational exposure was considered (Adam et al., 1981; Lew et al., 1983; Rigel et al., 1983; Elwood et al., 1985b; Dubin et al., 1986; Holman et al., 1986; Østerlind et al., 1988b; Zanetti et al., 1988; Beitner et al., 1990; Grob et al., 1990; Nelemans et al. 1993). The RRs in the highest categories of exposure were generally between 1.5 and 2.5. Only one study has shown a negative association with recreational exposure: MacKie & Aitchison (1982), in Scotland, observed an RR of 0.4 (95% CI 0.2-0.9) for the highest category of hours a week in outdoor recreation. Their statistical model, however, included socioeconomic status and history of sunburn, both of which may measure sun exposure; thus overadjustment of the estimate of RR is likely. All measures of number or frequency of vacations in sunny places were positively associated with risk of melanoma. The RRs for the highest category of this variable ranged from 1.2 to 5 and the finding was statistically significant in six of eight studies (Lew et al., 1983; Elwood et al., 1985b, Østerlind et al., 1988b, Zanetti et al., 1988; Beitner et al., 1990; Nelemans et al., 1993).

Sunburn

Fifteen of seventeen studies of melanoma in which sunburn was recorded (see table 23 in IARC, 1992) showed a statistically significant, moderately to strongly positive association with a history of sunburn (MacKie & Aitchison, 1982; Lew et al., 1983; Elwood et al., 1985a; Green et al., 1985; Sorahan & Grimley, 1985; Elwood et al., 1986;

Holman et al., 1986; Holly et al., 1987; Østerlind et al., 1988b; Zanetti et al., 1988; MacKie et al., 1989; Weinstock et al., 1989; Beitner et al., 1990; Elwood et al., 1990; Nelemans et al., 1993) (see table 23: IARC, 1992). Twelve of these studies showed RRs greater than 2.0 for the highest category of sunburn. Positive associations were obtained for both sunburn in childhood and sunburn at any age. The greater consistency of the relationship of melanoma with sunburn compared to that with other exposure variables may indicate a specific association with sunburn per se or simply that sunburn is a more accurately measured indicator of sun exposure.

Presence of other sun-related skin conditions

Cutaneous microtopography

Severity of sun damage to the skin as measured by cutaneous microtopography was strongly associated with risk of melanoma in Western Australia. The RR for the most severe grade of damage was 2.7 (95% CI 1.4-5.0; p-value for trend=0.003; Holman et al., 1984b). There was no similar relationship, however, in a study in Denmark, in which similar methods were used (Østerlind et al., 1988b).

Freckling of the skin has been shown to be associated with an increased risk of melanoma in several studies (see for example, Elwood et al., 1986, 1990, Østerlind et al., 1988b; Dubin et al., 1986).

Solar keratoses and other skin cancers

The risk of melanoma was significantly increased in association with a past history of nonmelanocytic skin cancer with RRs of 3.7 (95% CI 2.1-6.6) in Australia (Holman et al., 1984b) and 3.8 (1.2-12.4) in the USA (Holly et al., 1987). Relative risks for a history of solar keratoses or "actinic tumours on the face" were similarly high (Green & O'Rourke, 1985; Dubin et al., 1986).

Exposure to artificial sources of UV

Several studies have reported increased risks of cutaneous melanoma in users of sunlamps or sunbeds (IARC, 1992). In the most recent of these studies (Walter et al., 1990), the relative risks for any use of sunbeds or sunlamps were 1.9 (95% CI 1.2-3.0) in men and 1.5 (95% CI 1.0-2.1) in women. Relative risk increased with increasing duration of use: for more than 12 months use the relative risks were 2.1 (0.9-5.3) in men and 3.0 (1.1-9.6) in women. Positive associations were found in two of four other case-control studies in which these exposures were studied (Swerdlow et al., 1988; MacKie et al., 1989; see also IARC, 1992). Sun exposure is a potential confounding variable in studies of sunlamps and sunbeds but has not been taken into account. Specifically it was considered by Walter et al. (1990). Exposure to a group of other artificial sources of UV, including plan printers, laboratory equipment emitting UV, insect tubes, black lights and photocopiers, was not associated with melanoma in one case control study in Australia (Holman et al., 1986) but for a similar group plus welding the RR was 2.2 (95% CI 1.0-4.9) in Canada (Elwood et al., 1986). Siemiatycki (1991) found no association between arc welding or other occupational exposure to UV in a study of occupation and cancer in Canada.

A number of case-control studies have examined the association between melanoma and exposure to fluorescent lighting. Only the first such study found a statistically significant positive result (Beral et al., 1982). Six subsequent studies found little or no evidence of a positive association (IARC, 1992).

8.5.3 *Cancer of the lip*

Cancer of the lip is defined as cancer of the vermilion border and adjacent mucous membranes and thus excludes cancers of the skin of the lip (WHO, 1977). Most are SCC and occur on the lower lip (Keller, 1970; Lindqvist, 1979), a site more heavily exposed to the sun than the upper lip (Urbach et al., 1966). The inclusion of adjacent oral mucosa in the definition of cancer of the lip raises the possibility of confounding of tobacco and alcohol use (well established causes of cancer of the mouth; Tomatis, 1990).

The incidence of cancer of the lip is much more common in men than women. Among men in the USA, it is some 20 times more common in whites than blacks and it is rare in black and Asian populations worldwide (Parkin et al., 1992). Incidence of and mortality from cancer of the lip are substantially lower in migrants to Australia and Israel, who come from places with potentially lower sun exposure, than those born in these countries (Armstrong et al., 1983; McCredie & Coates, 1989; Steinitz et al., 1989).

The incidence of cancer of the lip is higher in rural than urban areas (Doll, 1991) and descriptive studies have consistently reported higher incidence or mortality rates of this cancer in men with outdoor occupations such as farmers, agricultural labourers and fishermen. (Atkin et al., 1949; Clemmesen, 1965; Gallagher et al., 1984; Olsen & Jensen, 1987; Lynge

& Thygesen, 1990). Four case-control studies of varying quality have examined the association between outdoor work and cancer of the lip. Keller (1970) compared 301 men with cancer of the lip with 301 oral cancer controls. Crude RRs for employment as a farmer or in any outdoor work were 4.0 and 2.6 respectively. The use of patients with oral cancer as controls allowed a rough adjustment for confounding with tobacco and alcohol use in this study. Spitzer et al. (1975) compared 339 men with cancer of the lip with 199 matched population controls. The relative risk for any outdoor work was 1.52 and, for employment as a fisherman, 1.50 ($p < 0.05$ in both cases). Pipe smoking but not alcohol drinking was controlled in the analysis. The other two studies also showed a positive association between outdoor work and cancer of the lip (Lindqvist, 1979; Dardanoni et al., 1984) but did not control for smoking and alcohol use and showed other methodological difficulties (IARC, 1992).

8.5.4 *Ocular cancers*

Ocular melanoma and other ocular cancers are dealt with in Chapter 10.

8.5.5 *Other cancers*

Observations of increasing mortality with increasing latitude have formed the basis of suggestions that cancers of the breast, colon and prostate may be prevented by increasing exposure to the sun (Garland & Garland, 1980; Gorham et al., 1989, 1990; Garland et al., 1989, 1990; Hanchette & Schwartz, 1992), perhaps through proposed anti-carcinogenic actions of vitamin D (Eisman et al., 1980; Colston et al., 1989; Schwartz & Hulka, 1990; Ainsleigh, 1993). Variation with latitude in medical care, death certification practices, diet and other lifestyle factors are alternative explanations for the latitude gradients in these cancers. These observations, therefore, can be taken only to raise hypotheses about indirect anti-carcinogenic effects of UV which require testing by other means.

8.5.6 *Action spectrum*

There are few data from which the action spectrum of UV carcinogenesis in humans can be inferred. For practical purposes, therefore, reliance is placed on action spectra which have been determined in experimental animals (see chapter 7).

If, as is argued below, it is accepted that the formation of cyclobutylthymidine dimers is a step in the production of mutations that are associated at least with BCC and SCC, then it would be reasonable to accept the action spectrum for production of thymidine dimers in humans as possibly indicative of the action spectrum for production of nonmelanocytic skin cancer (figure 8.1). This action spectrum was determined by Freeman et al. (1989) who irradiated untanned gluteal skin of 30 caucasian volunteers with 1 or 2 MED of narrow band UV at 275 nm, 282 nm, 290 nm, 296 nm, 304 nm, 334 nm and 365 nm. At least five subjects were irradiated at each wavelength. Following irradiation, shave biopsies were taken of the irradiated skin, DNA extracted and incubated with Micrococcus luteus endonuclease to determine the frequency of endonuclease sensitive sites which indicate the presence of thymidine dimers. Figure 8.1 shows that the effectiveness of UV in producing dimers increased from 275 nm to a peak at 296 to 304 nm and then fell by four orders of magnitude to the lowest measured level at 365 nm. This fall is quite consistent with that observed in the relative effectiveness of UV for carcinogenesis in mouse skin over the same wavelength range. The authors reported, also, that observations had been made at 385 nm and 405 nm and that these wavelengths were "largely ineffective" in net production of dimers.

Some indication of the effectiveness of UVA in causing skin cancer could be obtained from the experience of people exposed to high doses of UVA from sunbeds or in tanning salons. There is some evidence to suggest that these exposures are associated with an increase in risk of nonmelanocytic skin cancer, cutaneous melanoma and ocular melanoma (see above). In none of the studies carried out, however, has exposure to mainly UVA sources been distinguished from sources that emit both UVA and UVB. In addition, confounding with sun exposure is a possibility in all these studies.

8.5.7 *Dose-response*

In theory, the best way to estimate the dose-response relationship between UV and cancer in humans would be to measure the lifetime exposure to the sun of each member of a population and relate this measurement, by way of a cohort or a case-control study, to their probability of developing skin cancer. In practice this is very difficult. First, measurement of lifetime exposure to the sun generally requires recall of amount and pattern of sun exposure and use of protective measures against the sun for as long as 40 or more years in the past.

Second, exposure in early life may be particularly important in determining risk of skin cancer, at least, and this is to a large extent outside the range of accurate recall. Third, while problems of recall could be solved by conduct of a cohort study, such a study would require

Figure 8.1 Action spectrum for the formation of pyrimidine dimers in human skin on exposure to UV between 275 nm and 366 nm as measured by the formation of micrococcus luteus endonuclease sensitive sites (ESS). Each point (•) represents one subject, circled points indicate two subjects with identical dimer yields. ph=photon, kb=kilobase. (Reprinted in modified form with permission from Freeman et al., 1989).

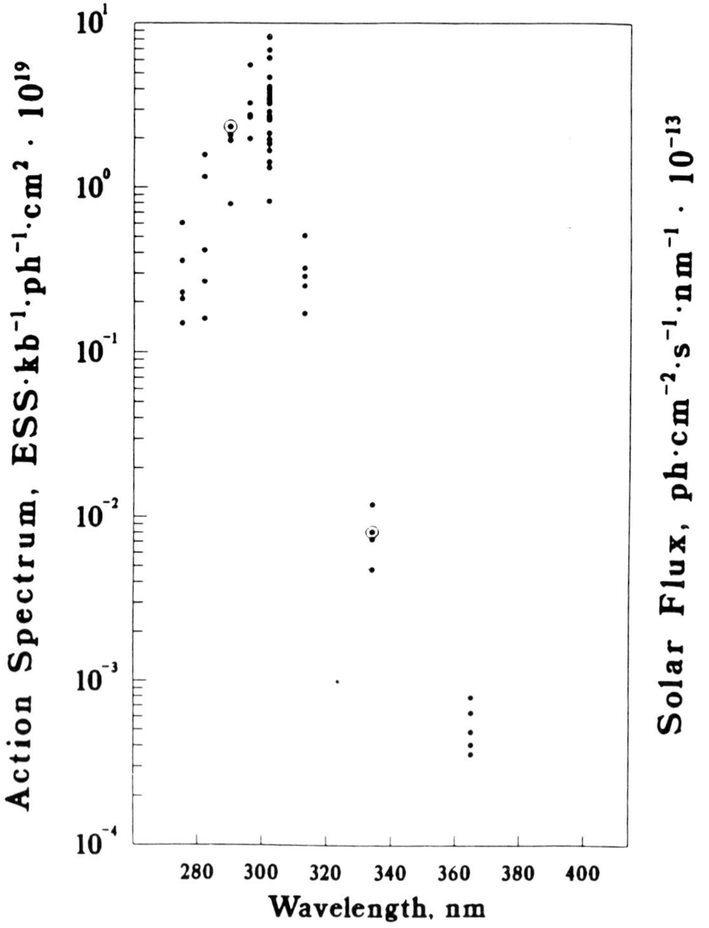

measurements of sun exposure beginning in the first few years of life and repeated periodically throughout life to the age at which UV-related cancers become common. Such a study would be logistically and economically impracticable. The whole process is complicated by the fact that a simple measure of lifetime exposure may be insufficient for adequate description of dose-response. The evidence that period and pattern of exposure may be important determinants of some UV-related cancers (see below) means that to model incidence correctly as a function of exposure it would be necessary to collect data on dose-rate of UV and its variation throughout life.

One attempt has been made to estimate the dose-response relationship between UV and SCC and BCC in a retrospective cohort study of Chesapeake Bay watermen (Strickland et al., 1989). The watermen work mainly in traditional fishing tasks that are regulated by law and have undergone few changes in the past 80 years. They presented, therefore, better prospects than most populations for the accurate recall of past sun exposure. Briefly, 808 caucasian subjects among 1 250 licensed watermen aged 30 years or more participated in an interview and skin examination. Present skin cancers were identified at examination and a history of past skin cancer was taken and; as far as possible, histological confirmation of the diagnosis was obtained for both present and past skin cancer. Totals of 47 SCC in 35 subjects, 60 BCC in 33 subjects and 344 solar keratoses in 202 subjects were identified. About a half of the SCC and BCC had been diagnosed before the survey examination while over 90% of the solar keratoses were diagnosed at the examination. Histological confirmation was available for at least one lesion in 51% of subjects with SCC, 72% with BCC and 13% with a solar keratosis (Vitasa et al., 1990). The average annual exposure of facial skin to solar UVB was estimated for each subject by the combination of data from a personal history of mainly occupational outdoor exposure from 16 years of age to the interview, estimates of ambient UV radiance in the area in which the watermen lived and worked, based on the US network of Robertson Berger meters (Berger & Urbach, 1982), and field measurements of individual exposure to UVB under working conditions as recorded by polysulphone film dosimeters. Annual average ambient UVB for the area was estimated at about 1.14×10^6 J m^{-2} or 3260 MED assuming 350 J m^{-2} to be equivalent to 1 MED. Personal annual average exposure of facial skin ranged from about 1% to 8% of ambient UVB, i.e., 33 to 260 MED a year.

The dose-response relationships obtained are shown in figure 8.2. They were derived from the following mathematical model:

$$\text{prevalence} = (\text{exposure})^a (\text{age})^b$$

or, equivalently,

$$\log(\text{prevalence}) = a \log(\text{exposure}) + b \log(\text{age}).$$

While prevalence is stated in the above expressions and the y axis in figure 8.2 is labelled as prevalence, it is believed that the figures are cumulative incidence proportions in which each subject with more than one of a particular type of lesion was counted only once. Only cumulative incidence of SCC appeared to increase with increasing estimated exposure to solar UVB. The value of a for SCC was 1.7. It should be noted however, that 4 subjects with SCC among 64 men in the lowest sun exposure category were excluded from the regression because of the anomalously high incidence in this group and because of the possibility that these subjects may have been hypersusceptible to UV. Apart from all having solar keratoses, however, they did not consistently show phenotypic features of high susceptibility to UV and it was not possible on any basis, therefore, to remove hypersusceptible subjects from the higher dose categories. The values of a for BCC and solar keratoses were -0.2 and 0.005 respectively. It was suggested that because of the high sun exposure of all men in the study the cumulative incidence of BCC may have reached a saturation point at the lowest level of sun exposure such that further increases in exposure did not lead to further increases in incidence.

An alternative approach to estimating dose-response relationships has been to examine the relationship, geographically, between incidence or mortality of skin cancers in whole populations and estimated or measured ambient UV (Armstrong, 1993). This work has been done in the context of estimating the increase in skin cancer that might be expected from some increment in ground-level UV caused by depletion of stratospheric ozone. It has made the fundamental assumption that the observed geographical variations in incidence or morbidity rates of skin cancer is due largely to geographical variations in UV. The results have commonly been expressed in terms of the biological amplification factor (BAF) defined as follows (de Gruijl and van der Leun, 1980).

There are substantial uncertainties regarding the dose-response relationships shown in figure 8.2. First, the estimates of dose were based on exposure of the face only, excluded dose in the first 16 years of life and did not take account of dose-rate or pattern of exposure. Second, there is likely to have been appreciable underascertainment of cancers diagnosed before the survey and high proportions of all lesions were not confirmed histopathologically. Third, the exclusion of four men with SCC must have

Figure 8.2 Relationship of cumulative incidence of nonmelanocytic skin cancers and solar keratoses to individual estimated average annual exposure of the face to UVB since 16 years of age. O, solar keratosis; △, SCC; □, BCC. (Reproduced with permission from Strickland et al., 1989).

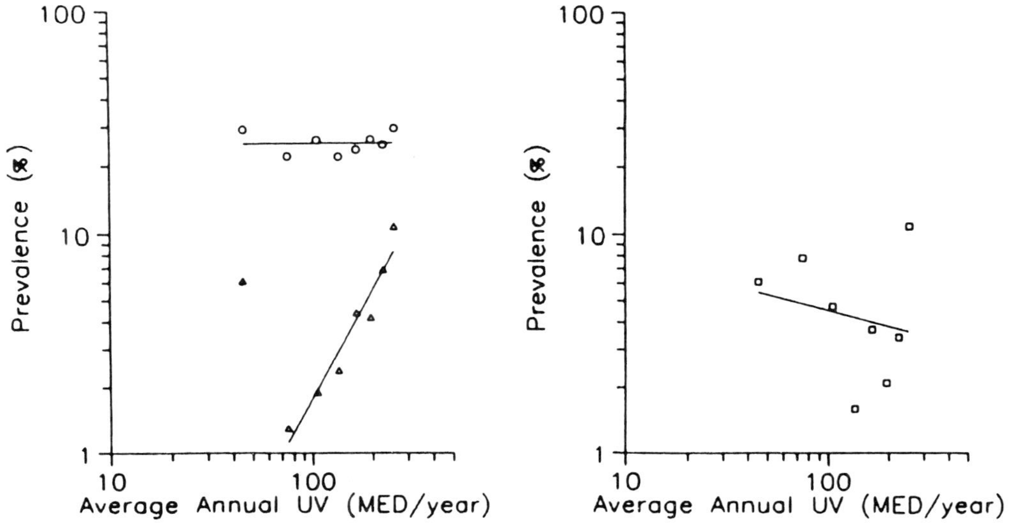

had an appreciable effect on the value of *a* for SCC. Fourth, no mention is made of having controlled in the analysis for potential negative confounding between cutaneous sun sensitivity and sun exposure. Such confounding might be expected to reduce the slope of the dose-response relationships. Finally, no measure of precision was given for the values of a; given the small numbers of subjects with SCC and BCC, those for these two cancers must have had quite wide 95% confidence intervals. This study gives only a hint, therefore, as to what the dose-response relationship between solar UVB and nonmelanocytic skin cancer might be at one end of the human exposure range. No similar observations are available for cutaneous melanoma.

$$BAF = (dI/I)/(dD/D)$$

where dI equals a small increment in the existing incidence of skin cancer, I, which results, in the steady state, from a small increment dD in the existing biologically effective ambient level, D, of solar radiation (i.e., spectral dose weighted by the action spectrum for production of skin cancer).

The best known and most commonly used geographical relationships between skin cancer incidence and ambient UV used for dose-response estimation are those established from data on nonmelanocytic skin cancer collected in a special survey in the USA in 1977 and 1978 and UV measurements collected through the US network of Robertson-Berger meters (Scotto et al., 1983). Corresponding relationships were later established between melanoma incidence measured by the US SEER cancer registries and the Robertson-Berger meter data (Scotto and Fears, 1987). The relationship for melanoma is shown in figure 8.3. In this figure, the logarithm of age-adjusted annual incidence of melanoma is plotted against the logarithm of the annual average Robertson-Berger meter counts at each location. The lowest annual average meter count was 95×10^4 units at Seattle and the highest, Albuquerque, New Mexico, at 197×10^4 units. These values translate, approximately, into 0.75×10^6 and 1.56×10^6 J m^{-2} respectively. The estimated slopes of the regression lines were 0.7 in males and 0.8 in females which are also the estimated BAFs for melanoma from these data.

Table 8.2 summarises the most recent estimates of the BAFs for nonmelanocytic skin cancer (BCC and SCC) and cutaneous melanoma from data in the USA and Scandinavia. These estimates were based on various action spectra: the response spectrum of the Robertson-Berger meter (Scotto et al., 1983; Scotto & Fears, 1987; Pitcher & Longtreth, 1991), the CIE reference spectrum of McKinlay and Diffey (1987), Moan et al.

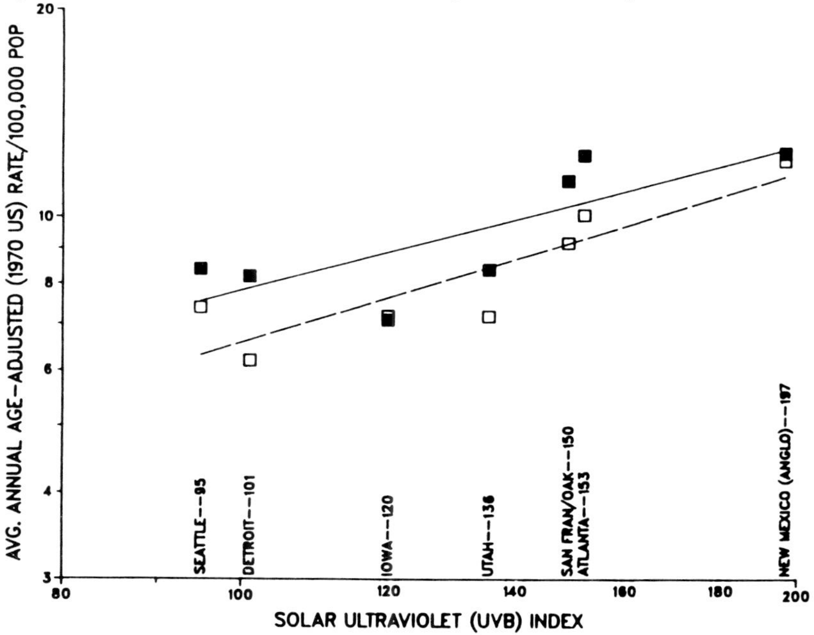

Figure 8.3 Relationship of average annual age-adjusted incidence of cutaneous melanoma in whites in seven areas of the United States in 1978-81 to average annual ambient UV as measured by Robertson-Berger meters. ■, males; □, females. (Reproduced with permission from Scotto & Fears, 1987).

(1989), Moan and Dahlbach, (1992), and the Sterenberg-Slaper action spectrum for UV radiation of skin cancer in albino hairless mice (de Gruijl and van der Leun, 1991). Generally, the BAF for BCC lay between about 1.5 and 2.0. For SCC and melanoma, there was much greater variation in estimates. Those for SCC were between about 2.0 and 4.0 when based on the US data but between 1.0 and 2.0 when based on Norwegian data. Similarly, BAFs for melanoma were between 0.3 and 0.5 when based on US data but between about 1.0 and 3.0 when based on Scandinavian data. While an attempt had been made to adjust the US estimates for confounding with population constitutional sensitivity to the sun and sun-related behaviour, even the unadjusted estimates (ranging from 0.6 to 1.0; Scotto & Fears, 1987; Pitcher & Longstreth, 1991) were considerably less than those for Scandinavia. The most likely reasons for the differences between the estimates is differences in their error.

This approach to estimation of dose-response has assumed, among other things, that: the correct action spectrum has been used to weight spectral UV irradiance when producing a single figure for ground level UV in each area; all members of the populations giving rise to the incidence rates have lived their whole lives in their present environment; the skin cancer incidence rates have been measured accurately and, in particular, that their error does not correlate with ambient UV radiance; and that possible confounding of ambient UV with constitutional sensitivity to the sun and sun-related behaviour is either unimportant or has been taken adequately into account. None of these assumptions is likely to be correct in any of the estimates of BAF made so far and the estimates are all likely, therefore, to be inaccurate (Armstrong, 1993).

It should be noted that even if dose-response relationships between UV and skin cancer incidence determined at the population level are accurate, they may not reflect dose-response relationships at the individual level. This is because of the averaging of exposure and risk that occurs at the population level. The actual population exposure of the skin at any level of ambient UV is an average of many different exposures and the actual population incidence of skin cancer is an average of many individual risks of skin cancer. The association of individual risk to individual exposure may be quite complex (as has been postulated for melanoma; Armstrong, 1988) but at the population level this could still translate into a simple exponential or power relationship between ambient exposure and incidence.

No attempts have been made to estimate the dose-response relationships for UV and cancers other than skin cancers that may be caused by UV.

Table 8.2 Recent estimates of the biological amplification factors (BAF) for nonmelanocytic skin cancer and cutaneous melanoma based on geographical correlations between average annual ambient UV and skin cancer incidence or mortality.

Authors	Region	Sex	BAFs for BCC Incidence	BAFs for SCC Incidence
Nonmelanocytic skin cancer				
Scotto et al, 1983	USA (8 centres)	M	1.3-2.6[a]	2.1-4.1
		F	1.1-2.1	2.2-4.3
de Gruijl & van der Leun 1991	USA (8 centres)	MF	1.4	2.5
Moan et al 1989	Norway (6 areas)	M	1.5-2.0[a]	1.2-1.5
		F	1.6-2.1	1.6-1.8
Melanoma				
Scotto & Fears, 1987	USA (7 areas)	M	0.4[c]	
		F	0.5[c]	
Pitcher & Longstreth, 1991	USA 215 SMAs	M		0.4[d]
		F		0.3[d]
Moan & Dahlback, 1992	Norway	M	1.9	
		F	3.2	
	Finland	M	1.3	
		F	2.2	
	Sweden	M	1.9	
		F	2.3	

a Exponential model used in which the value of the BAF varies with ambient UV, thus range of values given.

b Same data as used by Scotto et al (1983) except that a power model was used instead of an exponential model and the most recent action spectrum for UV carcinogenesis in mouse skin was assumed.

c Adjusted for population estimates of ethnic origin, pigmentary characteristics, use of sunscreens, and hours per week of outdoor exposure.

d Adjusted for population estimates of ethnic origin, household income, outdoor occupation and education.

8.5.8 *Effects of pattern of exposure*

There are a number of aspects of the epidemiology of cutaneous melanoma in European populations that appear inconsistent with a simple relationship between it and sun exposure (English & Armstrong, in press). First, in many populations, melanoma occurs as commonly in women as in men, although men are more likely to work outdoors; second, there is a relative peak in incidence in middle life, which is not the pattern to be expected from life-long exposure to an environmental agent; third, it most frequently occurs on the back in men and lower limbs in women, sites which are not maximally exposed to the sun; finally, melanoma is more common in indoor than outdoor workers and in those of higher socioeconomic status than those of lower status.

These observations led to postulation of the "intermittent exposure hypothesis" for the relationship of sunlight to melanoma. This hypothesis states that incidence of melanoma is determined as much (or more) by the pattern of sun exposure as by the total accumulated dose of sun exposure and, specifically, that infrequent or intermittent exposure of untanned skin to intense sunlight is particularly effective in increasing incidence of melanoma (Armstrong, 1988). If, as seems plausible, this postulated effect of intermittency of sun exposure is due to protective thickening and pigmentation of the epidermis with more continuous sun exposure, then intermittent exposure would be maximally effective if it occurred at intervals longer than the time it takes for the skin to return to its prior level of sensitivity after a single episode of sun exposure (two to three weeks).

The epidemiological evidence, summarised above, that risk of melanoma is apparently not increased with total or occupational exposure to the sun but is increased with increasing non-occupational exposure to the sun, in particular increasing time spent in sun-related vacations in populations with otherwise comparatively low sun exposure (Klepp & Magnus, 1979; Lew et al., 1983; Elwood et al., 1985b; Østerlind et al., 1988b; Beitner et al., 1990; Zanetti et al., 1992), and episodes of sunburn (IARC, 1992) is consistent with this hypothesis.

There are less grounds for believing that pattern of UV is important in causing nonmelanocytic skin cancer than there are for melanoma. Specifically, nonmelanocytic skin cancer as a whole, and BCC and SCC separately, are more common in men than women (Kricker et al., 1990; Parkin et al., 1992; Marks et al., 1993) and, in the largest, well-collected, population-based incidence series available, they showed steadily increasing incidence rates with age, except for a downturn in older age-groups possibly due to underascertainment (Scotto et al., 1983). On the other hand, recent series of BCC have shown unexpectedly high proportions on the trunk (Kricker et al., 1990; Magnus, 1991) and, as reviewed above, the relationship of nonmelanocytic skin cancer with occupational exposure to the sun is not at all clear. Moreover, there is some evidence of an association between sunburn and other indicators of intermittent exposure and BCC (Hunter et al., 1990; Kricker et al., 1991b).

8.5.9 *Interactions between UV and other agents*

5-methoxypsoralen and 8-methoxypsoralen (methoxsalen)

Methoxsalen, 5-methoxypsoralen and some other psoralens (hereafter referred to collectively as psoralens) are used in combination with UVA (referred to as PUVA) for the treatment of psoriasis and to produce repigmentation in vitiligo. A working group of International Agency for Research on Cancer concluded in 1987 that there was sufficient evidence that PUVA (defined as 8-methoxypsoralen plus long-wave UV radiation) causes cancer in humans, based mainly on evidence of its association with SCC.

Recent studies have confirmed and extended this conclusion. Stern & Lange (1988) reported on 5 to 10 year follow-up of patients treated with PUVA in the USA. In 13 384 person years of follow-up of 1 380 people, 100 people had developed 391 SCC and 94 had developed 218 BCC. There were statistically significantly increasing risks of both BCC and SCC occurring more than 58 months after entry into the cohort with increasing number of treatments with PUVA. Risk of BCC rose to 6.9 (95% CI 3.2-13.1) with 260 or more treatments and risk of SCC rose to 50.1 (95% CI 24.9-89.5). Therapeutic exposure to ionizing radiation, high doses of tar and UVB was unrelated to number of treatments with PUVA and, therefore, did not confound the observed dose-response relationship. Lindelöf et al. (1991) reported on follow-up for an average of 6.9 years of 4 799 Swedish patients treated with PUVA. Risk of SCC increased with increasing number of treatments with PUVA. In those who received 200 or more treatments, the relative risk, with reference to the general Swedish population, was 30.7 (14.7-56.5) in men and 18.5 (0.5-103.2) in women. BCC were not recorded in this study.

Cases of melanoma have been reported in patients treated with PUVA but the rates of melanoma in US and Swedish PUVA cohorts were little higher than those expected on the basis of population incidence rates. In the US cohort the relative risk was 1.46 (95% CI 0.3-7.3; Gupta et al.,

1988), while in the Swedish cohort it was 1.1 (0.2-3.2) in men and 0.8 (0.1-3.0) in women (Lindelöf et al., 1991).

It is not possible in any of these studies to estimate what the risk of skin cancer would have been if the patients had been treated with UV alone. It would seem reasonable to assume, however, on the basis of the evidence from experimental animals (see above) that administration of psoralens potentiated the effect of UV. In addition analysis of clinical data even suggests that this carcinogenicity of PUVA exceeds that of UVB treatment by an order of magnitude (Slaper, 1987).

Ionizing radiation

Ionizing radiation causes nonmelanocytic skin cancer, mainly BCC, generally after a long latent period (Shore, 1990; Fragu et al., 1991; Hogan et al., 1991; Sadamori et al., 1991; Møller et al., 1993). Incidence in the atomic bomb survivors was related strongly to exposure, although not for those closest to the blast (Sadamori et al., 1991). There is evidence that ionizing radiation and UV may act synergistically in causing skin cancer. In a study of skin cancer following irradiation of the scalp for ringworm, Shore et al. (1984) found a substantial excess of BCC in white subjects. In blacks, no skin cancers were observed when 13 would have been expected from the rate on the UV-shielded scalp in whites. This lack of skin cancers in irradiated blacks suggest that UV radiation contributes more than additively to the production of these cancers in irradiated whites. This inference is supported by the observation that the excess of BCC around the UV-exposed fringe of the scalp in irradiated whites was some four to five times higher per unit dose and area than that on the UV-shielded hairy scalp (Shore et al., 1984). Further, Modan et al. (1993) observed, in a separate cohort of people irradiated for ringworm of the scalp, that sunbathing increased the risk of skin cancer 2.6 times (95% CI 1.1-6.1). All except one of 39 cancers were BCCs and 60% were on the scalp, thus suggesting that the ionizing radiation had also contributed to their causation. However, no formal analysis of interaction was reported from this study.

Other agents

One or more SCCs occur in 30% to 50% of patients with epidermodysplasia verruciformis, a rare chronic skin disease in which there are multiple benign skin lesions caused by a variety of different types of human papilloma viruses (HPV; Quan & Moy, 1991). HPV DNA sequences have been identified in the SCC occurring in these patients and most of the cancers occur on sun-exposed sites. This coincidence suggests that the UV interacts with the virus in causing these cancers. Benign warts are also increased in frequency in renal transplant patients and it is possible that they, with UV, are involved in causing the excess of nonmelanocytic skin cancers that occur in these patients (Bouwes-Bavinck, 1992). These cancers, too, occur mainly on sun-exposed sites.

8.5.10 *Mechanisms of UV carcinogenesis*

Precursor lesions

Solar keratoses are very strongly related to risk of nonmelanocytic skin cancer (Kricker et al., 1991a) and it is a matter of clinical observation that SCC often occurs in lesions which, previously, had the clinical appearances of solar keratoses. There is evidence that solar keratoses are, themselves, caused by exposure to the sun. Thus solar keratoses could be the visible expression of an early, UV-caused, mutational step in the pathway to skin carcinogenesis.

Analogously with solar keratoses, benign melanocytic naevi are commonly observed in clinical or histopathological contiguity with melanomas and have been found, epidemiologically to be strongly related to risk of cutaneous melanoma (Holman & Armstrong, 1984a; Armstrong & English, 1988). Naevi may, therefore, represent an early, UV-caused, mutational step in the development of melanoma. In this regard, it is interesting to note that the most active development of naevi occurs during the first 15 years of life, thus providing a possible link to early life sun exposure as suggested by migrant data (see above). The appearance of naevi in children who have received chemotherapy for cancer may indicate that they can be caused by mutagens other then UV (Hughes et al., 1989; Baird et al., 1992; Green et al., 1992).

DNA damage

The evidence of much increased incidence rates of BCC, SCC cutaneous melanoma and tumours of the anterior eye in patients with xeroderma pigmentosum (XP) (see above) strongly suggests that unrepaired, UV-induced photoproducts in DNA form part of the genesis of these cancers. Almost all forms of XP have an inherited deficiency in excision repair of DNA photoproducts (Kraemer et al., 1987). The position is made somewhat less clear, however, by the existence of two other inherited syndromes involving deficiency in DNA excision repair, trichothiodystrophy and Cockaynes syndrome, that are not associated with increased incidence rates of skin cancer (Bridges, 1990; Barrett et al., 1991).

There is evidence also that low levels of DNA repair may be associated with skin cancer in the general population, although there is some disagreement in the results so far obtained . Munch-Petersen et al. (1985) studied 29 patients with multiple skin neoplasms, 19 with multiple BCC only and 10 with both BCC and squamous lesions (SCC, solar keratosis, or Bowen's disease), and 25 control subjects with roughly the same age and sex distributions. Patients with both BCC and squamous lesions had much higher UV-induced DNA synthesis in lymphocytes, as measured by incorporation of [3H]thymidine following irradiation with a Philips, TUV, 6 watt lamp (peak emission at 254 nm), than did controls. Patients with multiple BCC were not different from controls. The authors attributed this difference to possible defects in the DNA ligation process. Roth et al. (1987) studied the rate of loss of dithymidine dimers in DNA of cultured fibroblasts that had been irradiated with a Philips 6-V germicidal lamp with peak emission at 254 nm. Dimers were measured with a monoclonal antibody highly specific for the conformational change in DNA caused by the dimers. No significant difference was seen between 16 BCC cases and 30 controls in the rate of loss of dimers. In ten melanoma patients, however, the mean percentage of bound antibody at 60 minutes was 50.5 (SD 18.2) compared with 29.8 (SD 5.7) in controls ($p=0.001$) thus suggesting that average dimer repair capacity was less in the melanoma patients than the controls. Alcalay et al. (1990) compared 22 patients with a history of one (13 patients) or more BCC in the past with 19 healthy volunteers. Each subject was irradiated at two locations on the lower back with 1 MED of UV from a 150 W xenon arc solar UV simulator from which wavelengths < 295 nm had been removed by a 1 mm WG 320 filter. Shave biopsies of skin were taken from one of the sites immediately and the other 6 hours after irradiation and the concentrations of pyrimidine dimers in DNA measured by the micrococcus luteus endonuclease assay. Dimer yields immediately after irradiation were similar in BCC patients and controls but, after 6 hours, the proportion of dimers that had been repaired was 22% in the BCC patients compared with 33% in the controls ($p=0.06$). Wei et al. (1993) measured DNA repair capacity in 88 patients with a history of one or more histologically confirmed BCCs and 135 control subjects. Repair capacity was measured by assaying the capacity of lymphocytes to repair UV-induced damage in DNA of a nonreplicating recombinant plasmid. Damage was induced by irradiating the plasmid with either 3500 J m^{-2} or 7000 J m^{-2} of UV at 254 nm. The BCC cases had a significantly lower mean DNA repair capacity ($p=0.047$) than controls only when 29 controls with a family history of BCC or who themselves had an actinic keratosis were removed from the comparison.

It now seems highly likely that UV can mutate the p53 tumour suppressor gene in human skin and that UV-induced mutations in this gene may be involved in the aetiology of some human cancers. First, a recent study has shown that mutations that are strongly suggestive of a UV effect, CC-TT changes at dipyrimidine sites, could be found in 17 of 23 (74%) samples of sun-exposed normal skin in Australian skin cancer patients compared with 1 of 20 (5%) samples of skin from sites not exposed to the sun (Nakazawa et al., in press). Focal overexpression of p53 protein has also been observed in normal, sun exposed skin adjacent to BCC in 37 of 39 subjects but only in one keratinocyte in 14 samples of buttock skin from the same subjects (Shea et al., 1992). Second, several studies have found mutations at dipyrimidine sites in the p53 gene in 36% to 56% of BCC (Rady et al., 1992; Molès et al., 1993; Ziegler et al., 1993). In three similar studies of SCC one found these mutations in 14 (57%) of 24 cases (Brash et al., 1991) one in two of 10 cases (Pierceall et al., 1991) and, the other, none of 13 (Molès et al., 1993). The more detailed findings of these five studies are summarised in table 8.3. Mutations were found in the p53 gene, following examinations of varying extent, in 46% of BCC and SCC, the majority of which (88%) were base substitutions or one or two base deletions at dipyrimidine sites (the proportion expected by chance is 75%). The highest proportions of these mutations resulted from C $\rightarrow$ T, CC$\rightarrow$ TT and C $\rightarrow$ A base changes which is consistent with what would be expected if they had been caused by UV (Brash et al., 1991). Several studies have found p53 protein by immunostaining (evidence of overexpression of possibly abnormal p53 protein) in from 42% to 83% of BCC and 56% to 65% of SCC (Barbareschi et al., 1992; Shea et al., 1992; Stephenson et al., 1992, Ro et al., 1993) and are thus reasonably consistent with the observations as to prevalence of mutations.

The position with respect to p53 mutation is much less clear for other cancers possibly caused by UV. A number of studies have reported on the prevalence of detectable p53 protein in primary melanomas: the proportions have varied from 3.6% to 97% (see, for example, Stretch et al., 1991; Akslen & Mϕrkve, 1992; Lassam et al., 1993; Ro et al., 1993). There has been only one report of a p53 mutation in melanoma, a C $\rightarrow$ T transition in codon 248 of the gene in the melanoma cell line SK-MEL-13 (Volkenandt et al., 1991). The comparative lack of evidence of expression of p53 protein in melanocytic naevi (Yu et al., 1992; Lassam et al., 1993) would suggest that if p53 gene mutation is important in the genesis of melanoma it is not the earliest mutation. The protein product of p53 was detected in 12 of 18 (67%) choroidal melanomas (Tobal et al., 1992) but none of 7 choroidal naevi. The DNA of exons 5, 7 and 8 of the p53 was sequenced from two of the strongly positive choroidal melanomas: a mutation was found in each, one G $\rightarrow$ T and one C $\rightarrow$ G.

Mutations in the ras oncogenes appear to be less frequent than in the p53 gene in nonmelanocytic skin cancers. Mutations were sought in one or more codons of Ha-ras, Ki-ras and N-ras in 77 BCC and found in five (6%) (van der Schroeff et al., 1990; Lieu et al., 1991; Campbell et al., 1993). There were two mutations, one in a dipyrimidine site, in codon 61 of Ha-ras and three mutations at dipyrimidine sites in codon 12 of Ki-ras; two mutations were C $\rightarrow$ A, one was C $\rightarrow$ T and one was A $\rightarrow$ T. These mutations were also sought in 79 SCC and found in 7 (9%) (van der Schroeff et al., 1990; Corominas et al., 1991; Lieu et al., 1991; Campbell et al., 1993). There were three mutations in dipyrimidine sites in codon 12 of Ha-ras, three, but none in dipyrimidine sites, in codon 61 of Ha-ras and one at a dipyrimidine site in codon 12 of Ki-ras; three mutations were C $\rightarrow$ A, one was C $\rightarrow$ T and three were T $\rightarrow$ A. Overall, 8 of 12 (67%) mutations were at dipyrimidine sites. There is nothing about the pattern of base changes that would favour UV as the cause of the mutations. The comparative rarity of ras gene mutations in nonmelanocytic skin cancers is supported by a study of 26 such tumours in Japanese patients with xeroderma pigmentosum (Ishizaki et al., 1992). Only one mutation was found, an A $\rightarrow$ T change in codon 61 of Ki-ras.

Mutations in ras oncogenes have been demonstrated in some human cutaneous melanomas. In three series totalling 59 primary melanomas (van't Veer et al., 1989; Shukla et al., 1989; Albino et al., 1991), ras gene mutations were found in 11 (19%). The mutations occurred in codon 61 of N-ras (6), codon 13 of N-ras (4), codon 12 of Ki-ras (3) and codon 12 of Ha-ras (1) (two mutations were found in each of 3 melanomas). Ten of the 13 mutations (77%) were at dipyrimidine sites and nine were C $\rightarrow$ A, three C $\rightarrow$ T, one T $\rightarrow$ C and one T to A or G (IARC, 1992). The pattern of base changes is not such as to suggest that UV was responsible for the mutations. Mutations were sought but not found in codons 12, 13 and 61 of Ha-ras, Ki-ras and N-ras in up to 68 uveal melanomas (Mooy et al., 1991; Soparker et al., 1993).

Oxidative processes

Oxidative effects are an important consequence of exposure to UV, especially UVA (see Chapter 6) and if they are involved in mediating its carcinogenic effects in humans it might be expected that anti-oxidant vitamins would reduce the risk of UV-related cancers. There is some evidence of such effects, mainly for cutaneous melanoma. Risk of melanoma was slightly but not significantly reduced by high intakes of vitamin E and carotene and high plasma concentrations of -carotene and -tocopherol in a case-control study in the USA (Stryker et al., 1990). More persuasively, a nested case-control study in a cohort study in Finland

Table 8.3 Summary of results of detection of mutations in the p53 gene of BCC and SCC (Brash et al, 1991; Pierceall et al 1991; Rady et al., 1992; Molès et al., 1993; Ziegler et al., 1993).

Mutations Detected	BCC	SCC
	(60)[a]	(46)
Any mutation	52%	39%
Base substitutions or 1 or 2 base deletions at a dipyrimidine site	45%	35%
Types of base substitutions or 1 or 2 base deletions at dipyrimidine sites [b]	52%[c]	38%
C → T	13%	19%
CC → TT	13%	31%
C → A	10%	6%
C → G	3%	0%
T → C	3%	0%
T → A	3%	0%
G → C	0%	6%
C deleted	3%	0%
CC deleted		

a Total numbers of cancers examined.

b In consistency with the format adopted by Brash et al (1991) and Ziegler et al (1993), four base substitutions reported as G → A (Pierceall et al, 1991; Rady et al, 1992) were represented as C → T and two reported as G → T (Pierceall et al, 1991; Molès et al, 1992) were represented as C → A.

c Proportions of all point mutations at dipyrimidine sites.

showed significantly lower serum concentrations of -carotene and -tocopherol in 10 cases of melanoma and 18 controls (Knekt et al., 1991). Melanoma was the only cancer in this study to be associated with low levels of anti-oxidant vitamins. A similar result was obtained for -tocopherol in a case-control study of melanoma carried out in Moscow (crude relative risk for highest tertile of -tocopherol was 0.08, 95% CI 0.01-0.38; Zaridze et al., 1992); risk was not reduced by high serum concentrations of -carotene. As to nonmelanocytic skin cancer, in a hospital-based case-control study covering 53 cases of BCC and 35 of SCC, high intakes of vegetables were protective and cases had a significantly lower mean level of -carotene than did controls (Kune et al., 1992). It should be noted, however, that cases were on average, five years older than controls. No evidence was found for a protective effect of dietary carotenoids with vitamin A activity, vitamin C or vitamin E in a study of diet and BCC in a cohort of US nurses (Hunter et al., 1992).

Immune-suppression

UV has been shown to suppress immune functions in humans (see Chapter 9). In addition there are a number of lines of evidence that link immune suppression from other sources with skin cancer in humans.

As early as 1980 it was clear that renal transplant patients, who receive long-term immunosuppressive therapy, had an increased incidence of nonmelanocytic skin cancer (Kinlen et al., 1979; Hardie et al., 1980). Among 290 transplant patients in Queensland, Australia, it was estimated that the incidence of nonmelanocytic skin cancer was 21 times that in the general population Hardie et al., 1980); the ratio of BCC to SCC was reversed from 4:1 in the general population to 1:1.7 in the transplant patients suggesting that the incidence of SCC was particularly increased in them. Similar results were obtained in Canadian and Dutch series of transplant patients (Gupta et al., 1986; Hartevelt et al., 1990) In the Dutch study it was estimated that the incidence of SCC was 250 times higher than that in the general population and that of BCC 10 times higher.

There is evidence to suggest that the nonmelanocytic skin cancers occurring in renal transplant patients are caused by sun exposure. First their site distribution is similar to that of all nonmelanocytic skin cancers and strongly favours sun exposed sites (Hartevelt et al., 1990). Second, all 5 nonmelanocytic skin cancers found by Boyle et al. (1984) in 94 transplant patients occurred in the 17 patients judged to have high sun exposure. In a more thorough study based on 137 Dutch transplant patients, 20 of whom had SCC, 7 BCC and 9 both types of cancer, Bouwes-Bavinck (1992) found a relative risk for 20 000 or more cumulated hours of sun exposure compared with 10 000 or less of 97.5 (95% CI 6.6-1444) for SCC and 49.3 (2.8-878) for BCC thus suggesting that sun exposure had a strong effect on development of the transplant related skin cancers.

The incidence of cutaneous melanoma has also been observed to be increased in patients with renal transplants (relative risk 3.9, 95% CI 1.4-8.5; Hoover, 1977; Greene et al., 1981). All 14 renal transplant patients with melanoma reported by Greene et al. (1981) had fair complexions, light-coloured hair, light-coloured eyes and a tendency to freckle thus suggesting that there may have been an interaction between sun exposure and immune suppression in causing their melanomas. The rapid appearance of new melanocytic naevi has been reported in two renal transplant patients (Barker & MacDonald, 1988; McGregor et al., 1991). Melanoma incidence is also increased in patients with lymphohaematopoetic neoplasms which are associated with immune suppression (Greene & Wilson, 1985; Tucker et al., 1985b; Travis et al., 1991, 1992) and has been reported to be increased in patients with human immunodeficiency virus infection (McGregor et al., 1992; Reynolds et al., 1993). Rapid appearance of melanocytic naevi has also been reported in HIV infection (Duvic et al., 1989).

8.6 Conclusions

UV exposure of the skin has both beneficial and harmful effects. The beneficial effects include photochemical production of vitamin D and widely believed but poorly documented effects on general well-being. The harmful effects include sunburn, phototoxicity, photoallergy, benign abnormalities of melanocytes (freckles, melanocytic naevi and solar or senile lentigines) a range of other chronic abnormalities resulting from UV injury to keratinocytes, blood vessels and fibrous tissue, often described together as "photoageing", skin cancer (melanoma and non-melanocytic cancer) and possibly cancer of the lip.

The indirect epidemiological evidence that sun exposure causes cutaneous melanoma and non-melanocytic cancer is strong. Their incidence is less in darker-skinned ethnic groups than in those with lighter skins residing in the same geographic area and, within populations that are reasonably homogeneous ethnically, risk of skin cancer increases with decreasing pigmentation of the skin and reduced ability to produce a protective tan. Albinos, who lack cutaneous pigmentation, appear to have an increased risk of non-melanocytic skin cancer but not melanoma. The anatomic site distibution of SCC favours the head and neck and upper limbs, sites that are more or less continuously exposed to the sun when outdoors. This concentration is less pronounced for BCC and melanoma, but both are rare on sites that are rarely exposed to the sun.

Within countries covering an appreciable span of latitude, an inverse relationship within latitude and incidence of both non-melanocytic skin cancer and cutaneous melanoma has generally been observed. The incidence of both cancers is substantially lower in migrants from the United Kingdom (an area of low solar irradiance) to Australia (an area of high solar irradiance) than it is in persons of similar ethnic origin born in Australia. This difference is not observed for BCC and melanoma in those who migrate to Australia within the first ten years of life; this observation may suggest that sun exposure in childhood is particularly important in determining subsequent risk of skin cancer. Similar observations have been made for melanoma in migrants to other countries with high solar irradiance. Risk of melanoma has been shown to increase with increasing lifetime average ambient solar irradiance at an individual's places of residence.

The direct epidemiological evidence linking sun exposure and skin cancer is weaker. Estimated total sun exposure of individuals has not been consistently associated with risk of either non-melanocytic skin cancer or melanoma. Indicators of benign sun damage to the skin, however, are positively associated with risk of both types of skin cancer. Occupational sun exposure has been found to be weakly associated with non-melanocytic skin cancer in a few studies but not consistently associated, either positively or negatively, with melanoma. Non-occupational or recreational sun exposure is consistently and quite strongly associated with risk of melanoma whereas there are insufficient data to draw a conclusion regarding non-occuptional exposure and non-melanocytic skin cancer. The same is substantially true of history of sunburn although a few observations suggest that it is associated with non-melanocytic skin cancer.

Together, the indirect and direct evidence is sufficient to conclude that sun exposure causes both melanoma and non-melanocytic skin cancer.

Use of sunlamps or sunbeds has not been consistently associated with risk of non-melanocytic skin cancer in several rather poorly conducted studies. There is stronger evidence that it may be associated with risk of melanoma in a number of better studies but possible confounding of use of sunlamps and sunbeds with sun exposure has not been consistently controlled.

Cancer of the lip is much more common in white than black populations and is less frequent in migrants from areas of low ambient solar irradiance to Australia and Israel than in those born in these countries. It is associated with outdoor work but possible confounding with tobacco and alcohol use has not been adequately controlled in any study.

There are no data in humans from which the action spectrum for production of either non-melanocytic skin cancer or cutaneous melanoma can be inferred directly.

Problems in the quantitative measurement of the sun exposure of individuals have prevented the determination, in humans, of the relationship between individual dose of UV and risk of any form of skin cancer. The observed geographical relationship between ambient UV irradiance and incidence of skin cancers has been used to estimate the quantitative relationship between ambient UV irradiance and population risk of these cancers. Exponential or power relationships have generally given an adequate fit to the data, but provide rather variable estimates of the proportional increase in incidence of skin cancer per unit proportional increase in biologically effective UV irradiance. The accuracy of these estimates is uncertain, particularly because of difficulties in the accurate measurement of skin cancer incidence and difficulties in control of likely confounding with cutaneous sensitivity to the sun and sun-related behaviour.

A number of features of the epidemiology of melanoma suggest that infrequent or intermittent exposure of skin that is unadapted to sun exposure may be particularly important in its causation. This hypothesis is supported by the relatively strong evidence relating non-occupational (recreational) sun exposure and sunburn to melanoma. There is little evidence that pattern of sun exposure is important in the aetiology of non-melanocytic skin cancer but few directly relevant observations exist.

The much increased rates of all skin cancers in patients with xeroderma pigmentosum, who are deficient in the capacity to repair UV-induced DNA damage, suggest that direct UV damage of DNA may be a step in the causation of these cancers. This suggestion has been supported by observation of UV specific mutations of the p53 tumour suppressor gene in a proportion of patients with non-melanocytic skin cancer. No such evidence is available for melanoma. Oxidative and immune suppressant effects may also contribute to the capacity of UV to cause skin cancers.

9. HUMAN STUDIES: IMMUNE FUNCTION

9.1 Immune Function Assays

Several investigators have examined the effect of UV on contact hypersensitivity (CHS) responses to dinitrochlorobenzene (DNCB) or other contact sensitizers in humans (Hersey et al., 1983a, 1983b; O'Dell et al., 1980; Kalimo et al., 1983; Halprin et al., 1981; Friedmann et al., 1989; Sjovall et al., 1985; Yoshikawa et al., 1990; Vermeer et al., 1991; Cooper et al., 1992). Some of these studies are inconclusive because they used patients with skin diseases or recent UV-exposure, had insufficient subjects for statistical analyses, or used subjective assessments of CHS. Hence only 3 of these studies are discussed here.

Yoshikawa et al. (1990) exposed human buttock skin to 4 daily UV doses of 1440 J m^{-2} using a high pressure mercury vapour lamp (290-320 nm).Immediately after the last exposure, the irradiated site was sensitized with 2000 μg DNCB. The inner surface of the forearm was challenged 30 days later with 50 μg DNCB and CHS was assessed. In this study 40-45% of healthy irradiated adults failed to develop CHS. They designated these subjects UVB-S and suggested that, as in mice, susceptibility to UV is genetically controlled. Among biopsy proven skin cancer patients a much higher percentage (92%) of UV-exposed individuals failed to developed CHS. The UVB-S phenotype appeared to be a risk factor for the development of skin cancer. Suppression of CHS was also demonstrated in 50% of black-skinned individuals indicating that melanin does not protect against the deleterious effects of UVB on the development of CHS (Vermeer et al., 1991). Attempts to resensitize healthy UVB-S individuals through normal skin following primary sensitization to DNCB through irradiated skin were generally successful; however, 50% of skin cancer patients failed to respond to resensitization attempts suggesting that these patients developed immunological tolerance similar to that demonstrated in experimental animal models (Yoshikawa et al., 1990; Vermeer et al., 1991).

Cooper et al. (1992) exposed human buttock skin (using FS lamps) to 0.75 or 2 MEDs of UVB (1 MED = 291 J m^{-2} to 325 J m^{-2} depending on the individual) for 4 days and sensitized with 30 μg DNCB through irradiated skin immediately after the last exposure. Subjects were challenged 3 weeks later with 4 serial 2-fold dilutions of DNCB, the highest of which was 12.5 μg. In addition, some subjects were exposed to 4 MED (moderate sunburn) and sensitized 3 days later with DNCB. Analysis of overall individual responses revealed decreased frequencies of fully successful immunizations in all UVB exposed groups. Increasing doses of UVB resulted in a linear decrease in immunological responsiveness to DNCB. Only 5% of individuals exposed to 2 MED had strong positive responses as opposed to 73% of unexposed individuals. The rate of immunologic tolerance to DNCB (lasting up to 4 months) in the groups that were initially sensitized on skin receiving erythemagenic doses of UVB was 31% compared to 7% in controls. Similar results were observed with UVA (320-340 nm) exposure (Cooper, 1993). The differences in the Cooper and Yoshikawa studies may have to do with different sensitization and challenge regimens, and differences in methods used to quantitate the CHS response. Also, Cooper controlled for diminished levels of CHS that occur in menstruating women except during midcycle (Oberhelman et al., 1992) by sensitizing all female subjects 14 days after the onset of menses.

Despite differences in the 2 studies it appears that unresponsiveness following the application of a contact sensitizer on UV-exposed skin can be induced in some parts of humans following exposure to moderate levels of UV and that some individuals become immunologically tolerant to the sensitizer in a manner reminiscent of animal studies. Cooper et al. (1992) also demonstrated modulation (although not clear-cut suppression) of contact sensitivity to diphenylcyclopropenone (DPCP) in subjects exposed to 4 MED and sensitized 3 days later through unirradiated skin. A similar effect was not observed with the 2 MED exposure regimen, either because the dose was lower or the sensitization was immediately following the last exposure. Hence the systemic effects observed in mice may also occur in humans, although currently the experimental data to support such effects are minimal.

As in the mouse, UV treatment of human skin resulted in altered antigen presentation. UV caused depletion of Langerhans ($CD1a^{+}DR^{+}$) cells followed by an influx of $CD1a^{-}DR+$ macrophages that preferentially activate CD4+ cells (suppressor-inducer) which, in turn, induce maturation of CD-8+ suppressor T lymphocytes and deregulate lymphocyte activation (Baadsgaard et al., 1990; Cooper et al., 1986). Rasanen et al. (1989) reported a 70-80% suppression in the ability of epidermal cells exposed to 2000 J m^{-2} UVB in vivo to present PPD or HSV to lymphocytes in vitro. In these studies recovery was observed 3 and 7 days post exposure. The UV wavelengths responsible for induction of CD1a-DR+ cells were found to lie predominantly within the UVB band and to a lesser extent in the UVC band; UVA was a poor inducer of these non-Langerhans cell antigen presenting cells (Baadsgaard et al., 1987,1989). Hersey et al. (1983b) reported an increase in CD8+ T cells and a decrease in CD4+ T cells in subjects exposed for 1 hour/day for 12 days to natural sunlight and a suppressor T cell activity which lasted in many subjects for up to 2 weeks.

Filtration of solarium radiation through mylar prevented these changes suggesting effects were due to UVB (Hersey et al., 1988). Hence in humans as in mice, UVB appears to act by altering antigen presentation in ways that favours suppressor cells.

Robinson & Rademaker (1992) studied 61 patients with two or more BCC for occurrence of a further BCC. Patients were counselled to avoid sun exposure, however there was a clear distinction between those who reduced their sun exposure and those who did not. The numbers of new BCC occurring after 36 months was determined by regular examination of all patients. Plasma lymphocyte subpopulations were measured at 0, 6, 12 and 18 months. At 36 months an index of sun exposure was developed from questions on sun-related behaviour before and after entry to the study. All 35 patients with high sun exposure had low T helper to T suppressor cell (CD4/CD8) ratios. The mean number of BCCs occurring during follow-up was 5.5 in those with high sun exposure and low CD4/CD8 ratios, 2.2 in those with low sun exposure and low CD4/CD8 ratios and 1.1 in those with low sun exposure and high CD4/CD8 ratios. The difference between the first and the third groups was statistically significant. While there is total confounding between high sun exposure and low CD4/CD8 ratios in this study it is consistent with the possibility that the effect of sun exposure on risk of recurrent BCC was mediated by way of its effect on cell-mediated immunity.

UV from solaria suppressed natural killer(NK) cell activity in the blood of subjects exposed for 1 hr/day for 12 days and tested 1 and 7 days after exposure. NK activity returned to normal 21 days post exposure. Filtration of UV through mylar did not affect this response; hence effects on NK activity were attributed to UVA (Hersey et al., 1983a; Hersey et al., 1988).

9.2 Susceptibility to Tumours, Infectious and Autoimmune Diseases

As previously indicated Yoshikawa et al. (1990) found that suppression of contact sensitivity following UV exposure was more common among skin cancer patients than in healthy subjects. In their study only skin cancer patients developed an immunological tolerance. They suggested that individuals who were phenotypically sensitive to the immunosuppressive effects of UV were at greater risk of skin cancer.

Adverse effects of UV on 4 types of human infections have been reported. Smallpox lesions were made larger by exposure to sunlight (Finsen 1901). Lesions from Herpes Simplex Virus(HSV) types I and II were reactivated by exposure to UV (Spruance, 1985; Klein, 1986). Using the criteria established by Yoshikawa et al. (1990) for the UVB-S phenotype, Taylor et al. (1993) reported that 66% of individuals who had a strong history of HSV lip lesions provoked by sun exposure were UVB-S as compared to 40-45% in the general population and 92% in skin cancer patients (Yoshikawa et al., 1990). Also, exposure of immunosuppressed patients to sunlight led to an increased incidence of viral warts caused by papilloma virus, presumably due to UVB exposure (Boyle et al., 1984; Dyall-Smith & Varigos, 1985). Hence there is some indication that UV may exacerbate certain infections in humans.

Recent attention has been paid to the effects of UV on immune response in patients with human immune deficiency virus (HIV) because UV has been shown to activate HIV in vitro (reviewed by Zmudzka & Beer, 1990). It has been suggested that UV exposure could progress these patients to full blown AIDS by interfering with protective immunity, since Th1 responses appear to be protective against AIDS whereas Th2 responses are not (Shearer & Clerici, 1992). However, Warfel et al. (1993) found no difference in CD4+ cell counts in HIV patients before and after treatment with 50-60% of their MED for dermatological disease. More research in this area is needed to resolve these issues.

Finally, it has been known for some time that UV exposure adversely affects the clinical course of systemic lupus erythematosus, an autoimmune disease (Epstein et al., 1965); however, the relationship of UV in this immune response is unclear.

9.3 Conclusions

The above studies suggest that UV exposures at environmental levels suppress immune responses in both rodents and man. In rodents this immune suppression results in enhanced susceptibility to certain infections with skin involvement as well as some systemic infections. The mechanisms associated with UV-induced immunosuppression in rodents and man are similar. Also, host defense mechanisms which provide protection against infectious agents are similar in rodents and man as shown in figure 9.1. It is therefore reasonable to assume that exposure to UV may enhance the risk of infection and decrease the effectiveness of vaccines in humans.

Additional research is needed to substantiate these assumptions. In particular, experimental studies are needed in rodents and man to access effects on immune function parameters in a fashion that allows quantitative comparisons between the two species. Results of experiments on rodents showing the effects of UV exposure on the susceptibility to various infections could be used to extrapolate the risk of infectious disease in humans. Ultimately epidemiological studies on the effects of UV exposure on susceptibility to infection and vaccine effectiveness are needed to validate this hypothesis.

Figure 9.1 Parallelogram model of relationship between suppression of immune function and susceptibility to infection in humans and laboratory rodents following UVB exposure. ● data obtained experimentally show that UVB suppresses contact and delayed type hypersensitivity (CHS & DTH) in both humans, mice and rats, and enhances infectious diseases in mice and rats. O data which are not available because challenging humans experimentally with infectious agents in usually not possible; hence this point must be extrapolated from the other 3 points.

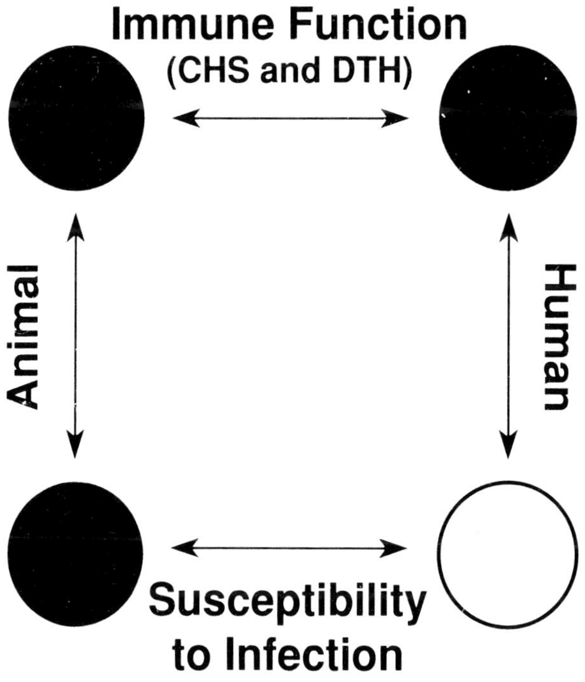

10. HUMAN STUDIES: THE EYE

10.1 Introduction

Since the early part of this century ophthalmologists have suggested an association between sunlight exposure and UV and the development of cataracts and other ocular effects (Widmark 1889, 1901; Hess 1907; Martin 1912; Birch-Hirschfeld, 1914; Verhoeff and Bell, 1916; Duke-Elder, 1926b); however, only in the past twenty years have epidemiological studies provided a scientific link. UV is probably one of a number of factors associated with the development of cataract. Despite the number of animal and human studies, many questions remain as to the validity of interpretations of past data and the biological and physical factors that influence the outcome of UV exposure of the eye.

10.2 The Eye

The eyeball is deeply set in a bony orbital cavity, and the upper bony ridge provides not only protection from mechanical injury but also serves as a shield from overhead sky light. The upper and lower eyelids (figure 10.1) also provide considerable protection by serving as "*shutters*" against bright light. The eyeball consists of three layers of tissue: (a) an outer protective layer, the sclera and cornea; (b) a middle layer of blood vessels, pigment cells and muscle fibres called the uvea; and (c) an inner, light sensitive layer called the retina.

The sclera, the outer posterior layer, is a tough, thick, opaque tissue formed of collagen fibres. The cornea, the anterior transparent part of the eyeball, consists of multiple layers. The surface epithelium continues with the surface epithelium of the conjunctiva. The epithelial cells are known to be constantly changing and the basal layer overlies the Bowman layer. The outermost epithelial cells undergo rapid turnover, having a lifetime at the surface of approximately 48 hours.

The main bulk of the cornea, the stroma, consists of highly organized collagen fibres in a pattern that makes the cornea transparent. The innermost layer, the endothelium, is a single layer of an active ion pump (Na-K) that maintains the hydration state of the stroma, an important factor for corneal transparency.

The middle layer of the eyeball consists of the iris anteriorly, the ciliary body, and the choroid. The iris is a diaphragm that adapts by

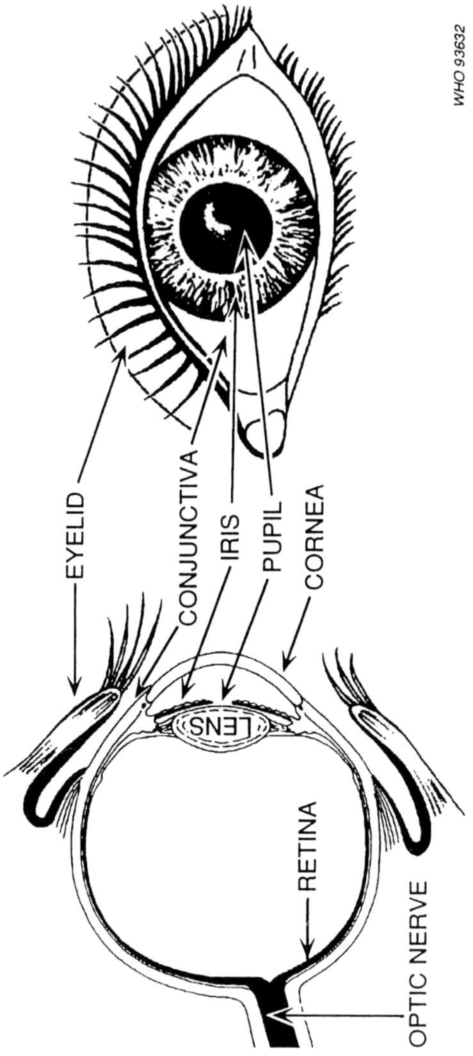

Figure 10.1 Schematic of the human eye

changing the pupillary size according to ambient light level. The iris is formed of mainly pigmented cells of various densities, blood vessels and smooth muscle fibres that are attached to the anterior part of the ciliary body. The smooth muscle fibres form the sphincter and dilator of the pupil.

As part of the middle layer lining the sclera, the choroid consists of a meshwork of blood vessels, nerves and pigment cells that contribute to the nutrition of the retina and support the function of the innermost layer, the retina, that contains the photoreceptors and the neuronal network.

The lens, embryologically of ectodermal (skin) in origin, consists of closely and orderly packed transparent elongated lens cells that are enclosed in a capsule. New lens cells are constantly formed at the so-called lens equator and old ones are displaced towards the centre of the lens. The lens is suspended to the ciliary body by fine ligaments. The lens shape can be changed by contraction or relaxation of the ciliary muscles. This change provides a focusing power to the eye that is called accommodation and is made possible by the elasticity of the young lens. The lens is avascular and obtains its nutrient from the aqueous fluid in front of it and the vitreous body that fills the posterior cavity behind it. Notably, the lens proteins cannot be renewed and therefore accumulate lesions inflicted on them throughout life.

The photoreceptors, the rods and cones of the retina, constitute the primary light receptor with rods functioning at low light levels (scotopic vision) and cones operating at high light levels (photopic vision). Thus the rod system subserves the function of retinal sensitivity, whereas cones provide colour vision, high resolution visual acuity and motion perception. The retinal pigment epithelium is essential for the maintenance of photoreceptor metabolism including, the transport, storage and regeneration of the visual pigments.

Visible light (400-760 nm) incident upon the eye is strongly refracted at the cornea, then transmitted through the aqueous humour in the anterior chamber to the lens where it is refracted further. After transmission through the vitreous gel-like structure, it finally reaches the light-sensitive receptors in the retina. It is these structures that are primarily damaged by UV and visible radiations. The neuronal layers perform the complex task of information processing. The primary visual signal is transformed and ultimately transmitted to the visual cortex in the brain, thus providing the image seen by the eye.

Most of the UV incident on the eye is absorbed in the tear film, the cornea and the lens. The lens and the tissues in the anterior part of the eye may however, be exposed to UV at wavelengths above 295 nm and the retina is exposed to a fraction of the incident UVA. Absorption of UV in the ocular media is given in Fig 10.2 (Sliney & Wolbarsht, 1980). Boettner & Wolter (1962) measured the transmission of direct forward scattering UV in the cornea, aqueous humour, lens and vitreous humour from freshly enucleated normal human eyes. The cornea absorbed all UV with wavelengths <300 nm, while above 300 nm some UV was transmitted through the cornea. About 60% of UV at 320 nm and 80% at 380 nm was transmitted through the cornea. The aqueous humour transmitted most incident UV (90% transmission at 400 nm) with no evidence of scattering.

Recently Barker and Brainard (1993) quantified the change in UV transmittance of the human lens with age. All of these studies clearly show the steady decrease in UV transmittance of the lens age. At birth there is a small window of transmission to the retina at 320 nm. This window almost disappears by the second decade due to an age-related yellowing of the human lens. As shown in Fig 10.3 the lens absorption is strongest in the 340-380 nm band with somewhat less absorption in the 310-320 nm range (Rosen, 1986; Barker and Brainard 1993). The human lens is unique in that it contains a UVA absorbing filter (O-beta of 3-hydroxykynurenine) which protects the retina.

10.3 Study Design

This chapter reviews the epidemiological evidence for a causal association between exposure to UV and development of specific eye diseases which have at some point been linked with exposure to UV. Two distinctive types of UV exposure assessments have been used in the epidemiological studies. Some studies have related the occurrence of eye disease to non-personal factors associated with place of residence, such as meteorological data on average annual UV dose or average annual hours of sunlight. Other studies have obtained estimates of exposure at the individual level (e.g. hours of sunshine exposure, lifetime exposure to UV) and related these to disease occurrence.

Three types of epidemiological studies have been used to investigate an association with UV exposure: geographical correlation studies, cross-sectional studies, and case-control studies. In the geographical correlation studies the prevalence of eye disease in different areas has been related to non-personal factors associated with place of residence. These studies are useful for generating hypotheses but of limited value in testing a particular hypothesis because observed correlations may result from confounding by

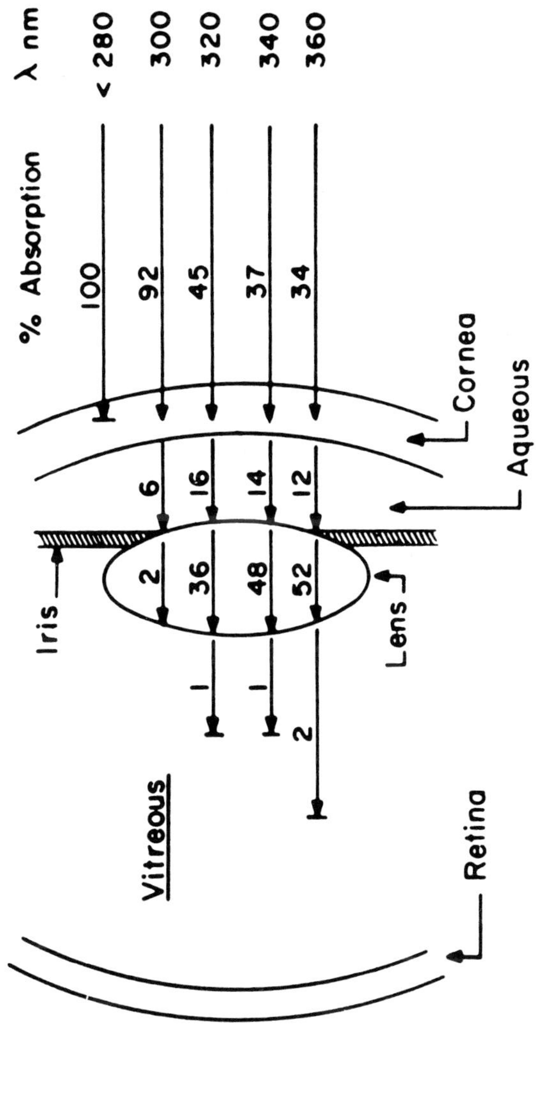

Figure 10.2 Schematic of absorption of UV in the ocular media. Values represent the percent of UV incident upon the corneal surface that are absorbed by various layers. From Sliney & Wolbarsht (1980), based on data from Boettner & Wolter (1962)

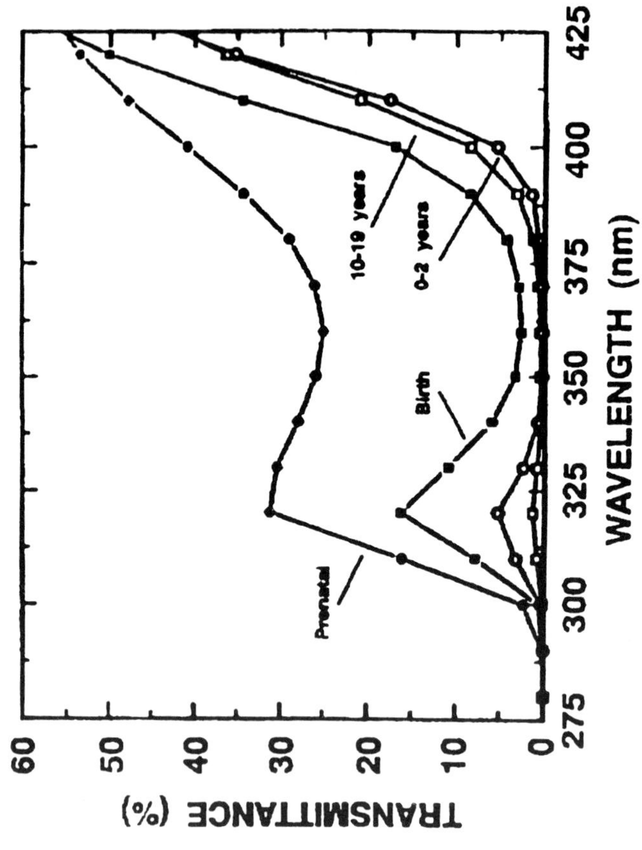

Figure 10.3 Spectral transmission of the human lens as a function of age (adapted from Barker & Brainard, 1993)

other factors which also vary geographically, and because the level of exposure for persons with the disease is not known.

The second, and most common type of study design, has been the cross-sectional study in which a population or occupational group is surveyed and disease prevalence measured. Cross-sectional surveys identify all persons with the disease, some of which are new cases while other persons may have had the disease for a period of time. Some cross-sectional studies have related non-personal factors associated with place of residence to disease status. Other studies have collected detailed information from each study participant on personal exposure to UV or indices of exposure (e.g. hours of exposure to sunshine, occupation) and related these exposures to disease status.

The third type of study design has been the case-control study, where differences in UV exposure between persons with the disease and those without have been compared. Cases have usually been drawn from a hospital or clinic. Controls have been drawn from other hospital or clinic patients or from the general population and have usually only included persons with good visual acuity, without the disease of interest, and without a disease that is associated with UV exposure. Some case-control studies have related disease status to non-personal factors associated with place of residence while others have used personal exposure information.

Data from both cross-sectional and case-control studies can be useful in confirming a hypothesis, but have a number of limitations. If there is an excess risk of death associated with the disease, as has been suggested for cataract (Minassian et al., 1992; Vitale et al., 1992), both types of study will be biased towards the survivors. In addition, disease status and prior exposure indices are measured at the same time and it may not be possible to differentiate between cause and effect, especially if the disease has a long latency period.

10.4 Diseases of the External Eye

10.4.1 *Photokeratitis and photoconjunctivitis*

Cases of photokeratitis and photoconjunctivitis have occurred between 0.5 and 24 hours after prolonged exposure to intense solar radiation, often in highly reflective environments (Wittenberg, 1986). The most severe cases are usually manifested as snow blindness, suggesting that UV is the cause of this condition.

The action spectrum for UV photokeratitis produced in the rabbit was first measured by Cogan and Kinsey (1946). Pitts (1974, 1978) in a series of laboratory studies on humans estimated the mean threshold of UVB (290-315 nm) for photokeratitis at 3500 J m^{-2}. These laboratory data are supported by Blumthaler et al. (1987), who estimated that the radiant exposures in clinically observed cases of photokeratitis ranged from 1200 to 5600 J m^{-2}. It is estimated that 100 to 200 seconds of direct, unattenuated exposure to 295-315 nm solar radiation will result in photokeratitis (Sliney, 1987; Wittenberg, 1986). Blotting out the solar disc would remove around 40% of the UV, still leaving a threshold of around 5.5 minutes. Sliney (1986) has estimated that the reflected levels of UV from light sand should be sufficient to cause a threshold photokeratitis within exposure periods of 6-8 hours centred around midday, and within 1 hour for UV reflected from snow.

Experimental data shows photokeratitis can be induced in animals by UVB exposure and that use of UVB absorbing contact lens or chromophores can prevent UVB induced photokeratitis in laboratory animals. Collectively, there is sufficient experimental and epidemiological evidence that exposure to intense UVB radiation causes photokeratitis and photoconjunctivitis.

10.4.2 *Climatic droplet keratopathy*

Climatic droplet keratopathy, among a variety of other names (Gray et al., 1992), is also known as spheroidal degeneration from its histological appearance. It is a degenerative condition usually affecting both eyes symmetrically, and restricted to the exposed interpalpebral band of the cornea. This condition is of major significance for vision in some parts of the world, reducing vision to blindness levels in older people. For example, in Mongolia it has been found in an initial survey to be the third cause of blindness (Baasanhu et al., in press).

Climatic droplet keratopathy occurs throughout the world, but is more common in areas with snowfall persisting late into the summer in the northern hemisphere, such as parts of northern Canada, Siberia and Mongolia, and in areas of sand and desert in other latitudes, including Somalia, the Arabian peninsula, Iran, and Australia. It is also particularly common on sea coasts where there is coral sand or the sand is impregnated with salt, such as the islands of the Red Sea (Gray el al., 1992).

In a cross-sectional study of Australian aborigines Taylor (1980a) found no correlation between the prevalence of climatic droplet keratopathy and ambient UVB levels, although the condition was more common among those working as stockmen. Johnson (1981) reported a geographical correlation with the calculated flux of reflected UV from snow and ice throughout the year in the eastern coast of Newfoundland and Labrador and the eastern Arctic of Canada.

In a cross-sectional study of Chesapeake Bay waterman study Taylor et al. (1989) examined the risk of climatic droplet keratopathy with chronic UVB exposure. Although a positive association was found (RR= 6.4, 95%CI=2.5-11.7) for those in the highest quarter of exposure compared to those with the bottom quarter, further analyses of this data (Taylor et al., 1992) showed the risk of climatic droplet keratopathy was also related to UVA.

There is strong evidence that the corneal degeneration is due to environmental factors. Circumstantial evidence exists that it is caused by solar UV, mainly reflected from ground surfaces such as snow and sand which are particularly reflective of UV. Histologically, the material deposited in the superficial corneal stroma as spheroidal droplets is most likely to be derived from a mixture of altered plasma proteins, including fibrinogen, albumin, and immunoglobulins (Johnson & Overall, 1978).

Other proposed aetiological agents such as low atmospheric humidity, low temperature or high temperature have been excluded. It is possible that particulate injury by wind-blown ice or snow or sand particles may contribute to the development of the condition by causing inflammation and therefore outpouring of additional plasma proteins from the blood vessels of the limbs.

10.4.3 *Pinguecula*

Pinguecula is a fibro-fatty degeneration of the interpalpebral conjunctiva. The pathological changes that occur in pinguecula are similar to actinic elastosis of the skin, a condition thought to be linked to sunlight exposure. This indirect evidence suggests that exposure to sunlight may be a risk factor for pinguecula.

Geographical variation in the occurrence of pinguecula has been reported, with higher prevalence in Arabs living near the Red Sea than in Eskimos from Greenland or Caucasians in Copenhagen (Norn, 1982). Johnson et al. (1981) in a study of pinguecula in Labrador found the size of pinguecula was correlated with the severity of climatic droplet keratopathy. Taylor et al. (1989) in the study of Chesapeake Bay watermen found a weak association for the presence or absence of pinguecula with exposure to UVA and UVB. The relative risk for the top quartile of exposure was 1.4 (95%CI=0.9-2.2), less than for climatic droplet keratopathy or pterygium. Karai & Horiguchi (1984) in a study of 191 Japanese welders found no difference in the occurrence of pinguecula between welders and controls.

It is concluded that there is currently insufficient epidemiological or experimental data for an assessment of the risk of pinguecula with exposure to UV.

10.4.4 *Pterygium*

Pterygium is a triangular shaped degeneration and hyperplastic process in which the bulbar conjunctiva encroaches on the cornea.

A geographical association between variation in the occurrence of pterygium and variation in sunlight exposure was first suggested by Talbot (1948). Based on observation of pterygium in New Zealand and South Pacific Islands Elliott (1961) suggested pterygium in these locations resulted from UV exposure.

Studies of non-personal factors associated with place of residence

In a study of pterygium patients in US Veterans Administration hospitals during 1957-59 Darrell & Bachrach (1963) related mean daily UV (319nm) levels to the ratio of pterygium to all hospital discharges. A trend was found between UV level and pterygium ratio for persons born in rural counties. A similar association with UV level was seen for persons residing in a rural county at the time of the hospital discharge. Cameron (1965) examined the global pattern of pterygium and reported an inverse gradient with latitude. In a study of Australian aborigines Taylor (1980a) found pterygium was correlated with ambient UVB level and hours of sunshine at place of residence. Data from Canada indicates that pterygium is also common in arctic and sub-arctic environments (Johnson et al., 1981). Moran & Hollows (1984) found a nonsignificant increase in the prevalence of pterygium among Australian aborigines residing in areas with higher ambient UV levels.

Studies with personal exposure measurements

Four studies have related occurrence of pterygium to personal measurements. Karai & Horiguchi (1984) examined 191 Japanese welders for the presence of pterygium. A trend of increasing risk of pterygium was found with years of employment as a welder, an indirect measure of cumulative occupational exposure to UV.

Booth (1985) undertook a hospital-base case-control study of pterygium in Sydney. No difference between cases and controls was found in subjective assessment of exposure to sunlight in work or sport. However, a family history of pterygium was found to be a strong risk factor.

Among Chesapeake Bay watermen, Taylor et al. (1989) found a dose-response relationship between risk of pterygium and exposure to UVA and UVB. The relative risk for the top quarter of UVB exposure was 3.1 (95%CI=1.8-5.3) compared to the lowest quarter. However, it is noted that pterygium was equally associated with ocular exposure to UVA and visible light.

Mackenzie et al. (1992) undertook a hospital-based case-control study of pterygium in Queensland. A strong dose-response relationship was found with closeness of place of residence to the equator, type of outdoor work environment (e.g. sandy) and amount of time spend outdoors. The most striking finding was the magnitude of risk associated with spending most of the time outdoors was stronger when related to childhood exposure (RR=17.2, 95%CI=6.2-47.6) than to adult exposure (RR=5.7, 95%CI=3.1-10.6). The risk associated with working at ages 20-29 in an outdoors environment of mainly sand or concrete was associated with a relative risk of 11.3 compared with indoor workers. Comeo (1993) has suggested that the cornea is acting as a side on lens focusing light and also UV across the anterior chamber to the nasal limbus. This hypothesis may explain why pterygia usually commence on the nasal side of the eye.

Evaluation of epidemiological evidence

While several geographical studies have reported an inverse trend with latitude, the common occurrence of pterygium in arctic and subarctic locations suggest that closeness to the equator does not fully explain the distribution of this disease.

The strength of the association with time spent outdoors reported by Mackenzie et al. (1992) suggests that the association may be causal. However, there is insufficient evidence to show that the observed association with UV exposure is not, in part, due to confounding. The findings from three of the studies lend support to a hypothesis that irritation by particulate matter is associated with pterygium. The Australian aborigines live in a dry, dusty environment and welders are occupationally exposed to a range of particles. Similarly, the Queensland study found highest risk among those who worked in sandy locations. The particulate matter hypothesis is also supported by a report (Dhir et al., 1967) of higher prevalence of pterygium among Punjabi Indians working in sawmills (an indoor occupation) in New Delhi and British Columbia than Punjabi farmers (an outdoor occupation). Similar findings of increased risk of pterygium among sawmill workers in Thailand and Taiwan have been reported (Detels & Dhir, 1967). The evidence of possible confounding by particulate matter is inconsistent, with the Chesapeake Bay watermen study finding an association with sunlight exposure in a location that was neither hot, dry or dusty.

It is not possible, based on available epidemiological data, to assess the risk of pterygium with exposure to UV because of possible confounding of observed associations by exposure to particulate matter or other factors.

10.4.5 *Hyperkeratosis, carcinoma-in-situ, and squamous cell carcinoma of the conjunctiva*

These conditions probably form a gradation of development and cannot necessarily be distinguished clinically. Invasive squamous cell carcinoma is often said to arise from a pre-cancerous lesion. Epithelial dysplasia and carcinoma-in-situ look the same, and are sometimes keratinized and present as leucoplakia in which case the term actinic keratosis may be applied (Naumann & Apple, 1986; Garner, 1989). The main argument for an actinic causation is that these tumours usually present in the exposed area of the eye between the lids (the interpalpebral fissure) and under conditions where they may be expected to be exposed to solar radiation.

Xeroderma pigmentosum is a recessively inherited syndrome characterized by clinical and cellular hypersensitivity to solar radiation and a defect in the capacity to repair UV-induced damage in DNA (Fitzpatrick, et al., 1963). Among reports of 337 patients with xeroderma pigmentosum for whom ocular findings had been described, Kraemer et al. (1987) identified 88 ocular tumours of which 73 were specific to the corneal-scleral limbus (34), the cornea (24) or the conjunctiva (15). Of the non-melanomas for which histopathological type was specified, 28 were squamous cell carcinomas and 12 were basal cell carcinomas. Among 64 patients with ocular neoplasms whose age was stated, half the neoplasms had occurred before 11 years of age. While the eyelids are a site of preference for basal cell carcinoma, this tumour rarely, if ever, arises in the conjunctiva in otherwise normal individuals.

Squamous cell carcinoma of the conjunctiva is an uncommon tumour. Garner (1989) reviewed all cases of tumours at the limbus sent over a 40 year period for examination to the Institute of Ophthalmology, London. The total was only 636 tumours, of which 73 were squamous carcinomas. This amounts to less than 2 cases per year coming to the Pathology Laboratory, even though Moorfields Eye Hospital which the Laboratory serves, attracts patients from all over the country and from overseas.

Lee & Hirst (1992) attempted to provide population-based figures and estimate the incidence of these tumours in metropolitan Brisbane (latitude 30° south). They surveyed the histological records of all ocular surface tumours examined in the pathological laboratories over the previous 10 years, serving a population of more than 745,000 in 1989. There were 139 cases of which 79 were corneal epithelial dysplasia, 28 carcinomas-in-situ and 32 were squamous cell carcinomas. There was a strong male preponderance. The incidence ranged from 1 per 100,000 in 1980 to 2.8 per 100,000 in 1982. This is well below the rate for squamous cell carcinoma of the skin and melanoma of the skin in Queensland as a whole. On the other hand, it is a substantially higher rate than that recorded in London where the pathological laboratory referred to also covers a much larger population.

Squamous cell carcinoma of the conjunctiva has been reported to form a greater proportion of eye tumours in Africans living in areas close to the equator (Templeton, 1967) than in the south of Africa (Higginson & Oettlé, 1959), and much higher than in Baltimore (39^0N). The incidence (0.3 per 100,000) in Uganda (0^0) has been reported to be twice that in Denmark (55^0N) despite the potential underascertainment in Africa (Templeton, 1967).

It is extremely rare for a neoplasm to arise *de novo* in the corneal epithelium, where it may be called a corneal intra-epithelial neoplasm. Most such intra-epithelial sheets are connected at the corneo-scleral limbus to a conjunctival lesion, such as a papilloma or a leucoplakia over a pterygium or pinguecula (Waring et al., 1984). The only available evidence for an UV aetiology is the location of the lesion within the interpalpebral fissure, and the fact that it may arise from a lesion which is itself associated with UV. Three cases of corneal intra-epithelial neoplasia have been recently reported in people aged 31 to 38 who wore contact lenses and were considered to have had substantial exposure to artificial and solar UV (Guex-Crosier & Herbort, 1993).

10.5 Diseases of the Lens

10.5.1 *Cataract*

For the purpose of this review, a cataract is defined as an opacity of the lens of the eye. The three major types of cataract are cortical, nuclear and posterior subcapsular (PSC). When a lens opacity interferes with vision, a clinically significant cataract is present. If left untreated, cataract will often progress to blindness. Cataract causes half of the world's blindness.

Definitions of cataract and methods used to assess the presence and severity of cataract have not been uniform in epidemiological studies of cataract. Many studies include lens opacities that are not necessarily accompanied by a decrease in visual acuity. Some have combined all three major types of lens opacities into a single "cataract" category, while others have investigated associations for specific types of opacity. Methods of assessing the presence and sometimes the severity of opacities range from reviews of existing charts to clinical examinations using written definitions of cataract, and the use of standardized grading systems that have been found to be highly reliable.

Occupational case series

When cataracts result from occupational exposure to UV, it may be difficult to differentiate between the contribution of occupational and non-occupational factors to the development of the disease. Lerman (1980) described the onset of lens opacities in three persons who worked in a dental clinic and were exposed to UV (300-400 nm) from a dental curing unit. The lens damage varied from posterior subcapsular cataract in the dentist, who was reported to have received the highest dose, to zonular type opacities in one of the dental assistants. However, any retrospective reconstruction of the actual ocular exposure has a large degree of uncertainty, and the results from such an exercise must be interpreted with caution.

Studies in which UV exposure was inferred from place of residence

Selected studies of humans exposed to solar UV are presented in tables 10.1 and 10.2. Studies were selected for inclusion in the tables on the basis of the scientific quality of the published report and the overall contribution of the paper to the evaluation of the UV-cataract hypothesis. The tables do not include the relative risks for other factors, which in some instances are higher than for sunlight or UV exposure.

Hiller et al. (1977) investigated sunlight and cataracts using data from the large sources (blindness registries in 14 states and the cross-sectional Health and Nutrition Examination Survey (HANES) of 35 geographic areas of the US) and US Weather Bureau geographical data on annual hours of

TABLE 10.1 SELECTED HUMAN CATARACT STUDIES WITH SUNLIGHT OR UV EXPOSURE BASED ON RESIDENCE

AUTHOR	POPULATION	MEASURE OF OUTCOME	MEASURE OF SUNLIGHT EXPOSURE	ASSOCIATIONS OBSERVED	COMMENTS
Hiller et al. (1977, 1983, 1986)	MRA: 9110 persons registered as blind in 14 US States; whites;	Blind from cataract, visual acuity (VA) 6/60	Average hours of sunlight ≤ 2400 vs 3000+	RR= 3.3 (age 65-74)	Adjusted for age and sex; blind registry data
	NHANES: 3580 persons; probability sample of US population;	Lens opacity and VA ≤ 6/7.5	Average hours of sunlight ≤2400 vs 3000+	RR= 2.7 (age 65.74)	Adjusted for age and sex
	NHANES data	Lens opacity and VA ≤ 6/9	Average daily UVB count in area of residency 6000 vs 2600	RR= 1.58 (age 45-74, p<.05)	Adjusted analysis
	NHANES data	Nuclear and cortical opacity	Average daily UVB count in area of residency 6000 vs 2600	RR= 3.6 for cortical opacity; no association with nuclear opacity	Adjusted analyses; pure opacity types only
Taylor (1980b)	Survey of 350 Australian Aborigines	Lens opacity with good vision, poor vision or blindness	Average daily sunlight hours in area of residence: 9.5+ vs ≤ 8	RR= 4.2 (95% CI=0.9-18.9[1]	Unadjusted for age or potential confounding factors
			Annual mean UVB rrdiation level for area of residence: 3000 vs 2000	RR= 1.8 (95%ci=0.9-3.4)[1] [1] 95%CI estimated from published data	
Hollows & Moran (1981)	Survey of 64,307 Aborigines and 41,254 non-Aborigines, Australia	Lens opacity and VA < 6/6	Average daily UVB count in 5 zones of Australia: 3000 vs 1000	Significant positive correlation between prevalence of lens opacity and UVB counts in Aborigines; no association in non-Aborigines	Wide age bands; unadjusted analyses
Brilliant et al. (1983)	Survey of 27,785 Nepalese; national probability sample; lifelong residents;	Lens opacities or aphakia	Average daily sunlight hours: 12 vs 712 vs 7-9	RR= 3.8 (p<.001)	Adjusted for age and sex; RR decreased with increasing altitude; sun blocked by mountains at high elevations
			12 vs 712 vs 7-9	RR= 2.6 (p<.005)	
Cruickshanks et al. (1993)	Cross-sectional survey of 4926 persons, Wisconsin, USA	Nuclear, cortical and PSC opacities	Average annual ambient UVB exposure	UVB exposure associated with cortical opacities in men (RR=1.36, 95%CI=1.02-1.79) but not women, not associated with nuclear or PSC opacities	Adjusted for other risk factors; measure of exposure represents average potential exposure at residency; also Table 9.2

TABLE 10.2 SELECTED HUMAN CATARACT STUDIES WITH INDIVIDUAL UV EXPOSURE ASSESSMENT

AUTHOR	POPULATION	MEASURE OF OUTCOME	MEASURE OF SUNLIGHT EXPOSURE	ASSOCIATIONS OBSERVED	COMMENTS
Collmann et al. (1988)	Clinic-based case control study of 113 cases and 168 controls, North Carolina, USA; whites	Nuclear, cortical and PSC opacities	Average annual sunlight exposure, based on residential history and amount of time spent in sun	No significant association with any type of opacity	Low power to detect association; matched on age and sex
Taylor et al. (1988)	Cross-sectional survey of 838 watermen, Maryland, USA	Nuclear and cortical opacities	Cumulative ocular exposure to UV since age 16, based on life history and ocular exposure model	Dose-response relationship in which a doubling of cumulative UVR exposure increased risk of cortical opacity by 1.60 (95%CI=1.01-2.64). RR= 3.30 (95%CI=0.90-9.97) for highest vs lowest quartile. No association between ocular exposure to UVR and nuclear opacity	High exposure study population; detailed ocular exposure model
Bochow et al. (1989)	Clinic-based case-control study of 168 cases and 168 controls, Maryland, USA	PSC cataract (surgical patients)	Cumulative ocular exposure since age 16, based on life history and exposure model	Increased levels of UVB exposure associated with increased risk of PSC cataract	Adjusted analyses; association present when adjusted for cortical cataract
Dolezal et al. (1989)	Clinic-based case-control study of 160 cases and 160 controls, Iowa, USA	Cataract (scheduled for surgery)	Lifetime sunlight exposure, based on life history, amount of time in sun and use of glasses and hat	No association between lifetime sunlight exposure and risk of cataract; use of head covering reduced risk of cataract in males (RR=0.48, 95%CI=0.25-0.94)	Only partially adjusted for potential confounding factors; crude index of exposure, low power
Italian-Am. study (1991)	Clinical-based case-control study of 1008 cases and 469 controls, Italy	Nuclear, cortical, PSC and mixed opacities	Work location in the sunlight; leisure time in the sunlight; use of glasses and hat	Cortical and mixed opacities associated with work location in sunlight (RR=1.75, 95%CI=1.15-2.65), leisure time in sunlight (RR=1.45, 95%CI=1.09-1.93). Cortical, PSC and mixed opacities associated with use of a hat in summer (RR=1.80, 95%CI=1.17-2.47). No association between sun exposure indices and nuclear opacities	Adjusted for other risk factors; crude indices of exposure; also Table 9.1
Leske et al. (1991)	Clinical-based case-control study of 945 cases and 435 controls, Massachusetts, USA	Nuclear, cortical and PSC mixed opacities	Work in sunlight; leisure time in sun; residence and travel to areas of high sun exposure, use of hat and sunglasses	Work in sunlight significantly reduced risk of nuclear opacity (RR=0.61, 95%CI=0.37-0.99); no significant associations between exposure and cortical or PSC opacities	Analyses adjusted for other risk factor
Cruikshanks et al. (1993)	Cross-sectional survey of 4926 persons, Wisconsin, USA	Nuclear, cortical and PSC opacities	Leisure and work time outside; use of glasses and hat	No associations with cortical opacities; reduced risk of nuclear and PSC opacities amount men for outdoor leisure time in winter; use of hats and sunglasses significantly increased risk of PSC opacity in women	Adjusted for other factors; crude indices of exposure; also Table 9.1

sunlight in each geographical area. Above the age of 65 the prevalence of cataract increased with annual hours of sunlight, with the highest prevalence found in locations with 3000+ annual hours of sunshine. At ages 45-64 there was some evidence of an association with hours of sunshine but the gradient was weaker. Below age 45 there was little association between annual hours of sunshine and prevalence of cataract. In a further analysis of HANES data Hiller et al. (1983) reported a correlation between average daily UVB levels and prevalence of cataract. Analysis of HANES data by type of cataract (Hiller et al., 1986) revealed UVB levels at location of residence were associated with pure cortical cataract but not with pure nuclear or posterior subcapsular cataract.

The prevalence of cataract among Australian aborigines was found to be correlated with annual ambient UVB level at place of residence (Taylor et al., 1980b). Hollows & Moran (1981) found the prevalence of cataract was highest among aborigines living in the north of Australia, an area with high average daily UVB radiation. Mao & Hu (1982) studied age related cataract in seven rural areas of China and found the prevalence of cataract was correlated with annual direct solar radiation.

Residents of rural villages in Nepal had a prevalence of cataract related in different zones of the country to average hours of sunshine (Brilliant et al., 1983). The prevalence was higher in the plains where there were 12 hours of direct sunshine compared to the mountains with 7-9 hours per day. Factors such as use of glasses and hats modify personal ocular exposure to UV and should be assessed.

Age and sex adjusted prevalence for all types of cataract in persons aged 40 years and older was found to be 60% greater in Tibet than in Beijing (14.6% versus 9.1%, $p>0.001$) (Hu et al., 1989). The authors suggested a relationship with higher UV at the higher altitudes of Tibet, but confounding factors could not be excluded and prevalences were higher in women than men.

Studies with personal exposure measurements

A number of studies have collected information from each study participant and estimated personal exposure to either sunlight or UV. Factors such as use of glasses and hats should be assessed. The characteristics of selected studies are outlined in Table 10.2.

In a cross-sectional study of cataract in the Punjab related prevalence of cataract to work environment Chatterjee et al. (1982) found a suggestion of lower cataract incidence among men whose main work location was outdoors (RR=0.7, 95%CI=0.5-1.1).

Collman et al. (1988) examined lifetime exposure to sunlight in a clinic-based case-control study of cortical, nuclear or PSC. Lifetime exposure to sunlight was estimated from intensity of solar radiation in area of residence, years of residence and average amount of time spent outdoors during daylight hours. A non-significant risk (RR=1.1) of cataract was found for the highest category of lifetime exposure to sunlight.

Personal exposure history and ambient UVB data were combined to estimate an individual's lifetime annual ocular exposure to UVB after age 15 in a cross-sectional study of Chesapeake Bay watermen (Taylor et al., 1988). This included information on occupational and leisure exposures, type of work surfaces, seasons, and use of head wear and eyewear. A moderate association with a trend of increasing risk with exposure to UVB was seen for cortical cataract, with a RR of 3.3 (95%CI=0.9-10.0) for the top quarter of exposure relative to the bottom quarter. A nonsignificant association was also found between exposure to UVA (320 -340 nm) and prevalence of cortical cataract. Little evidence was found for an association between UVA or UVB exposure and nuclear cataract. It is noted that UVA and UVB exposures were highly correlated and that the study would not have been able to differentiate between the effects of UVA and UVB. Further analyses suggested a significant difference between the cumulative lifetime ocular exposure among cases of cortical cataract compared to non-cataract controls. No threshold or latency period was observed.

In a clinic-based study of PSC cataracts in Maryland, cases were persons who underwent PSC extraction in an ophthalmic practice (Bochow et al., 1989). Controls, matched on age, sex, and type of referral were chosen from other patients on the appointment book of the same ophthalmic practice who did not have a PSC cataract or a previous cataract extraction. Annual and cumulative ocular UVB exposures were estimated for each individual using the same method as the studies of Chesapeake Bay watermen. Thirty-nine percent of cases had a pure PSC cataract, the remaining 61% had mixed PSC and other cataracts. Almost half the controls had a non PSC cataract (nuclear, cortical or other lens opacity). UVB exposure was significantly associated with PSC cataracts. Both the average cumulative exposure and average annual exposure were higher in cases than controls, after adjusting for steroid use, eye colour, education, diabetes and presence of cortical cataracts.

In a hospital-based study of cataract patients in Iowa Dolezal et al. (1989) found little evidence of an association between individual lifetime sunlight exposure and cataract. Mohan et al. (1989) in a similar study of cataract in New Delhi examined a range of environmental factors, including occupation. An increase in cloud cover was significantly associated (RR=0.8, 95%CI=0.7-0.9) with cataract when adjusted for each of the other environmental variables. The study did not quantify individual lifetime exposure to sunlight or UV.

In a study of cataract patients in a Massachussetts hospital, Leske et al. (1991) investigated occupational exposure to sunshine. No association was found for PSC cataract (RR=1.3, 95%CI=0.7-2.3), cortical cataract (RR=0.9, 95%CI=0.6-1.3), or mixed cataract (RR=0.8, 95%CI=0.6-1.1) among those with at least 2 hours of exposure to bright sunshine per day for at least 2 months. The risk of nuclear cataract was reduced (RR=0.5, 95%CI=0.3-0.9).

A hospital-based study from Italy (Italian-American Cataract Study Group, 1991) found an excess of pure cortical and mixed cataract (RR=1.8, 95%CI=1.2-2.6) and a nonsignificant deficit of nuclear (RR=0.6) and PSC cataract (RR=0.8) among those with a work location in the sunlight. Leisure time spent in the sunlight was associated with an excess of cortical and mixed cataract (RR=1.4, 95%CI=1.1-1.9) and a nonsignificant deficit of posterior subcapsular cataract (RR=0.6).

In an Indian clinic-based study of cataract and history of severe diarrhoeal diseases Bhatnagar et al. (1991) found an elevated risk of cataract (RR=2.1, 95%CI=1.2-3.6) for outdoor occupations compare with indoor occupations. However Zaunuddin & Saski (1991) found no relationship between hours of exposure to sunshine and prevalence of nuclear or cortical cataract in Sumatra (0^0 latitude). In Beaver Dam, Wisconsin, Cruickshanks et al. (1993) found no association between average annual exposure to UVB and cortical, PSC or nuclear cataract. Wong et al. (1993) surveyed fishermen in Hong Kong. A sun exposure score was calculated based on daily sunlight exposure, and protection from use of a canopy, hat, and glasses. The highest grades of cataract of all types considered together were more common in subjects with the highest sun exposure scores, but none of these associations was significant at the 5% level. A population-based case-control study (Shibati et al., 1993) reported an increased risk of cortical cataract among men aged 40-50 years who spent 5 or more hours per day outdoors compared with those who spent less time outdoors (RR = 6.89; 95%CI = 1.22-39).

Evaluation of epidemiological evidence

An association has been demonstrated between prevalence of cataract and residence in areas at low latitudes, with long hours of sunlight or high ambient UV radiance in several studies undertaken in different parts of the world. However, in each study, the observed association may be confounded by other possibly causal factors. Certain of the earlier studies did not classify the lens opacities into types of cataract.

Cortical cataract was examined separately in four studies. Only one study assessed individual exposure. Taylor et al. (1988) found a dose-response relationship with exposure to UVB radiation. The relative risk for the highest exposure category was three times that for the lowest exposure category. It is unlikely that the exposure assessment was able to distinguish between UVA and UVB exposure. The other two used simple measures of sun-related behaviour. Leske et al. (1991) found no association between exposure to bright sunshine and cortical cataract, while in the Italian-American Cataract Study (1991), a work location in the sunlight was related to cortical and mixed cataract. The Italian study also found an association between leisure time outdoors and cortical and mixed cataract. The other two studies showed non-significant trends in opposite directions. More recently, Cruickshanks et al. (1993) found annual UVB exposure was associated with cortical opacities among men, but no association was found for women.

Four studies report risk estimates for posterior subcapsular (PSC) cataracts. Bochow et al. (1989) measured individual exposure and found PSC cataract patients had higher annual and cumulative exposures to UVB than controls, even after allowing for the effects of several other factors. The other two studies used simple measures of sun-related behaviour and showed non-significant trends in opposite directions. Leske et al. (1991) found elevated risk for pure PSC cataract patients compared to controls. However, the Italian-American Cataract Study (1991) reported reduced risk for pure PSC cataract patients with a work location in the sunlight or who spent leisure time in the sunlight. Cruickshanks et al. (1993) found no association between annual UVB exposure and risk of PSC cataract.

Five studies provide risk estimates separately for nuclear cataracts. These studies are consistent in showing no association between UV exposure and nuclear cataract (Taylor et al., 1988; Dolezal et al., 1989; Leske et al., 1991; The Italian-American Cataract Study, 1991; and Cruickshanks et al., 1993). Collectively these studies are consistent in showing no association between UV exposure and nuclear cataract.

All of the published epidemiological studies of UV and cataract have been challenged by the enormous difficulty of determining ocular exposure in different climates. As noted previously, the cornea and lens are seldom directly exposed to light rays from much of the sky; hence the sunlight scattered from the ground and the horizon determine the actual accumulated UV dose.

These studies clearly demonstrate that UV is at least one aetiologic factor in cataractogenesis. However, extrapolation of strong associations found in a mid-latitude population where no serious nutritional problems are present (e.g. Taylor, et al., 1988) to a tropical population in less developed regions, may not be valid, since the contribution of UV relative to other factors such as malnutrition and dehydration may be far more important.

10.5.2 *Exfoliation syndrome*

The exfoliation syndrome (pseudoexfoliation of lens capsule) consists of abnormal material deposited on or arising from various parts of the anterior eye. This condition was originally described from Finland by Lindberg (1917). In the Nordic countries it contributes to a high proportion of glaucoma in the older population. This appears as a round area in the centre of the anterior lens capsule, corresponding to normal pupil size, on which bluish-grey flakes are deposited. This is surrounded by a clear zone, which in turn is surrounded by a peripheral band of involvement as well. On the border of the pupil it looks like "dandruff". Similar material is trapped in the pores of the trabecula meshwork and may be seen on the ciliary processes, on the zonulas, surrounding the conjunctival vessels and in retro-orbital tissues. It is a basement membrane material, akin to amyloid in some respects, although many histochemical studies do not support this identification.

The prevalence varies enormously from country to country, and even within countries. The highest prevalence was found in the Navajo Indians of New Mexico, in which 38% were over 60 years of age. At the other extreme, only 2 cases have ever been recorded in Eskimos, and these were two Greenlanders, possibly of mixed ancestry, aged over 70 years (Ostenfeld-Åkerblom, 1988). The average prevalence in central Europe is around 2% on the basis of figures from several authors (Forsius, 1988).

The possibility of environmental factors was proposed by Taylor (1979) based on observations of exfoliation in Australian aborigines. The distribution of exfoliation was linked to annual global radiation and to climatic droplet keratopathy.

Exfoliation syndrome sometimes occurs in other areas of high UV, and high prevalence of climatic keratopathy. Examples include Somalia, Djibouti and Saudi Arabia. There is, however, considerable evidence to suggest that UV is not the main factor associated with the development of exfoliation. The geographic distribution does not consistently correspond with that of climatic keratopathy. There may be wide differences in prevalence of exfoliation syndrome at similar latitudes. For example, it is frequent in parts of East Africa, but rare in West Africa. Similarly it may be seen at high prevalence in the Lapps of Finland and Sweden, but not in Eskimos at the same latitude. The prevalence may vary within the same country. A total of 4,042 patients aged over 50 were examined in clinics in 6 areas in different parts of France over a 2 week period. The prevalence was high in Brittany (20.6% in those over 60 years) and extremely rare in Picardy at a similar latitude (Colin et al., 1985). Exfoliation is usually more frequent in females than males. It is found in parts of the eye, such as the ciliary body and in the orbit, remote from the influence of light. Forsius (1988) has reviewed the evidence for genetic aetiology for the condition.

The present conclusion is that environment, at least in the form of UV, is not the primary cause. There is not a consistent direct relationship with solar radiation. There is at least a major racial or genetic predisposition, but it is possible that light or some other environmental factor activates or induces the development of the exfoliation syndrome in those who are genetically predisposed.

10.5.3 *Anterior lens capsule*

In 1989 a previously unrecorded condition was reported from Somalia (Johnson et al., 1989). This consisted of alterations of the pupillary area of the anterior capsule of the lens. The first stage appeared to be an opalescence of the capsule, which then became a plateau-shaped elevation above the surrounding contour of the anterior lens. In its most developed form it was a bagging of the anterior lens capsule and contents through the pupil, appearing like a hernia. This condition was invariably associated with climatic droplet keratopathy, but not necessarily with cataract. In fact, there appeared to be an inverse relation with cataract.

The absolute association with climatic keratopathy suggests that it also may be due to excessive UV exposure. Attempts to secure histology on extracted lenses with this condition were difficult because the lens capsule so frequently tore from the rest of the lens as it was extracted by the cryoprobe. The capsules examined showed thinning and splitting of the layers, and death of many of the nuclei of the epithelial cells. However, there were no controls from the same geographical and ethnic area of the same ages for comparison.

10.6 Diseases of the Choroid and Retina

Among adults, only extremely small amounts of UVA and UVB at wavelengths below 380 nm reach the retina, because of the very strong absorption by the cornea and lens. Less than 1% of radiation below 340 nm and 2% of radiation between 340 and 360 nm reaches the retina (Barker and Brainard, 1993). Even in early childhood the highest spectral transmittance reaches about 4% in the UVB and is generally of the order of 1%. However, because of the biological activity of the shorter wavelengths of UVB, the biological importance of the small amount of this radiation that does reach the retina cannot be completely neglected. As children age, UV is increasingly absorbed by the cornea and lens, and the proportion reaching the retina decreases. This suggests firstly, that exposure to UV during childhood may be of more importance than exposure to UV during adult life, and secondly, that exposure to longer wavelength radiation (e.g. visible light) may be of more importance in adulthood.

10.6.1 *Uveal melanoma*

Exposure to solar radiation is considered to be causally associated with the development of cutaneous malignant melanoma (IARC, 1993). There is a possibility that exposure to UV may also cause melanoma of the uveal tract. There is no separate ICD code for intra-ocular melanoma, so descriptive studies have generally been based on cancer of the eye (ICD-9 190), of which it has been estimated that 80% are intra-ocular melanomas (Østerlind, 1987). In the case-control studies cases of uveal-tract melanomas were confirmed histologically, but also included tumours of iris and ciliary body with those of the choroid.

The incidence of cancer of the eye is higher among white than black or Asian populations residing at the same latitude. For example, in US whites the incidence rates are 0.7 per 100 000 person years in males and 0.6 in females compared with 0.2 in both sexes in blacks (Parkin et al., 1992). Among people of European ancestry, risk of ocular melanoma was observed to be least in those of southern European ethnic origin; for example, in comparison with an RR of 1.0 in those of southern European origin, the RR in people of northern European origin was 6.5 (95% CI 1.9-22.4; Seddon et al., 1990). Risk of ocular melanoma was observed to be increased in those with light eye colour, with RRs of 1.7 to 2.1 (Gallagher et al., 1985; Tucker et al., 1985c; Holly et al., 1990), but not when ethnicity was taken into account (Seddon et al., 1990). Kraemer (1987) found five cases of ocular melanoma among reports of 337 patients with xeroderma pigmentosum for whom ocular findings had been described. The defect in this condition is failure to repair DNA after damage by UV.

There is no evident latitude gradient in incidence of ocular melanoma in white populations of the northern hemisphere or Australia (IARC, 1992) and, within the USA, its risks in those born in southern parts of the country, where ambient solar radiation is highest, has variously been reported to be more (Tucker et al., 1985c), less (Seddon et al., 1990) or the same (Schwartz & Weiss, 1988; Mack & Floderus, 1991) as that in those born elsewhere in the country. Similarly Gallagher et al. (1985) in Canada found no association with latitude of residence.

Two studies have examined place of birth and risk of uveal melanoma, but the findings are inconsistent. Tucker et al. (1985) found an excess of cases were born south of latitude 40^0N, whereas Seddon et al. (1990) found a deficit.

Indicators of personal sun exposure have been inconsistently associated with risk of cancer of the eye or ocular melanoma. A small rural excess in incidence of cancer of the eye has been reported (Doll, 1991). Two descriptive studies reported an association with farming (Saftlas et al., 1987; Gallagher, 1988) but this was not found in several other such studies (Milham, 1983; Office of Population, Censuses and Surveys, 1986; Vågerö et al., 1990) or two case-control studies of ocular melanoma (Gallagher et al., 1985; Seddon et al., 1990). Some high exposure activities such as gardening (RR 1.6, 95% CI 0.7-1.6) and taking sunny vacations (RR 1.5, 95% CI 1.0-2.3, for highest category) were significantly associated with increased risks of ocular melanoma in one case-control study (Tucker et al., 1985c) but no similar associations with personal sun exposure at work in leisure time, or in vacation were found in three other studies (Gallagher et al., 1985; Holly et al., 1990; Seddon et al., 1990). Indeed, Gallagher et al., (1985) found an elevated risk for government workers, a predominantly indoor managerial group. The lack of use of protective eyewear (sunglasses, visors, headgear) was associated with an increased risk of ocular melanoma in one study (Tucker et al., 1985c) with an RR for infrequent or rare use of 1.6 (95% CI 1.2-2.2). Weak evidence of a similar effect was found by Seddon et al. (1990).

No statistically significant association has been observed between ocular melanoma and a personal history of skin cancer in several studies of cancer registry or other data (Østerlind et al., 1985; Tucker et al., 1985a; Holly et al., 1991; Lischko et al., 1989; Turner et al., 1989).

There is evidence of associations between exposure to sunlamps and some other artificial sources of UV and risk of ocular melanoma in the three case-control studies in which they have been examined. Tucker et al. (1985c) found a relative risk of 2.1 (95% CI 0.3-17.9) for frequent use of sunlamps compared with no use (p=0.10 for trend over four categories of use); Holly et al. (1990) found a relative risk of 3.7 (95% CI 1.6-8.7) for ever having an exposure to "artificial UV or black light" and with welding burn, sunburn to eyelids, or snow-blindness, RR 7.2 (95% CI 2.5-20.6); and Seddon et al. (1990) found a relative risk of 3.4 (95% CI 1.1-10.3) for frequent or occasional use of sunlamps compared with never used. In one of these studies, there was also a strong association with employment as a welder (RR 10.9, 95% CI 2.1-56.5; Tucker et al., 1985c). No similar association was found by Seddon et al. (1990) but an increased risk in welders (RR 8.3, 95% CI 2.5-27.1) was found in an occupational study of French Canadians (Siemiatycki, 1991).

Overall, the epidemiological studies do not provide convincing evidence of an association between exposure to solar UV and uveal melanoma. None of the studies has developed a practical assessment of individual cumulative ocular exposure to UVB. They have all used various simple estimates of sun-related behaviour.

On the other hand, the use of a sunlamp, an artificial source of UV, was significantly associated with uveal melanoma in the two case-control studies that examined their use. Another study found elevated risk of uveal melanoma with exposure to UV or black lights. Collectively, these studies suggest frequent use of a sunlamp may be associated with a 2-4 fold increase in risk of developing uveal melanoma. Sunlamp use can produce over five-fold more DNA damage per unit of erythema than the sun (Nachtwey & Rundel, 1981).

The large number of ocular melanomas in xeroderma pigmentosum patients also means that exposure to UV cannot be ruled out as a causative factor.

10.6.2 *Age-related macular degeneration*

Age-related macular degeneration (AMD) is one of the leading causes of blindness in the industrialized world. Visual loss can occur because of the development of geographic atrophy (loss of the outer retinal segments and retinal pigment epithelium), retinal pigment epithelial detachment or sub-retinal neovascularization (exudative AMD). Prior to visual loss AMD is characterized by the presence of drusen (lipofuscin and other material deposited between the retinal pigment epithelial cells and Bruch's membrane and appearing as yellow-white nodules with distinct and indistinct edges on retinal examination).

There is evidence for association of AMD with UV exposure. Photochemical retinal damage can occur from prolonged exposure to high intensity light. Whether such damage is directly related to AMD is unknown. Although aged Rhesus monkeys have drusenoid deposits, no good experimental animal models for AMD currently exist.

In a case control study, Hyman et al. (1983) found no association of AMD and light exposure based on residential history. They also found no association of AMD to occupational light exposure.

In studies based on individual exposure data; the results are equivocal. The initial evaluation of the association of AMD and UV exposure in the cross-sectional study of Chesapeake Bay watermen revealed no statistically significant association (West et al., 1989). However, a reanalysis based on the small number of cases of AMD with exudative disease or geographic atrophy suggested an association with 20 year exposure to blue light but not UVA or UVB (Taylor, 1992).

The Beaver Dam Eye Study found an association of late stage AMD (exudative AMD or geographic atrophy) and summer leisure time outdoors (RR=2.2 CI=1.1-4.2). It was also suggested that an association existed in men only between early stage AMD and summer leisure time outdoors. The magnitude of the risk estimates were unchanged after adjusting for numerous possible confounding factors (Cruickshanks et.al. 1993).

It can be concluded that there are very limited data demonstrating an association of AMD with UV exposure. The finding of an association with blue light exposure is consistent with the wavelengths of visible light reaching the retina and needs further investigation.

10.7 Conclusion

The causal links between UVB exposure and various ocular conditions were evaluated on the basis of the following definitions:

Sufficient evidence for a causal association indicates that positive associations have been observed between human exposure to UV and the effect in which chance, bias and confounding could be ruled out with reasonable confidence.

Limited evidence for a causal association indicates that positive associations have been observed between exposure to UV and the effect for which a causal interpretation is considered to be credible, but chance, bias or confounding could not be ruled out with reasonable confidence.

Inadequate evidence for a causal association indicates that the available studies are of insufficient quality, consistency, or statistical power to permit a conclusion regarding the presence or absence of a causal association between UV and the effect, or no data were available.

Evidence for lack of causal association indicates that there are several adequate studies covering the range of exposure that humans are known to encounter which are consistent in not showing a positive association between UV and the effect.

There is sufficient evidence to link photokeratitis to acute ocular exposure to UVB.

Sufficient evidence exists to link the production of cortical and PSC cataracts to UVB exposure in animals. There is limited evidence to link cortical and PSC cataract in humans to chronic ocular exposure to UVB. Inadequate evidence is available to link PSC cataract in humans to chronic UVB exposure. Insufficient data have been collected upon which to evaluate the risk of cataract associated with childhood exposure to UVB. Half the world's 35-million blind people are blind because of cataract. The proportion of cataract that results from UVB exposure is unknown, but may be as high as 20%.

There is limited evidence to link sunlight exposure of the eye to the development of pterygium. It is unclear whether the observed association is specific for UV. The contribution from other environmental factors remains unclear.

There is limited evidence to associate climatic droplet keratopathy with UV exposure and insufficient to link pinguecular and cancers of the anterior ocular structures. Insufficient evidence exists to link uveal melanoma to ocular exposure to solar UV radiation. However, several epidemiological studies have suggested that the use of sunbeds (an artificial source of UV) is associated with uveal melanoma.

There is inadequate evidence of an association between ocular UV exposure and acute solar retinitis, age-related macular degeneration, acceleration of pigmentary retinopathies and exfoliation syndrome.

11. EFFECTS ON PLANT AND AQUATIC ECOSYSTEMS

11.1 Introduction

Human populations may be affected by direct and indirect consequences of increased solar UVB on aquatic food webs. Because more than 30% of the world's animal protein for human consumption comes from the sea (in many developing countries this percentage is even larger), a substantial decrease in biomass production would diminish fishery resources in the face of growing world populations. Reductions of leaf area, fresh and dry weight, lipid content and photosynthetic activity were typically found in UVB sensitive plant species. Additionally, alterations of leaf surface, epicuticular waxes, diffusion of water vapour through the stomata have been reported. For previous comprehensive publications see Caldwell et al. (1989), Wellmann (1991) and SCOPE/UNEP (1993).

11.2 Effects on Terrestrial Plants

11.2.1 *UV penetration into the leaf*

UVB has a direct effect on photosynthesis. Reductions in photosynthesis often accompany changes in leaf pigmentation, anatomy, and leaf thickness. After exposure to enhanced UVB, the internal light regime of leaves was altered (Bornman & Vogelmann, 1991). In a recent study, *Brassica campestris* (origin: northern latitudes) was subjected to 6.3 kJ m^{-2} day^{-1} of UVB and responded by increasing leaf thickness by 45% and UVB screening pigments by 21% relative to controls (Bornman & Vogelmann, 1991). Chlorophyll content (per leaf area) and photosynthetic activity decreased while scattered light within the leaves of UV-treated plants increased. Since the distribution of photosynthetically active radiation was altered at different depths within leaves after UV, these changes can also be expected to have an indirect effect on photosynthetic capacity.

In a study on a group of 22 diverse plant species (including herbaceous and woody dicotyledons, grasses and conifers), widely varying UVB penetration was found. For instance, epidermal transmittance of the herbaceous dicotyledons ranged from 18% to 41% with penetration up to 140 μm, while conifer needles excluded a large percentage of the incident UVB. Penetration of UVB into leaves of the woody dicotyledons and grasses was in between that of the herbaceous dicotyledons and conifers (UNEP 1989).

11.2.2 *Changes in growth*

The growth of many plant species is reduced by enhanced levels of UVB. The main components of plants affected by UVB are shown in figure 11.1 (UNEP 1989). The ozone filter technique was used to simulate a relative solar UVB enhancement of 20% by providing 54.4 kJ m^{-2} day^{-1} (unweighted) or 5.1 kJ m^{-2} day^{-1} of biologically effective radiation (UVB_{BE}) through one cuvette and 45.3 kJ m^{-2} day^{-1} (unweighted) or 3.6 kJ m^{-2} day^{-1} UVB_{BE} through the other cuvette (Tevini et al., 1991b). These were average values measured from May 1990 to August 1990 and are equivalent to an ozone depletion of approximately 10%. Plant height, leaf area, and the dry weight of sunflower, corn, and rye seedlings were significantly reduced, while oat seedling remained almost unaffected (Tevini et al., 1991b). The reduction of hypocotyl growth of sunflower seedlings under artificial UVB irradiation is associated with a UV dependent destruction of the growth regulator indole-3-acetic acid (IAA) and the formation of growth inhibiting IAA photoproducts. The inhibition of elongation in UV-irradiated sunflower seedlings might also be due to the action of peroxidases working as IAA-oxidase, causing a decrease in cell wall extensibility of the hypocotyl epidermis (Ros, 1990). Shading of shoot apex was shown to reduce UVB induced reduction in growth of Vigna seedlings (Kulandaivelu et al., 1993).

11.2.3 *Effects on plant function*

When high UVB irradiances were used in combination with low levels of white light, such as commonly found in growth chambers, effects on photosynthesis were generally deleterious. However, even in the presence of higher levels of white light in green houses and in the field, reductions in photosynthesis of up to 17% were reported in the UVB sensitive soybean cultivar Essex when supplied with UVB equivalent to an 18% ozone depletion (Murali & Teramura, 1987). Solar UVB also reduced net photosynthesis in sunflower seedlings by about 15% when a 12% ozone depletion was simulated by using the ozone filter technique (Tevini et al., 1991c). One reason for the reduction in overall photosynthesis might be due to stomatal closure by enhanced UVB.

Recent studies reveal the effects of UVB radiation on tropical plants. Rice is among the most important tropical crops in the world. Sixteen rice *(Oryza sativa L.)* cultivars from several different geographical regions when grown for 12 weeks in greenhouses with supplemental levels of UVB exposure equivalent to 20% ozone depletion over the equator (15.7 kJ m^{-2} day^{-1} UVB_{BE}) showed alterations in biomass, morphology, and photosynthesis. Approximately one-third of all cultivars tested showed a

Figure 11.1 A generalized model for the effects of UVB radiation on plants. Presumed targets of UVB on growth, stomatal function and thylakoid structure are indicated by arrows (UNEP, 1989).

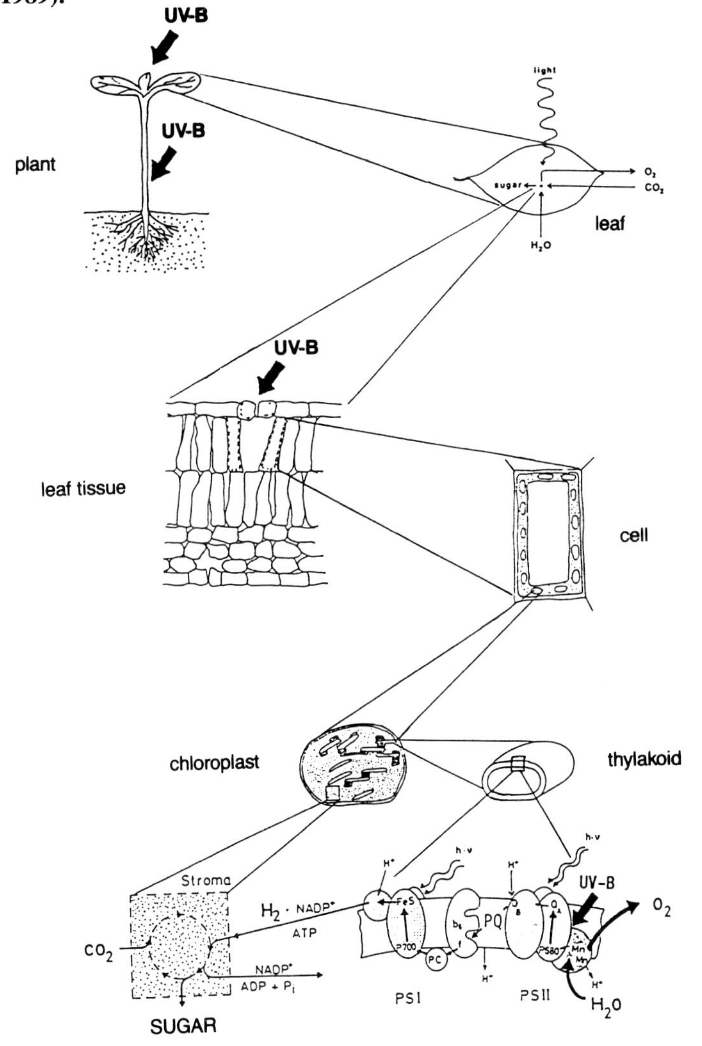

statistically significant decrease in total biomass with increased UVB exposure. Photosynthetic capacity declined for some cultivars, but only a weak relationship existed between changes in photosynthesis and biomass with increasing UVB exposure. In one of the rice cultivars tested, total biomass significantly increased by 20% when grown under enhanced levels of UVB exposure. Therefore, despite the fact that the effects of UVB are generally damaging, in some cases, it has been reported to have a stimulating effect. Such positive growth effects are presently not easily explainable. Results from this experiment indicate that 1) a number of rice cultivars are sensitive to increases in UVB exposure; 2) the diversity exhibited by rice in response to increased levels of UVB suggests that selective breeding might be successfully used to develop UVB tolerant rice cultivars. Other preliminary screening studies on rice seedlings also corroborate these observations (Coronel et al., 1990).

In a three year field study (Sullivan & Teramura, 1991), photosynthetic capacity was generally reduced in loblolly pine trees exposed to supplemental levels of UVB simulating a 16% and 25% ozone depletion (11.5 and 13.6 kJ m^{-2} UVB_{BE}). Absolute reductions varied from 0 to 40% between the seed sources and with needle age. For example, photosynthesis was significantly reduced by up to 40% in needles which had been exposed to UVB for an entire season, but only 19% on recently expanded needles. These reductions, however, were only transient in some plants because they could not be detected following the dormant winter period. This suggests that UVB repair mechanisms may exist. Measurements of chlorophyll fluorescence and the photosynthetic response to light indicated that the quantum yield was significantly reduced in some cases by direct effects on photosystem II. No significant effects were observed on stomatal conductance of transpiration, and chlorophyll concentrations were not generally altered by UVB exposure.

In vitro studies, using isolated chloroplasts, indicate that UVB-induced damage to photochemical reactions is greater in C_3 plants (*Dolichos lab lab, Phaseolus mungo,* and *Triticum vulgare)* than in C_4 *(Amaranthus gangeticus, Zea mays,* and *Pennisetum typhoides*). Such differences are associated with the polypeptide composition of the thylakoids (Kulandaivelu et al., 1993).

Studies in growth chambers with the ozone filter for attenuating solar UVB report significant reductions in net photosynthesis (measured under saturating light conditions) on a leaf area and whole plant basis in sunflower seedlings, when grown for three weeks at a daily maximum temperature of 28°C or 32°C under a 20% higher UVB level compared to controls (5.1 kJ m^{-2} day^{-1} UVB_{BE} vs. 3.6 kJ m^{-2} day^{-1}). These represent average values from May 1990 to August 1990 and are equivalent to approximately a 10% ozone depletion. In contrast, net photosynthesis was lower in maize seedlings only during the earliest stages of development at both temperatures (Tevini et al., 1991c).

11.2.4 *Species competition*

Enhanced UVB exposure can cause changes in the growth of plants without necessarily decreasing plant production. Such changes include reduced leaf length, increased branching, and increased number of leaves (Barnes et al., 1990). These changes seem to be general among different crop and weed species. Both graminoid and broad-leaf species respond in this fashion, with graminoids generally more responsive. Although these growth form changes do not lead to changes in the production of monocultures, in mixed species these alterations can lead to a change in the balance of competition for light.

Multi-year field studies had shown that the balance of competition between wheat and wild oat (a common weed) began to favour wheat when mixtures of these species were subjected to increased UVB irradiation (Barnes et al., 1988). In a recent study involving canopy light microclimate assessments and a detailed canopy radiation interception model, it was shown that the shift in growth-form of the two species was sufficient to quantitatively explain the change in the competitive balance (Ryel et al., 1990). Thus, in many cases where plants are not necessarily depressed in overall growth by increased UVB exposure, changes in growth-form can have ecologically meaningful consequences. The direction of competitive balance changes are not easily predicted at present. However, altered competitive balance also has important implications for mixed-crop agriculture and species composition of nonagricultural ecosystems.

11.2.5 *Plant diseases*

Certain diseases may become more severe in plants exposed to enhanced UVB levels. Sugar beet *(Beta vulgaris)* plants infected with *Cercospora beticola*, and receiving 6.9 kJ m^{-2} day^{-1} UVB_{BE}, showed large reductions in leaf chlorophyll content, and fresh and dry weight of total biomass. In another study, three cucumber *(cucumis sativus)* cultivars were exposed to a daily UVB dose of 11.6 kJ m^{-2} UVB_{BE} in a greenhouse before and/or after infection with *Colletotrichum lagenarium* or *Cladosporium cucumerinum*, and analyzed for disease development (Orth et al., 1990). Two of the three cultivars were disease resistant and the other was disease susceptible. Pre-infection treatment with UVB led to greater disease development in the susceptible cultivar and in one of the disease resistant cultivars. Post-infection treatment did not alter disease development. The increased disease development in UVB irradiated plants was found only on the cotyledons and not on true leaves, suggesting that the effects of UVB on disease development in cucumber vary according to the cultivar, timing of UVB exposure, and tissue age.

11.2.6 *UV-protection systems*

Epidermal pigments

UVB induces flavonoid production (Wellmann, 1971), and may regulate the synthesis of UV protective pigments (Braun & Tevini, 1991). In a study using two important crops (rye and oat), UV-fluence and wavelength dependent accumulation of isovitexin derivatives in the epidermal layer of rye seedlings prevented damage to chloroplast functions. In contrast, photosynthetic function was low without the accumulation of screening pigments (Tevini et al., 1991a). Because the epidermal layer of oat seedlings already accumulates large amounts of UV-absorbing pigments during early development, the photosynthetic apparatus is better protected than rye seedlings against UVB (Braun, 1991). This inherently higher flavonoid production occurs even in absence of UVB irradiation, and appears to be constitutive in nature. UVB induction of flavonoids was demonstrated in two species of columbines, *Aquilegia caerulea*, growing in alpine environments, and *Aquilegia canadensis*, which grows at lower elevations (Larson et al., 1990). In both species, flavonoid content increased upon UVB irradiation, even though the alpine species accumulated higher amounts in the UVB-free controls when compared to A *canadensis* after UVB irradiation. This demonstrates that plants which are already genetically adapted to higher UVB environments can further increase their adaptation capacity.

Photorepair

A second protective mechanism in plants is photoreactivation. The UV-induced production of DNA pyrimidine dimers can be repaired by DNA photolysase. This enzyme was shown to increase with UVB irradiation in *Arabidopsis* (Pang & Hays, 1991) but also by visible light via phytochrome in bean seedlings (Langer & Wellmann, 1990). This inducibility means that *de novo* synthesis of DNA photolysase itself is a target for UV damage. Thus, the repair capacity of the cell may be reduced in the presence of increasing UVB (Wellmann, 1991).

11.3 Effects on Aquatic Ecosystems

Aquatic ecosystems contribute more biomass (104 Gt a^{-1}) than all terrestrial ecosystems (100 Gt a^{-1}) combined. Recent work on UVB effects has concentrated on inhibition mechanisms and field studies in the subpolar waters of Antarctica, because of its high biomass production and the occurrence of the ozone hole over this region.

Phytoplankton organisms orient within the water column using external factors. Mobility and orientation mechanisms are impaired by UVB exposure. Most organisms do not possess UVB receptors, and so cannot avoid deleterious effects of enhanced UVB that produces higher intensities deeper into the water column. New action spectra indicate that, in addition to DNA, other targets absorb UVB including proteins of the photoreceptor and photosynthetic apparatus. The inability of phytoplankton to adjust their position within the water column causes massive inhibition of photosynthesis. In only a few cases have UVB inducible screening pigments been identified.

11.3.1 *Effects on phytoplankton*

Recent UVB aquatic research has concentrated on phytoplankton and the Antarctic ecosystem. As shown in figure 11.2, phytoplankton is at the base of the aquatic food chain/trophic structure and serves as food for primary consumers (e.g., larvae of fish and shrimp), which in turn are consumed by secondary and tertiary consumers (e.g. fish). The production of phytoplankton has been estimated at about 6 x 10^{14} kg (UNEP, 1989). A loss of 10% would far exceed the gross national product of all countries in the world, assuming any reasonable price for biomass on the market. table 11.1 gives the estimated annual biomass production for plankton and fish.

Table 11.1 Estimated annual biomass production at different levels in marine food web and possible loss after 10% decrease at the phytoplankton level (adapted from UNEP 1989 report)

Type	Annual Production (in million tonnes)	10% loss
Phytoplankton	600,000	60,000
Zooplankton	60,000	6,000
Small fish	6,000	600
Large fish	600	60

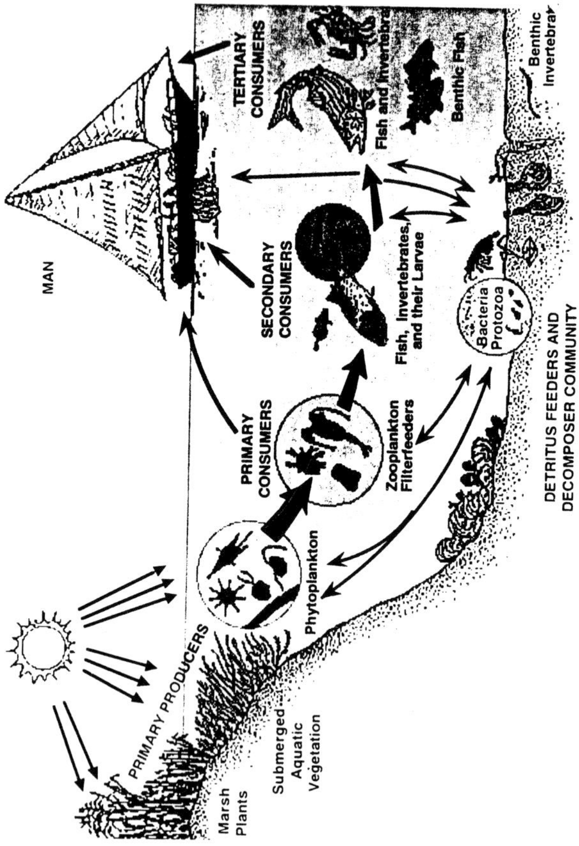

Figure 11.2 Example of the biological food web in a marine ecosystem, which starts with the primary producers; the biomass they produce in utilized by the primary consumers, which in turn serve as food input for the next level in the food web (UNEP, 1989).

Concentrations of phytoplankton in subpolar waters may be 10^3 to 10^4 times greater than concentrations of phytoplankton found in tropical and subtropical seas (Jeffery & Humphrey, 1975). Any significant increase in UVB could well diminish growth and productivity of phytoplankton, subsequently affecting all higher trophic levels in the aquatic food web. Therefore, it is not surprising that a majority of recent research has looked at the effects of increased UVB exposure in Antarctic waters. Ongoing research activities include investigations of both direct (physiological and behavioural) and indirect (trophic implications) effects.

Phytoplankton dwell in the top layers of the water column (the photic zone) because of their requirement for solar energy (Ignatiades, 1990). Their position within the column is maintained by precise orientation strategies using light, gravity and other external factors as guides. Phytoplankton in the photic zone would be exposed to any increase in solar UV. Most phytoplankton organisms do not possess UVB photoreceptors to guide them away from harmful UV, a situation similar to humans. Previous work demonstrated that mobility/orientation mechanisms in response to light are impaired by solar UV (Häder & Worrest, 1991; Baker & Smith, 1982). The ability of phytoplankton to adjust their position within the water column, in response to constantly changing conditions, may even be affected at ambient UVB levels. Although ambient UVB fluxes may cause damage to some species of phytoplankton, it should be emphasized that there are uncertainties regarding the magnitude of these effects. These included problems of extrapolating laboratory findings to the open sea and the nearly complete absence of data on long-term effects and ecosystem responses. Likewise, there is a need to investigate adaptation mechanisms. Before effects of exposure to solar UVB can be predicted, information is required on seasonal abundances and vertical distributions of marine organisms, vertical mixing, and the penetration of UVB into appropriate water columns.

In their natural habitats, organisms are exposed to a wide range of UVB intensities. This radiation has been shown to affect growth, photosynthesis, nitrogen incorporation, and enzyme activity (Döhler & Alt, 1989; Döhler, 1990).

11.3.2 *UV increase and primary biomass production*

Recent results indicate that orientation mechanisms responsive to both light and gravity are affected by solar UV in a number of ecologically significant phytoplankton groups (Häder & Lui, 1991). Action spectra inhibitory effects are different from the DNA absorption spectrum and the action spectra calculated for higher plants, suggesting that UV exposure affects these organisms by a different mechanism. Proteins essential for specific functions such as orientation and photosynthesis are the primary targets of UVB.

Biochemical analyses conducted to reveal the molecular targets of UVB inhibition show that specific photoreceptor proteins are degraded. Simultaneously photosynthetic pigments (responsible for converting solar energy) are bleached and destroyed by radiation (UNEP, 1989). The results of these biochemical studies are further supported by spectroscopic investigations showing losses in pigmentation.

In order to evaluate the effects of enhanced UV, the vertical movement of natural phytoplankton was analyzed in 3m Plexiglas columns (Eggersdorfer & Häder, 1991). Most organisms moved to the surface during daytime hours, although some species avoided periods of intense UV during the midday hours by moving slightly down in the water column. However, this avoidance response is not sufficient to protect organisms under conditions of increased UVB irradiation (UNEP, 1989).

The UVB irradiance in Antarctic waters significantly increased during the occurrence of the ozone hole (Bidigare, 1989; Lubin et al., 1989; Karentz & Lutze, 1990). However changes in marine productivity accompanying UV flux changes have not been determined. Recent measurements show that UVB penetrates 65 meters deep into clear Antarctic waters (UNEP 1991). Consequently, measurements of photosynthetic biomass production in Antarctic waters under the ozone hole show a pronounced decrease in productivity by up to 25% (Holm-Hansen, 1990).

Field studies indicate that photosynthesis is impaired first, followed by decreases in protein concentration and changes in pigment composition. As a result, a dramatic decrease in photosynthetic oxygen production can be measured after exposure to solar radiation (Smith et al., 1980). Other spectral bands, such as UVA and visible radiation, may contribute to photosynthetic inhibition (Smith et al., 1980). Likewise, photosynthetic inhibition has been detected in macroalgae at their natural depth (Bittersmann et al., 1988; Nultsch et al., 1990).

In contrast to higher plants only a few photoplanktons produce UV absorbing substances (Carretto et al., 1990; Karentz et al., 1991b). However, all of these mycosporine-like amino acids have maximal absorption in the UVA range and only secondary peaks in the UVB. It is not clear whether the production of these potentially screening substances can be induced by exposing organisms to UV (Raven, 1991). One exception is cyanobacteria where a UVB inducible pigment has been found within the slime sheath surrounding the organisms, which absorbs up to 88% of the incident UVB (Garcia-Pichel and Castenholz, 1991).

11.4 Conclusion

Field and laboratory experiments on plant responses to increased UVB radiation underscore the concern for agriculture, forestry and natural ecosystems as the stratospheric ozone level is depleted.

Growth and photosynthesis of certain crop plants can be inhibited even under ambient levels of UVB radiation. Certain environmental factors, both biotic (e.g. plant diseases and competition with other plants) and abiotic (e.g. carbon dioxide, temperature, heavy metals, and water availability) can alter UVB effects in plants. This increases the difficulty in making any quantitative predictions. Plants in temperate regions and certain tropical species were found to be adversely affected by enhanced UVB radiation.

Marine ecosystem which provides the primary food for human consumption (in some countries) has been shown to be more sensitive to UVB than terrestrial plants. One consequence of loss in phytoplankton is reduced biomass production which would be propagated throughout the whole food web. The marine phytoplankton is a major absorber of atmospheric carbon dioxide. Any reduction in this population would decrease the uptake of carbon dioxide and so augment the greenhouse effect.

12. HEALTH HAZARD ASSESSMENT

12.1 Introduction

For the vast majority of people, the sun is the single largest source of exposure to UV. In some cases solar exposure will be elective such as from sunbathing, in others it will be adventitious as a result of outdoor recreational and/or occupational activity. Exposure may also occur from artificial sources of UV, either deliberately for example during medical treatment or the use of a sunbed for cosmetic purposes.

The health risks associated with exposure to UV include those of both acute and chronic effects and will vary according to the nature of the exposure. Factors important in assessing such risks include: the biologically-effective irradiance of the UV incident on the person exposed; the duration and frequency of occurrence of exposures; and the individual sensitivity of the person to UV as determined by genetic and other factors.

International guidelines on protection against UV given in chapter 13 are based on available scientific data (IRPA/INIRC, 1991). The guidelines define occupational exposure limits (ELs) below which it is expected that nearly all people may be repeatedly exposed without adverse effects. The Els are intended to be used to evaluate potentially hazardous exposures from, for example, solar radiation, arcs, gas and vapour discharges, fluorescent lamps and incandescent sources. The Els are generally below levels which are often used for the UV exposure of patients required as part of medical treatment and below levels associated with sunbed exposure. IRPA/INIRC recommend that, where they are to be incorporated in regulations, the ELs should be considered as absolute limits for the eye, but only as advisory for the skin. This is because of the wide range of susceptibility to skin injury depending on skin type. The values were developed by considering lightly pigmented populations, with greatest sensitivity to sunburn and non-melanocytic skin cancer. In recommending similar limits, Threshold Limit Values (TLVs), the American Conference of Governmental Industrial Hygienists (ACGIH 1993) indicate that conditioned, tanned, individuals can tolerate skin exposure in excess of the exposure limits without sunburn effects, but that conditioning may not protect individuals against skin cancer. ELs are not intended to apply to exposure of pathologically photosensitive individuals, to people concomitantly exposed to photosensitising agents or to neonates.

The threshold for adverse acute effects may be exceeded in certain people without exceeding the exposure limit. The risk of skin cancer increases with cumulative exposure over time. Therefore, it is recommended that all exposures should be reduced as far as is reasonably practicable.

An estimate of the risk of cumulative exposure to UV can be expressed in terms of the cumulative incidence (I) of non-melanoma skin cancer in the form of the equation (Schothorst et al., 1985; Diffey 1988).

$$I = \gamma\, A\, H^{\beta}\, a^{\alpha} \qquad 12.1$$

where I is the total number of cases per 100,000 of the population in the age group up to age 'a' years:

H is the annual carcinogenic-effective radiant exposure at the skin surface:

A is the fraction of the body surface area exposed:

γ, β and α are numerical constants reflecting the genetic susceptibility of the exposed population, the biological amplification factor and the age dependence of the cumulative incidence respectively.

The above equation applies only to situations where the annual effective exposure remains constant year by year. This will not be the case, for example, for workers whose job may result in additional occupational exposure during their working lives (Diffey 1988). In these circumstances the cumulative incidence I can be represented by the equation (Slaper et al., 1986).

$$I = \gamma\, A\, H_e^{\beta}\, a^{\alpha} \qquad 12.2$$

where H_e is given by

$$H_e = H + H_o(a-a_s)/a$$

H is the annual effective radiant exposure of solar UV:

a_s is the age at which the occupational exposure began:

H_o is the annual effective radiant exposure from occupational exposure.

In the following sections estimates of personal exposures likely to result from different situations are considered and, where the availability of data permits, examples of estimates of quantitative risk are provided. The exposure situations include elective exposure to solar UV, from medical treatment and from the use of sunbeds, as well as adventitious exposure resulting from solar radiation and from artificial sources of UV.

12.2 Elective Exposures

12.2.1 *Medical exposure*

UV is used in medicine for both the diagnosis and treatment of disease. The highest and most extensive medical exposures to UV result from phototherapy and photochemotherapy.

Medical treatment using UV carries the risk of acute side effects and long term risks of chronic effects, in particular skin cancer. The acute side effects of UVB phototherapy exposure include; reddening, swelling, blistering and desquamation of the skin. The acute effects following PUVA treatment include itching, skin pain and nausea (Green et al., 1992).

Chronic effects include those on both the eyes and the skin. However, the eyes of patients are generally well protected during PUVA treatment and only one case of PUVA induced cataract in humans appears to have been reported (Cyrlin 1980). Structural changes in the skin, akin to those characteristic of long term damage resulting from solar radiation exposure, have been observed as a result of both UVB and PUVA phototherapy.

The risk of skin cancer from ultraviolet phototherapy has been reviewed by Green et al. (1992). They conclude that data on the association between UVB phototherapy and skin cancer are very poor. Only one case control study has been reported and no correlation was found between UVB phototherapy and skin cancer in 85 patients who had received UVB phototherapy for up to 25 years. The association between PUVA treatment and skin cancer in psoriasis patients has been reported in ten studies. However, only one study (Stern et al., 1979) indicated that PUVA acted as an independent carcinogen, the risk of developing skin cancer being 6-12 times that of a population survey. The results of other studies point to PUVA acting in the role of a co-carcinogen, other factors involved being a family history of skin cancer and treatment with antipsoriatic medication. Comparisons and interpretations of data from US and European studies have been complicated by differences in the exposure regimens used.

12.2.2 *Phototherapy of seasonal affective disorder (SAD)*

Typical treatment consists of sitting in front of a panel of fluorescent lamps and exposing the face, with the eyes open, to an illuminance of about 2500 lux for 2 to 6 hours per day during the winter months. This is equivalent to a daily erythemally-effective radiant exposure of up to 40 J m^{-2} (Diffey 1993). An annual cumulative exposure of up to 24 MEDs results, which, if continued for several decades is estimated to result in a risk of non-melanoma skin cancer of about 1.5, compared with someone (typical indoor worker) minimally exposed.

12.2.3 *Sunbeds*

Among lightly pigmented people, a suntanned skin is unfortunately still socially desirable. The establishment of the 'suntanning industry' has enabled the acquisition of a 'suntan' irrespective of the availability of solar radiation. Suntanning is caused by UV and as with exposure to the sun, there are attendant risks in using sunbeds.

Adverse health effects of sunbed use include acute effects on the skin, longer term structural damage of the skin and increased risk of skin cancer (Roza et al., 1989). Provided that appropriate protective eyewear is worn, adverse health effects on the eyes will be avoided. The extent to which adverse, but relatively transient skin effects occur is demonstrated by the results of a survey of the use of sunbeds in the United Kingdom (Diffey 1986). Questionnaire replies from over 1000 sunbed users indicated that the incidence of acute adverse effects was substantial; 28% of users complained of itching and about 8% developed a skin rash or had felt nauseous at some time during or immediately after exposure. The incidence of such effects was higher among women taking oral contraceptives than in women who were not. No conclusion could be drawn about other medications as few individuals were taking them. The survey also revealed that 50% of sunbed users in the United Kingdom are female and aged between 16 and 30 years. 43% of users had skin types I and II, the most sensitive to the adverse effects of UV and the ones least likely to tan well.

Structural damage to human skin from exposure to UVA, such as demonstrated experimentally in mice (Kligman et al., 1987, Bissett et al., 1989) might be expected in people as the result of excessive use of sunbeds. Increased skin fragility and blistering (Farr et al., 1988; Murphy 1989) and atypical melanocytic lesions (Jones et al., 1987) have been observed in people who have used UVA sunbeds excessively. In some people, photodermatosis and polymorphic light eruption, is readily caused by exposure to UVA radiation from a sunbed (Rivers et al., 1989). Certain photo-aggravated dermatoses, such as lupus erythematosus, are exacerbated by the use of UVA sunbeds (Stern and Docken 1986). The use of certain medications such as antihypertensives and antibiotics (Hawk 1984) and topical application of certain products, including perfumes, body lotions, etc., may produce a photosensitising effect on exposure to a sunbed.

Some localised skin and systemic changes in immunological reactions result from exposure to UV and, of particular relevance to sunbeds, from exposure to UVA. There is also evidence that exposure to UV can accelerate the growth of human viruses (e.g. Otani and Mori 1987, Perna et al., 1987), including human immunodeficiency virus (HIV) (Zmudzka and Beer 1990). At present, the significance of these observations with respect to the health of people exposed to UV from sunbeds is unclear.

The risk of non-melanocytic skin cancer in northern Europeans who sunbathe and who use sunbeds has been estimated by Diffey (1987) using a mathematical model of skin cancer incidence that makes allowance for childhood, occupational and recreational solar radiation exposure. The model takes into account the fractions of total skin surface area that might normally be exposed during everyday activities and the larger fraction, normally unexposed, but exposed during sunbathing and sunbed use. The annual effective radiant exposures resulting from different activities and exposure scenarios used as the basis for risk calculations are expressed as representative minimal erythemal doses (MEDs) in table 12.1.

Table 12.1 Representative annual minimal erythemal doses (MEDs) for various exposure scenarios in northern Europeans (Diffey, 1987, 1993a).

Scenario	Annual MEDs
Outdoor worker	270
Indoor worker (including weekend exposure)	90
Sunbathing holiday in Mediterranean area for 2 week period in summer	50-100
UVA sunbed (low pressure fluorescent lamps, 30 x 30 minute sessions *	20

* Recommended maximum number of sessions per year (IRPA/INIRC, 1991a) with estimated exposure of 0.7 MED per session (Diffey, 1987).

Diffey (1987) concluded that the increased risk of non-melanocytic skin cancer associated with the use of a UVA sunbed for 10 sessions per year is negligible. However, frequent use of a sunbed, for example once per week from the age of 20 years will result in an estimated doubling of the risk of non-melanocytic skin cancer by age 45 years.

Several studies have reported increased risks of cutaneous melanoma in users of sunlamps and sunbeds (IARC 1992).

12.2.4 *Sunbathing*

A significant contribution to the risk of non-melanocytic skin cancer that results from sunbathing (Diffey, 1987). In these calculations it was assumed that the subjects were indoor workers who began sunbathing at age 20 years, and that their annual exposure up to age 16 years is one half that of an outdoor worker. An indoor worker who does not sunbathe is estimated to have a 2-3% risk of non-melanoma skin cancer by age 70. Annual two week vacations spent sunbathing at Mediterranean latitudes (~40°N) will increase this risk by a factor of about 5. Sunbathing for four weeks annually is estimated to result in a 10-20 fold increase in cumulative risk compared with non-sunbathers. It should be stressed that sunbathing during vacation periods was assumed to take place for nearly the whole day on every day of vacation. This is unlikely to be the case for most holiday makers and so the estimated risk factors for most people taking holidays in a sunny climate are likely to be one-third to one-half of those given.

12.3 Adventitious Exposures

12.3.1 *Outdoor exposures*

Studies using personal dosimeters to monitor exposure of individuals to UV have shown that, on average the carcinogenic-effective UV exposure (excluding vacation exposure) of outdoor workers is about 3 times that of indoor workers (Holman et al., 1983; Larko and Diffey 1983; Schothorst et al., 1985). Assuming that up to the age of 16, indoor and outdoor workers receive the same carcinogenic-effective radiant exposure and that both receive equivalent vacation exposures, the relative risk for non-melanoma skin cancer for outdoor workers is estimated to be 3.7 times that for indoor workers (Diffey 1987). However, recent population studies have found only small differences in skin cancer incidence between outdoor and indoor workers (see chapter 8).

Armstrong & Kricker (1994) have estimated the proportion of cutaneous malignant melanomas that is caused by sun exposure. The estimated proportions varied from 0.97 in males and 0.96 in females in Queensland, Australia, when the incidence on the whole body was compared with the incidence on unexposed sites, to 0.68 when the incidence in people born in Australia was compared with that in migrants to Australia from areas of lower sun exposure. A comparison of whites and blacks in the US in which the incidence in blacks was taken as the incidence in unexposed whites, gave estimates of 0.96 in males and 0.92 in females. It was estimated that some 59,000 (65%) of about 92,000 malignant melanomas worldwide in 1985 were caused by sun exposure.

12.3.2 *Artificial sources*

General public exposure

Exposure of the general public to potentially hazardous levels of UV from artificial sources is unlikely. However, an area that merits note is the increased use of tungsten halogen lamps for lighting. Very high filament temperatures combined with quartz envelopes results in the emission of significantly higher levels of UV compared with conventional incandescent lamps (Césarini & Muel, 1989; McKinlay et al., 1989). For many applications of such lamps the presence of a glass filter effectively attenuates the potentially harmful UV. However, for some others, and particularly when such lamps are incorporated in desk-top luminaires, no protective filter is present, and significantly high levels of erythemally effective UV have been measured. However, for lamps of similar design and having nominally the same power, there is a wide range of emitted levels of UV, (for example, between 2 and 56 mW m^{-2} effective, in the beam of the lamp at 30 cm distance)

Occupational exposure

Sources that emit UV are used for a wide range of applications in the workplace. High intensity discharge sources should be, and often are, contained in interlocked enclosures thus obviating hazardous exposure of people. Hazard evaluation surveys generally consist of measurements of the effective exposure levels of UV and comparison with recommended guidelines on limiting exposure. This approach addresses the adverse acute effects of exposure, but very few risk assessments have been carried out in relation to chronic effects. The risk of non-melanocytic skin cancer for any occupational situation can be calculated using multivariant analysis, provided the effective exposures related to the occupation are known. However, although data on levels of exposure exist for some occupational situations there is generally a paucity of such data. Where estimates of skin cancer risk have been made, they have related to specific occupational exposure situations (Diffey 1988, 1989) or broadly with respect to general (fluorescent) lighting (Lytle et al., 1993).

Examples where occupational exposure to UV from artificial sources may occur include; electric arc plasma welding, the drying and curing of inks, resins, plastics and paints; printing, graphics arts, copying (using photographic processes) and photography, photoetching, projector lamps operation, medicine, scientific laboratory work, tanning and salon work and UV associated with general lighting fluorescent lamps and desk-top and other luminaires incorporating tungsten halogen lamps.

Welders are likely to be the largest occupational group with potential exposure to UV (IARC 1992). The UV effective irradiance levels around an operating welding arc can exceed recommended exposure guideline levels by several orders of magnitude, and the occurrence of acute effects of exposure, photokeratitis and erythema, is common (Eriksen 1987).

Many industrial photoprocesses use high intensity discharge lamps that emit copious quantities of UV. However, most of these sources are effectively shielded and interlocked to prevent human exposure. Some sources emit leakage radiation and, under these circumstances, a detailed measurement survey is required to assess the degree of hazard.

Medical physiotherapists involved in the phototherapy of patients are occupationally exposed to UV and an analysis of probable risk has been published (Diffey 1988). During a working life of 40 years, the additional risk of non-melanoma skin cancer for a member of this group is estimated to be around 25% compared with that for non-exposed workers.

General lighting

Low pressure mercury vapour fluorescent lamps are ubiquitous in the workplace and the home and concern has been expressed regarding the potential role of the UV they emit in the aetiology of malignant melanoma. Epidemiological data on exposure to general lighting fluorescent lamps and malignant melanoma are few and inconsistent. IRPA/INIRC (1991) concluded that UV exposure from indoor fluorescent lighting should not be considered as a malignant melanoma risk.

The exposure levels associated with the use of general lighting fluorescent lamps have been measured in a number of studies (Cole et al., 1986; McKinlay & Whillock, 1987; Muel et al., 1988 and Lytle et al., 1993). Exposure data vary considerably depending on the types of lamps examined and the exposure conditions considered. A recent study (Lytle et al., 1993) serves to illustrate estimates of the risk associated with long term exposure to unfiltered general lighting fluorescent lamps used in the United States. It was estimated that 50 years exposure to typical unfiltered levels of UV from fluorescent lamps added approximately 4% (1.6 - 12%) to any risks associated with exposure to solar UV.

13. INTERNATIONAL GUIDELINES ON EXPOSURE TO ULTRAVIOLET RADIATION

A number of national and international organizations have promulgated guidelines or standards on exposure to UV. Most are based upon the same basic criteria of ACGIH (1993) and IRPA/INIRC (1991).

The basic exposure limit (EL) for both general public and occupational exposure to UV incident on the skin or eye is 30 J m^{-2} effective), when the spectral irradiance E_λ at the eye or skin surface is mathematically weighted with the hazard relative spectral effectiveness factor S_λ from 180 nm to 400 nm. This is given as follows:

$$E_{eff} = \Sigma\, E_\lambda \; S_\lambda \; \Delta_\lambda$$

where:

E_{eff} = effective irradiance W m^{-2}

E_λ = spectral irradiance from measurements in W m^{-2} nm^{-1}

S_λ = relative spectral effectiveness factor (unit-less)

Δ_λ = bandwidth of the calculation or measurement in nm

At 270 nm in the UVC range, S_λ is 1.0, but at 360 nm in the centre of the UVA range, its value falls to 0.00013, and continues to fall for longer wavelengths.

For the UVA, the total radiant exposure incident on the unprotected eye should not exceed 10^4 J m^{-2} (1 J cm^{-2}) within an 8 h period. The total 8 h radiant exposure incident on the unprotected skin should not exceed the values in table 13.1.

The radiant UV exposure incident upon the unprotected skin or eye within an 8-hour period should not exceed the values given in table 13.1. The limits apply to sources whose emissions are measured with an instrument having a cosine response detector oriented perpendicular to the most directly exposed surfaces of the body when assessing skin exposure and along (or parallel to) the line(s) of sight when assessing ocular exposure. Although no measurement averaging aperture is recommended, 1 mm is commonly used.

Table 13.1 International UV exposure limits and spectral weighting factor (IRPA/INIRC, 1991)

Wavelength[a] (nm)	EL ($J\ m^{-2}$)	EL ($mJ\ cm^{-2}$)	Relative Spectral Effectiveness S_λ
180	2,500	250	0.012
190	1,600	160	0.019
200	1,000	100	0.030
205	590	59	0.051
210	400	40	0.075
215	320	32	0.095
220	250	25	0.120
225	200	20	0.150
230	160	16	0.190
235	130	13	0.240
240	100	20	0.300
245	83	8.3	0.360
250	70	7.0	0.430
254[b]	60	6.0	0.500
255	58	5.8	0.520
260	46	4.6	0.650
265	37	3.7	0.810
270	30	3.0	1.000
275	31	3.1	0.960
280[b]	34	3.4	0.880
285	39	3.9	0.770
290	47	4.7	0.640
295	56	5.6	0.540
297[b]	65	6.5	0.460
300	100	10	0.300
303[b]	250	25	0.190
305	500	50	0.060
308	1,200	120	0.026
310	2,000	200	0.015
313[b]	5,000	500	0.006
315	1.0×10^4	1.0×10^3	0.003
316	1.3×10^4	1.3×10^3	0.0024

Table 13.1 International UV exposure limits and spectral weighting factor (IRPA/INIRC, 1991)

Wavelength[a] (nm)	EL ($J\ m^{-2}$)	EL ($mJ\ cm^{-2}$)	Relative Spectral Effectiveness S_λ
317	1.5×10^4	1.5×10^3	0.0020
318	1.9×10^4	1.9×10^3	0.0016
319	2.5×10^4	2.5×10^3	0.0012
320	2.9×10^4	2.9×10^3	0.0010
322	4.5×10^4	4.5×10^3	0.00067
323	5.6×10^4	5.6×10^3	0.00054
325	6.0×10^4	6.0×10^3	0.00050
328	6.8×10^4	6.8×10^3	0.00044
330	7.3×10^4	7.3×10^3	0.00041
333	8.1×10^4	8.1×10^3	0.00037
335	8.8×10^4	8.8×10^3	0.00034
340	1.1×10^5	1.1×10^4	0.00028
345	1.3×10^5	1.3×10^4	0.00024
350	1.5×10^5	1.5×10^4	0.00020
355	1.9×10^5	1.9×10^4	0.00016
360	2.3×10^5	2.3×10^4	0.00013
365[b]	2.7×10^5	2.7×10^4	0.00011
370	3.2×10^5	3.2×10^4	0.000093
375	3.9×10^5	3.9×10^4	0.000077
380	4.7×10^5	4.7×10^4	0.000064
385	5.7×10^5	5.7×10^4	0.000053
390	6.8×10^5	6.8×10^4	0.000044
395	8.3×10^5	8.3×10^4	0.000036
400	1.0×10^6	1.0×10^5	0.000030

[a] Wavelengths chosen are representative; other values should be interpolated at intermediate wavelengths.

[b] Emission lines of a mercury discharge spectrum.

The permissible exposure duration, t_{max}, for exposure (in seconds) to UV is calculated by:

$$t_{max} = 30/\ E_{eff}\ (W\ m^{-2})$$

Examples are provided in table 13.2.

Table 13.2 Limiting UV exposure durations based on exposure limits (IRPA/INIRC, 1991)

Duration of exposure per day	Effective irradiance	
	E_{eff} (W m^{-2})	E_{eff} (μW cm^{-2})
8 hours	0.001	0.1
4 hours	0.002	0.2
2 hours	0.004	0.4
1 hour	0.008	0.8
30 minutes	0.017	1.7
15 minutes	0.033	3.3
10 minutes	0.05	5

The EL's were developed considering lightly pigmented populations with greatest sensitivity and predisposition to adverse health effects from exposure to UV. The limits apply to UV exposure of the working population, but with some precaution also apply to the general public. However, some rare, highly photosensitive individuals exist who may react adversely to exposure at these levels. These individuals are normally aware of their heightened sensitivity. Likewise, if individuals are concomitantly exposed to photosensitizing agents, an enhanced reaction can take place. Many individuals who are exposed to photosensitizing agents (ingested or externally applied chemicals, e.g., in cosmetics, foods, drugs, industrial chemicals, etc.) may not be aware of their heightened sensitivity. Lightly pigmented individuals conditioned by previous UV exposure (leading to tanning and hyperplasia) and heavily pigmented individuals can tolerate skin exposure in excess of the EL's without erythemal effects. However, repeated tanning may increase the risk of accelerated skin aging and even skin cancer. Such risks should be understood prior to the use of UV for medical phototherapy or cosmetic exposures.

14. PROTECTIVE MEASURES

14.1 Introduction

It is widely accepted by scientific and medical authorities throughout the world that UV is potentially carcinogenic and capable of producing other undesirable health effects. It is sensible therefore to take steps to minimise UV exposure. Many risks in life are completely beyond our control such as contracting a rare disease. However, risks to health associated with exposure to UV from both natural and artificial sources can be substantially reduced by taking appropriate control measures.

Since UV exposure occurs externally, simple measures can be taken to reduce the exposures received. A high degree of protection can be afforded by protective clothing (including hats), UV protective eyewear (welding helmets, face shields, goggles, sunglasses, spectacles etc.) and by sunscreens for exposed skin. However, the degree of protection afforded can be reduced by ingestion of photosensitizing drugs or photoallergic/phototoxic reactions produced by chemicals or cosmetics in contact with the skin. Thus, education is also an important control measure.

14.2 Education

Concern about high incidences of skin cancer and eye damage have led to national educational campaigns in some countries to encourage people to protect themselves against excessive UV exposure from the sun and in the workplace. Educational programmes directed at both the workforce and the public are intended to create an awareness of the adverse health effects that can result from overexposure to UV.

Presently, in several different countries around the world, daily environmental UV levels are supplied to the general public in the form of UV indices. Their provision is intended to educate the public on the basic climatology of UV, increase awareness of the hazards of UV and provide information necessary to plan protection. In a report commissioned to investigate Canadian attitudes to Environment Canada's UV index (Environment Canada, 1993), it was found that 73% of Canadians were aware of the UV index, 91% believed UV affected human health, and most important, 59% of respondents who were aware of the UV index had changed their sun exposure habits.

Different countries have adopted their own national UV indices. Unfortunately, they are not all compatible. Clearly, international uniformity would help to prevent confusion.

Educational programmes aim to produce a change in knowledge and attitudes, then a change in behaviour and eventually a reduction in the incidence and mortality rates of skin cancer. A survey of sunscreen use on beaches in Brisbane, Australia found about 70% of females and males applied sunscreen. Half of the sunscreens provided the maximum protection (SPF 15+) and almost 90% used a waterproof formulation. However, the sunscreen was not applied over the entire body with over half neglecting ears and lower limbs (Pincus et al., 1991). Survey results show that sunburn is still occurring; in a randomly selected group of adults in Melbourne, Australia 16% reported sunburn over a summer weekend (Hill et al., 1992). With regard to skin cancers it is still too early to evaluate the effectiveness of current educational/publicity campaigns.

With respect to changes in behaviour, there is good reason to avoid exposure to the midday sun since it has been estimated that up to one third of the day's erythemally effective UV is received within the period one hour before noon to one hour after noon. Shade is a useful method of protection but its value should not be over-estimated, as one may be exposed to a quarter or more of the total solar UV while shaded from direct sunlight, depending on the prevailing exposure conditions.

14.3 Protection Factors

The concept of a protection factor is useful when attempting to quantify the UV protection that items such as sunscreens, clothing and eyewear can provide (Gies et al., 1992). To determine the protection factor, the following procedure is conducted. An effective dose (ED) of UV to the unprotected skin or eye is calculated by summing the incident solar spectral power over the wavelength range 280 to 400 nm. In order to determine the effective dose (ED_m) for the skin or eye when it is protected, the calculation is repeated with the spectral transmission of the protection item as an additional weighting. The protection factor (PF) is then defined as the ratio of ED to ED_m and is given by the following equation:

$$PF = \frac{ED}{ED_m} \quad \frac{\Sigma E_\lambda \cdot S_\lambda \cdot \Delta\lambda}{\Sigma E_\lambda \cdot S_\lambda \cdot T_\lambda \cdot \Delta\lambda}$$

where:

E_λ = spectral irradiance (W m^{-2} nm^{-1}) at wavelength λ

S_λ = relative spectral effectiveness

T_λ = spectral transmission of protective item at wavelength λ

$\Delta\lambda$ = wavelength interval or bandwidth (nm)

λ = wavelength (nm)

The inclusion of the spectral effectiveness function in the calculation ensures that sufficient weighting is given to the biologically effective wavelengths below 315 nm. A description of how the protection factors for fabrics, eyewear and sunscreens are determined is given in Roy and Gies (1993) and CIE (1991).

14.4 Clothing

Use of protective clothing provides one of the simplest means of reducing UV exposure. Hats have been shown to afford protection, to various degrees, to the forehead, scalp, ears and most of the neck. Their protective properties have been studied by Diffey and Cheeseman (1992). In this study hats were classified into four categories, small brim, medium brim, large brim and peaked cap. The protection afforded to different anatomical sites on the head and neck is shown in table 14.1.

Table 14.1 Sun protection for various anatomical sites on the head and neck provided by different types of hat (Diffey & Cheeseman, 1992).

	Typical sun protection factor*				
Style of hat	Forehead	Nose	Cheek	Chin	Back of neck
Small brim < 2.5 cm	15	1.5	1	1	1
Medium brim 2.5-7.5 cm	>20	3	2	1	1
Large brim >7.5 cm	>20	7	3	1.2	5
Peaked cap	>20	5	1.5	1	1

* In this table 'sun protection factor' is defined as the reciprocal of the fraction of UV exposure recorded relative to that of the unprotected head.

The degree of protection provided by clothing depends on the penetration of UV through materials and this can vary considerably. Fabrics which are visibly opaque tend to be more highly absorbent of UV, but the structure or weave of a material is the most important factor in determining its protective value. Colour and thickness are a poor guide to UV protection. The transmission properties of some fabrics commonly used in the manufacture of clothing for everyday wear are given in table 14.2 (Welsh and Diffey 1981). Here the protection factor is an estimate of the protection afforded against biologically effective solar radiation. A high protection factor is associated with a tightly woven material. UV is transmitted and scattered through the interstices of the material itself rather than penetrating the fabric.

Gies et al. (1992) have recently extended the concept of protection factor (PF) to fabrics and proposed the Ultraviolet Protection Factor (UPF). The UPF scheme, as shown in table 14.3, is designed to give the general public information on the amount of UV protection available from fabrics and clothing and is now in use in Australia. UPF is analogous to SPF and a fabric of UPF 10 would, in principle, provide a similar level of protection as a sunscreen of SPF 10.

Table 14.2 UVB transmission properties of common fabrics (from Welsh & Diffey 1981)

Fabric	Structure	Colour	Thickness (mm)	% of incident UV transmitted	Protection factor
Nylon-tricel	Woven	Black	0.1	0.15	750
Nylon-viscose jacquard	Woven	Black	0.2	0.20	500
Nylon	Woven	White	0.1	1.7	55
Nylon-terylene mixture	Knitted	Blue	0.2	11	9
Nylon-acetate jersey	Knitted	Pink	0.2	24	4
Polyester-slub viscose	Woven	Pink	0.5	9	14
Polyester-printed lawn	Woven	Red	0.2	7	11
Polyester-jersey	Knitted	Fawn	0.3	7	14
Polyester-jersey	Knitted	Cream	0.4	5	19
Polyester-jersey	Knitted	Black	0.3	8	12
Polyester-jersey	Knitted	Orange	0.3	5	23
Polyester-jersey	Knitted	Turquoise	0.5	16	6
Polyester-jersey	Knitted	Brown	0.7	1.6	68
Polyester-jersey	Knitted	Black	0.5	4.4	23
Polyester-brushed jersey	Knitted	Blue	0.4	5.2	19
Polyester-brushed jersey	Knitted	Green	0.4	6.0	16
Polyester-bouclette	Knitted	Orange	0.4	3.0	33
Polyester-bouclette	Knitted	Purple	0.4	2.0	51
Cotton-needlecord	Woven	Brown	0.5	< 0.1	> 1000
Cotton-denim	Woven	Blue	0.5	< 0.1	> 1000
Cotton-printed	Woven	Brown	0.3	< 0.1	>1000
Cotton-printed	Woven	Cream	0.3	2.7	36
Wool-jersey	Knitted	Fawn	0.7	0.7	150

Table 14.3 Summary of the ultraviolet protection factor scheme for fabrics

Ultraviolet protection factor UPF	Mean % UV transmission	Protection category
UPF 40+	less than 2.5	Maximum protection 40+
UPF 30 to 39	3.3 to 2.5	Very high protection
UPF 20 to 29	5.0 to 3.3	High protection

Whether a material is wet or dry is important in relation to its UV transmission properties. The spectral transmittances of some cotton and polyester-cotton samples are shown in figure 14.1. Measurements show that the variation of UPF for wet and dry fabrics is consistent for cotton, all examples showing a decrease in UPF when wet (Gies et al., 1992). The variation in UPFs between wet and dry was less consistent for polyester-cotton than for the cotton, some UPFs increasing for wet fabric, while others decreased.

14.5 Sunscreens

Sunscreens are physical and chemical topical preparations which attenuate the transmission of solar UV into the skin by absorption, reflection or scattering. Physical sunscreens (sunblocks), for example zinc oxide, titanium dioxide or red ferric oxide, function by reflecting and scattering and provide protection against a broad spectrum of UV and visible wavelengths. They are normally nontoxic and have few known adverse effects. Sunscreens based on chemical absorbers contain one or more colourless UV-absorbing ingredients which generally absorb UVB radiation more strongly that UVA. Para-aminobenzoic acid (PABA) and its derivatives, salicylates, cinnamates and camphor derivatives primarily absorb UVB and transmit UVA; benzophenones essentially absorb UV of wavelengths of less than 360 nm. The use of solely UVA absorbers (di-benzoyl-methane) is allowed in only certain countries. These chemicals are all based on benzene (Moseley 1988).

The application of any sunscreen normally changes the spectrum of UV that reaches the target cells. Although most sunscreens are designed to attenuate UV, some contain additives such as bergamot oil (containing

Figure 14.1 Percentage transmissions of wet and dry samples of cotton and polyester fabrics (from Gies et al., 1992).

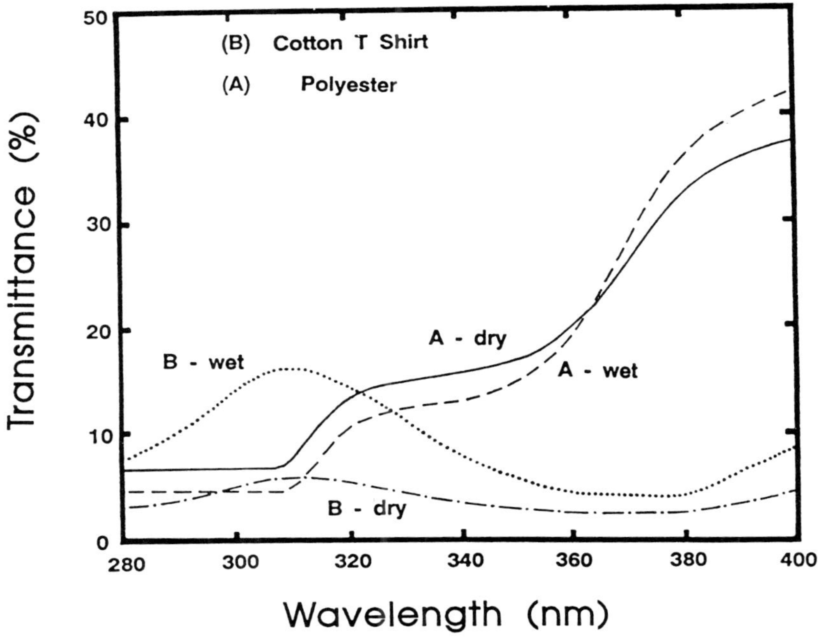

5-methoxypsoralen) to enhance pigmentation and photoprotection (Young et al., 1991). The role of such preparations remains controversial.

The generally accepted parameter for evaluating the efficacy of sunscreen preparations is the sun protection factor (SPF), which is defined as the ratio of the least amount of UV required to produce minimal erythema after application of a standard quantity of the sunscreen to the skin to that required to produce the same erythema without sunscreen application. Several countries have published recommendations for the efficacy testing of propriety sunscreens, e.g. the US Food and Drug Administration (1978) and CIE (1991).

Many factors influence SPF values; particularly important are the spectral power distribution of the source used for SPF testing and a clear definition of the end-point used for assessment (Urbach, 1989). Variations in these factors can lead to considerable differences in measured SPF values for the same product.

SPF values generally reflect the degree of protection against solar UVB radiation, but their protective capacity against UVA must also be defined. Several in-vivo and in-vitro methods have been proposed for defining protection against UVA but there is currently no international consensus on which is the most appropriate. However, this issue is currently being considered by a technical committee of the CIE.

Correctly used, sunscreens are effective in preventing sunburn. Actual SPF values depend critically on the thickness of the application and on other factors such as absorption into the skin, sweating and contact with water (for example while swimming).

If sun exposure causes skin cancer, it would be expected that the use of efficient sunscreens would prevent skin cancer. In animal experiments, sunscreens with a SPF of as low as 4 have been shown to be effective in preventing or delaying the onset of UV-induced skin tumours and cancers (Forbes et al., 1989). There is, at present, neither direct epidemiological nor laboratory evidence to suggest that they prevent melanoma or basal cell carcinoma. The few studies conducted to date suggest either no effect or a causal rather than a protective effect. For example, Holman et al. (1986) found a relative risk of melanoma of 1.06 (95% confidence interval 0.71-1.57) with 1-9 years use of sunscreens and 1.15 (95% confidence interval 0.78-1.68) with 10+ years of use relative to "never use". A statistically significant positive association of "often or very often" use of sun protection agents with melanoma (relative risk 1.8, 95% confidence interval 1.5-3.8) was found by Beitner et al. (1990). In their cohort study of basal cell carcinoma in US nurses, Hunter et al. (1990) found a higher risk in those who spent 8+ hours per week outside and used sunscreen than in those who spent the same time outside but did not use sunscreen.

These results cannot be taken at face value. First, there is likely to be negative confounding of the use of sunscreens with cutaneous sun sensitivity, people with highly sun sensitive skins are likely to use sunscreens more than people with less sensitive skin. Second, there is good evidence that the epidemiological studies have identified an enthusiastic suntanning population using sunscreens with minimal SPF to promote their suntan. Third, it is likely that people adopt or increase their use of sunscreens after their first skin cancer has been diagnosed, or their attention is drawn to their personal risk in some other way (for example, diagnosis of a solar keratosis). Thus present users of sunscreens are likely to be enriched with people at higher than average risk of skin cancer. While adjustment for confounding with skin sensitivity has been carried out in some studies (Holman et al. 1986, Hunter et al. 1990), this third issue has not been addressed in any published analysis. Fourth, relatively little information is available on the mutagenic and carcinogenic potential of various sunscreens. The US National Cancer Institute (1989) recommended the following six compounds to be evaluated for chronic testing in rodents by the US National Toxicology Program: cinoxate; 2-ethylhexyl 2-cyno-3,3-diphenyl-acrylate; 2-ethylhexyl para-methoxycinnamate; homosalate; methyl anthranilate; and oxybenzone. Neither epidemiological nor long term mammalian carcinogenicity data are available on these compounds. The results of in-vitro studies were assessed as either negative or inconsistent among systems or among batches of a compound (because of impurities). 2-ethylhexyl para-methoxycinnamate was implicated as a potential tumour initiator in one study in which hairless mice were painted with the compound over a nine-week period and subsequently treated with the tumour promoter, croton oil (Gallagher et al., 1984a). Subsequent work by Reeve et al. (1985), however, failed to confirm these results, and Forbes et al. (1989) found no evidence of tumour initiation by the compound in an initiation-promotion experiment in mice.

Sunscreens have been strongly promoted by the medical community such as in the United States, Canada, Australia, and Scandinavian countries. However, incidence rates of melanoma have risen steeply in recent decades, even after the introduction of sunscreens (Lee 1989, Jensen and Bolander 1980, Magnus 1977, 1986; Gallagher et al., 1986). The use of high SPF sunscreens is recommended by WHO and by the International Union Against Cancer (UICC) as a supportive part of a sun avoidance programme rather than its main thrust (Marks & Hill, 1992).

Both UVA and UVB have been shown to mutate DNA and cause skin cancers in animals (Staberg et al., 1983). UVA penetrates deeper into the skin than UVB and because of the energy distribution of sunlight and filtering by the outermost layers of the skin, melanocytes receive up to 70 photons of UVA for every photon of UVB. Sunscreens effectively block solar UVB. UVB is the normal stimulus for accommodation of the skin such as thickening and increased pigmentation.

Sunscreens suppress normal warnings of overexposure such as erythema and sunburn and allow excessive exposure to wavelengths of sunlight they do not block. Due to lack of these natural signs sunscreens create a false sense of security and individuals tend to stay in sun longer. In view of these behavioural changes which increases individuals UVA exposure it has been suggested that, because of the rising incidence of melanoma, UVA may be associated with its occurrence (Garland et al., 1992). While a recent study (Setlow et al., 1993) in fish reported melanoma induction by UVA, the role of UVA in the causation of human malignant melanoma has yet to be established.

Trans-urocanic acid, a natural compound of the stratum corneum which absorbs UVB and is used as an additive in some commercial sunscreen products, increased the yield of solar-simulated UV induced tumours in hairless mice (Reeve et al., 1989). The significance of this finding for human exposure has not been evaluated.

Reports on sunscreen protection against UV induced immunosuppression have been equivocal. Fisher et al. (1989) reported no protection of hairless mice against UV-induced systemic immunosuppression following application of Padimate 0 (a PABA ester and UVB absorber) or oxybenzone (a UVB/UVA absorber) with sun protection factors (SPF) of 6 or 15. Similarly SPF 15 octy-N-dimethyl-p-aminobenzoate (o-PABA) had no effect on UV-induced systemic immunosuppression; nor was susceptibility to UV-induced tumours altered in hairless mice (Reeve et al., 1991). In this study however, 2-ethylhexyl-p-methoxycinnamate (2-EHMC, SPF-15) was fully protective. Morison (1984) also reported protection of mice with PABA against both immunosuppression and susceptibility to UV-induced tumours. In recent studies (Wolf et al., 1993a, b), sunscreens with SPFs of 4-6, including o-PABA, 2-EHMC, and benzophenone all provided protection of mice against UV-induced local and systemic immunosuppression, although they were less effective in preventing systemic effects. Finally, in a human study, a sunscreen containing 8% octyl dimethyl PABA, 2% 2-hydroxy-4methoxybenzophenone, and 2% methoxydibenzoyl methane (SPF 15) did not protect against effects of solarium exposure on NK activity, recall antigen skin tests and immunoglobulin production in vitro in mitogen stimulated cultures (Hersey et al., 1987).

While further studies are still needed to clarify concerns raised about the ingredients and protectiveness of sunscreens, broad spectrum sunscreens which absorb both UVA and UVB with an SPF of at least 15 are still recommended as an effective means of personal protection against UV exposure.

14.6 Tanning Devices

Our modern lifestyle has suggested that having a tan is synonymous with good health. The increasing popularity of this symbol of health status and the inability to suntan during non-summer months, has led to the growth of an artificial tanning industry using sunlamps or sunbeds (combination of fluorescent lamp-shaped sunlamps into a bed). The dangers of excessive exposure to UV have been described earlier in this document. They range from mild erythema to severe burns of the skin from acute exposure, to skin cancer and skin ageing from long-term exposure. When eyes are exposed, damage can occur to the cornea, lens and retina, depending on the UV wavelength.

The first generation of sunlamps emitted primarily UVB and, if used correctly, were efficient tanning agents. Unfortunately, they also tended to cause a painful 'sunburn' and other undesirable side-effects. UVA lamps are now used and these, it is claimed, tan safely without burning. However, as the carcinogenesis action spectrum extends into the longer UVA spectral region, exposure to these lamps is not without risk.

Recommendations regarding the use of sunbeds

Following a thorough review of this topic, the IRPA/INIRC (1991a) issued recommendations on the use of sunlamps or sunbeds for cosmetic purposes as follows:

General

The use of sunbeds for cosmetic purposes is not recommended.

Specific

(1) People with skin types I and II should not use sunbeds. They are likely to be disappointed with the results of the exposures, they have

higher susceptibility to sunburn and have a higher risk of developing skin cancer.

(2) Any person with a large number of nevi (moles), a tendency to freckle, a history of severe sunburn especially in childhood, or a family history of malignant melanoma should not use a sunbed.

(3) Any person taking a medicine that is known to be photoactive should not use a sunbed. If in doubt, they should seek the advice of a physician.

(4) Any person who already has extensive skin "sunlight" damage, or who has had premalignant or malignant skin lesions, should not use sunbeds.

(5) Any person who has a skin disease should seek the advice of a physician before using a sunbed.

(6) Children should not use sunbeds.

(7) Sunbeds should not be used if perfumes, body lotions or sprays have been applied that day.

(8) Because the sensitivities of individuals vary greatly, it is advisable to limit the duration of the first session to about one-half of a regular session in order to establish the user's skin response. If following the first session any adverse reaction occurs, further use of the sunbed is not recommended.

(9) Regular exposure should not exceed two sessions per week with a maximum of 30 sessions per year or 30 minimum erythemal doses (MEDs) per year, whichever is the smaller erythemally effective exposure. An occasional break from the regularity of exposure is advisable.

(10) With respect to recommendation (9), the manufacturer of the sunbed should supply a schedule of exposure and recommended maximum exposure durations based on the emission characteristics of the sunbed.

(11) Appropriate protective eyewear should be provided by the manufacturer and should always be worn when using a sunbed.

(12) When the sunbed is being provided for use by a commercial operator, it is the responsibility of the operator to provide the person intending the use the sunbed with the appropriate information as summarized in recommendations (1) to (11) above.

14.7 Occupational Protection

Occupational exposure to UV should be kept to a minimum. Some UV sources emit a considerable amount of visible radiation, and in this case, the natural aversion response is evoked, so there is little chance of accidental over-exposure of the eyes. On the other hand, artificial sources emitting short wavelength UV radiation exist where accidental exposure is quite likely. While working outdoors, skin and eye protection should be used. Exposure outdoors during the periods of 2 hours either side of noon should be avoided.

Where UV levels, compared with the ELs and erythemal dose, are such as to constitute a hazard, protection against hazardous exposure may be achieved by a combination of engineering control measures; administrative control measures and personal protection. For artificial sources, wherever possible, priority should be given to engineering and administrative controls to reduce the requirement for personal protection.

Engineering controls

The principal and most effective engineering control measures are those intended to contain the radiation. Wherever possible UV from artificial sources should be contained within a sealed housing. If observation windows are required they should be made of suitably absorbent materials such as certain grades of acrylic and window glass. Where the exposure process is required to take place external to the source housing a screened area should be set aside where it may be carried out; an example of this is arc welding where screens must be provided to prevent exposure of people not involved with the welding process. Any such screened area should be subject to administrative control measures and persons working in the area should be adequately protected from UV as described below. Where a source of UV is normally enclosed during use but to which access is required, for example for maintenance, the housing should be fitted with safety interlocks. If anyone needs to gain access to the source while it is energized, the interlock should immediately switch off the power to the lamps and should not be able to be re-energized until the interlocks are re-engaged Many such sources are used for a variety of drying and curing purposes, particularly in the printing industry and all should be subject to strict engineering controls.

Administrative control measures

The principal administrative control measures are those that limit access to the source and provide information directed at making people aware of potential hazards associated with it. Access to an area where equipment emits UV should be limited to those persons directly concerned with its use. All persons concerned with the use of such equipment should be made aware of this and should be informed of the potential hazards. Appropriate hazard warning signs should be used to indicate the presence of UV and whenever possible warning lights may be used to show that equipment is energized. The user of a UV emitting source should keep as far from the source as possible. At large distances (greater than twice the greatest dimensions of the source) the irradiance (W m^{-2}) falls off as the square of the distance from the source. Closer to the source irradiance falls off approximately linearly with distance. Exposures should be kept to a minimum and the EL's recommended by IRPA/INIRC (1991) given in chapter 13 should not be exceeded. Particular care should be taken to prevent exposure of persons taking photosensitising medications or concomitantly exposed to photosensitisers in the environment.

Personal protection

The most effective way to protect the skin from UV is to cover it. In indoor occupational situations, the areas of the body most at risk are the face (and eyes) and neck, the forearms and the backs of the hands. The face can be protected by a shield and this should also provide eye protection. The arms should be covered by clothing with a low UVB transmission; in general materials that are visibly opaque are suitable (see section 14.4). Hands can be protected by wearing gloves. Face shields, goggles or safety spectacles which absorb UV should be worn where there is a potential eye hazard.

A range of suitable protective eyewear is commercially available (see figure 14.2). Welders should be protected by a helmet fitted with appropriate absorption filters. Some high pressure lamps are potential explosion hazards and the eyes and face should be protected against flying fragments of glass. Particular care should be taken to protect the eyes, face and hands when such lamps are being removed or replaced. The risk to outdoor workers such as agricultural workers, labourers, construction workers, fishermen etc from solar radiation exposure can be minimized by wearing appropriate tightly woven clothing, and most importantly a brimmed hat to reduce face and neck exposure. Sunscreens can be applied to exposed skin to reduce exposure further (see section 14.5).

Hazards from ozone

The absorption of short wavelength UV by oxygen in the air forms ozone, a powerful oxidising agent. The American Conference of Governmental Hygienists has published a threshold limit value for ozone exposure, 0.1 ppm, (ACGIH, 1993), and concentrations above this value should be avoided.

Levels of ozone may be reduced by providing adequate ventilation in the area in which the source is located. Very intense sources emitting short wavelength UVB, for example, high pressure linear and compact mercury and xenon lamps will normally require an extraction system to remove ozone.

14.8 Protection in Medicine and Dentistry

Protection of both patients and staff must be considered. When a patient is being exposed to UV for clinical purposes, sites not intended to be treated should be covered and the eyes protected.

In medical care, chlorpromazine and thioridazine are phenothiazine derivatives which are widely used as psychosedatives. As well as producing photosensitivity as a side-effect in some patients, these drugs may induce a similar type of reaction in hospital staff. Contact dermatitis may occur in staff handling phenothiazines or fouled laundry since metabolites of chlorpromazine are phototoxic (Moseley 1988). To avoid contamination, staff should wear protective clothing.

Problems may also occur in dentistry, both for patients and staff. The mouth is lined with a relatively thin squamous epithelium and so there may be considerable penetration of UV to underlying cells. Patients and staff with systemic lupus erythematous (SLE) have been reported to be at risk from lights used in dentistry (Moseley 1988). Both operating lamps and sources used to polymerise resins have been found to cause damage. In one case, a dentist, who was a known SLE sufferer, experienced a facial eruption after using a visible-light resin-curing source on a patient. Evidently, special care is required when lights are used on patients and a known history of SLE would be contraindicated for UV or visible light polymerisation.

14.9 Nutrition

Nutrition can provide the body with essential antioxidants and these molecules are distributed throughout the body. At the cellular level, they enter a number of endogenous photoprotective systems to control photochemical processes (Roberts et al., 1991). Quenchers which can negate specific reactive intermediates may be important as a defence mechanism against UV insult to the eye. Glutathione, due to the low energy of the SH (thiol) bond (65 kcal) is an efficient free-radical scavenger and singlet oxygen quencher. Ascorbic acid quenches free radical and superoxide reactions. α-Tocopherol quenches both singlet oxygen and free radicals. There are also various antioxidant enzymes present in the eye. Exogenous scavengers and quenchers may be able to prevent UV damage by interrupting transient intermediates which cause ocular damage. An approach is to increase the known endogenous quenchers, (antioxidants) ascorbic acid, α-tocopherol and β-carotene in the diet (Roberts et al., 1991).

14.10 Additional Protective Agents

Although it has been known that glutathione is a particularly effective quencher of excited state transients in the eye, until now there has been no success in increasing this endogenous sulphydryl compound in ocular tissues. There have recently been found (Roberts et al., 1991) a promising group of compounds, phosphorylated sulphydryls, which pass the blood retinal and blood ocular barrier, and appear to mimic the protective effect of the endogenous thiol glutathione. This offers a possible way of protecting the eye and other tissues from UV induced damage.

Protection from UV damage was reported in mice maintained on a diet supplemented with either carnosine (β alanylhistidine), an antioxidant known to have immunopotentiating properties (Reeve et al., 1993) or retinal palmitate in combination with canthaxanthin, a carotenoid (Gensler, 1989). Some protection was also afforded by retinal palmitate alone. Protection has been shown in healthy humans receiving a daily supplement of β-carotene (Fuller et al., 1992).

14.11 Eye Protection

In industry there are many sources capable of causing acute eye injury within a short exposure time, while in the natural environment acute injury is likely to occur mostly in situations where solar UV is reflected onto the eye, such as from snow while skiing. A variety of eye protection is available with various degrees of protection appropriate to their intended use (see figure 14.2). Those intended for industrial use include, welding helmets (additionally providing protection from intense visible and infrared radiation and face protection), face shields, goggles and UV absorbing spectacles. For use in the outdoor environment, they include (ski) goggles for extreme exposure conditions and sunglasses.

The appropriateness and selection of protective eyewear is dependent on the:

(1) intensity and spectral emission characteristics of the UV source,

(2) behavioural pattern of people near UV sources (distance and time are important),

(3) transmission properties of the protective eyewear material, and

(4) design of the frame of the eyewear to prevent exposure of the eye from direct unabsorbed UV.

In industrial exposure situations the degree of ocular hazard can be assessed by measurement and comparison with recommended limits for exposure (IRPA/INIRC, 1991) (see Chapter 13). Welders and nearby workers should routinely wear appropriate eye and face protection. For protection against other less intense sources of UV in the workplace tightly fitting goggles or spectacles with side shields may be appropriate, but consideration should also be given to the need for additional face protection. In general, protective eyewear provided for industrial use should fit snugly to the face, thus ensuring that there are no gaps through which UV can directly reach the eye and should have adequate mechanical construction to prevent physical injury.

For outdoor workers and the general public, the most hazardous source of UV exposure is the sun. Adequately designed (ski) goggles afford protection against exposure to solar UV at high altitudes and on snow, but for most other exposure conditions, good UV absorbing sunglasses are an adequate means of eye protection.

Transmission of UV through sunglasses varies considerably (Wester 1987, Gies et al., 1992), yet consumers are provided with little information about the protection afforded by them. Some countries have drafted standards limiting UV transmission through sunglasses and Gies et al.

(1990a) have proposed a UV eye protection factor (EPF) for sunglasses similar to the one developed for fabrics and sunscreens.

Figure 14.2 Various types of protective eyewear. (1) Goggles, regular ventilation; (2) Goggles, flexible fitting, hooded ventilation; (3) Goggles, cushioned fitting, rigid body; (4) Spectacles, metal frame with side shields; (5) Spectacles, plastic frame with side shields; (6) Spectacles, metal/plastic frame with side shields; (7) Welding goggles, eyecup type, tinted lenses; (8) Welding goggles, coverspec. type, tinted lenses; (9) Welding goggles, cover spec. type, tinted plate lens; (10) Face shield, with plastic or mesh window; (11) Welding helmet. (From WHO, 1989).

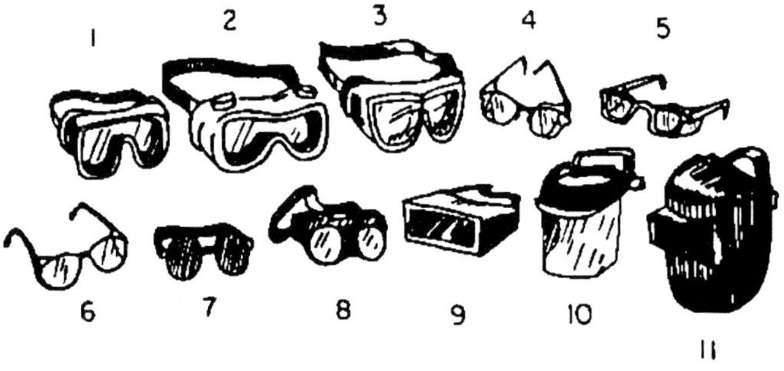

15. FUTURE RESEARCH

15.1 Introduction

At the United Nations Conference on the Environment and Development (UNCED) in 1992 it was declared under Agenda 21 that there should be activities on the effects of UV. Specifically:

(i) Undertake as a matter of urgency, research on the effects on human health of increasing UV reaching the earth's surface as a consequence of depletion of the stratospheric ozone layer;

(ii) On the basis of the outcome of this research, consider taking appropriate remedial measures to mitigate the above mentioned effects on human beings.

This report gives a thorough review of the health hazards of UV exposure. However, although it is known that the burden of UV-related diseases on human populations is high, the exact nature and extent of these diseases is still largely unknown.

There is great uncertainty about future trends in atmospheric ozone. For example the Antarctic holes and large depletions of ozone that have occurred recently were not predicted in any of the ozone depletion models. While agreements have been reached to reduce releases of CFCs into the environment, and this will have future benefit on the ozone layer, there is uncertainty about the extent of ozone depletion caused by chemical pollutants. What is apparent is that decreased ozone levels will persist for many years to come and the corresponding increases in UV intensities will result in more significant adverse health effects on all populations of the world for many decades to come (WMO 1993).

The health effects of UV are not restricted to fair skinned populations. UV exposure is thought to cause diseases of the eye and suppression of the immune system in all populations of the world. UV induced immune suppression may have adverse consequences on infectious disease immunization programmes, particularly in areas where the UV intensities are high. The possibility that UV will cause progression of various diseases such as for HIV positive patients still has to be elucidated. Many such important issues need to be resolved as a matter of urgency.

The WHO Task Group reviewing this monograph strongly supported action and coordination of UV research at the international level. In particular the Task Group supported the concept of the International

Research Programme on Health, Solar UV Radiation and Environmental Change (INTERSUN). INTERSUN is a collaborative effort between WHO, the United Nations Environment Programme (UNEP) and the International Agency on Cancer Research (IARC). The group recognised specific research needs in areas of exposure assessment, terrestrial plants, aquatic ecosystems, and human health effects related to the skin, immune system and eye. Some of these could be accomplished under the umbrella of INTERSUN, and some, at least initially, would require more basic laboratory research to be undertaken.

15.2 INTERSUN

The objectives and approach of INTERSUN are: to accurately evaluate the quantitative relationship between solar UV at the surface of the earth and human health effects; develop reliable predictions of health consequences of changes in UV; provide baseline estimates of the occurrence of health effects of UV in representative populations around the world; and develop practical ways of monitoring change in these effects over time in relation to environmental and behavioural change.

It is intended to establish field research centres covering a range of latitudes in both hemispheres in which will be measured: ground level UV irradiance; incidence of non-melanocytic skin cancer; incidence and mortality of malignant melanoma; immune function; biological markers of UV exposure and its' early carcinogenic effects; constitutional sensitivity to sun exposure; and present and past sun-related behaviour. In addition, in these centres there will be undertaken case-control or cross-sectional studies of relationships between skin cancers, cataract and immune response and constitutional sensitivity to the sun, lifetime exposure to the sun, and biological markers of UV exposure and early carcinogenic effects. Surveys should be repeated at 5-yearly intervals to allow trends in population measurements to be established.

Data collected at such centres would be used

- to describe quantitatively the relationship between ground level solar UV irradiance and the incidence of skin cancers and other health effects (particularly eye damage and effects on the immune system) of UV exposure in human populations.

- to estimate the change in occurrence of health effects of UV radiation that would result from change in ground level solar UV irradiance due to environmental change.

- to increase understanding of the relationship between personal risk of health effects of UV radiation and constitutional sensitivity to the sun and sun-related behaviour.

- to develop and validate appropriate ways of monitoring human exposure to UV and the occurrence of associated health effects.

- to develop a network of centres monitoring trends in ground level solar UV irradiance, sun exposure of populations, and the occurrence of health effects of UV radiation.

- to interpret these trends, as far as is possible, in relation to environmental change, changes in human behaviour, and the implementation of public policies aimed at ameliorating environmental change or human exposure to solar UV radiation.

- to provide a basis for development and evaluation of interventions to reduce the occurrence of adverse health effects of solar UV radiation.

In line with the above objectives and the gaps in knowledge needed to be filled to make a satisfactory health risk assessment, the following recommendations for future research are provided.

15.3 Solar and Personal UV Monitoring

The quantification of health detriment to an individual or to a population requires the assessment of exposure of the individual or the average exposure of a member of the exposed population. In interpreting epidemiological data the exposures of the groups comprising the study populations must be known. The requirements here are precise measurement data of the environment occupied by the exposed individuals combined with data on their exposure habits, derived from representative personal exposure measurements, skin damage or from questionnaires.

15.3.1 *Solar monitoring*

1. A comprehensive network of spectral and broad band monitoring stations is needed worldwide giving quality ground measurements of surface UV, to assess the effects of enhanced UVA and UVB radiation on exposed populations, and to document the impact of stratospheric ozone depletion on ambient UV. A long-term data record is important.

2. Quality and convenient monitoring data are needed as input to models and for model validation. Current models need to be further modified to account for cloud cover, gaseous pollutants and aerosols.

3. Common calibration and audit procedures should be developed and implemented for national and international monitoring programmes.

4. Monitoring activities should be coordinated with the efforts of other groups on a national and international scale. Close coordination is needed for inter-comparison studies and quality control/quality assurance efforts.

5. There is a need for global monitoring of UV radiation, with particular attention to long-term instrument stability and representative geographical deployment

15.3.2 *Personal monitoring*

Population studies using personal UV monitoring devices are needed to determine the fraction of the daily natural UV dose received by persons at risk. The daily amount of UV received by human skin varies greatly with occupation, behaviour, and local climatic and environmental conditions. Little is known about these factors and this seriously interferes with the interpretation of existing data on the relationship between UV and the development of skin cancer and of chronic skin and eye damage. Thus, the development of personal UV monitoring devices is important.

Small passive personal UV dosimeters or monitoring devices should be further developed and used to provide data on personal exposures. Biomarkers for UV exposure and skin cancer risk should be further developed, e.g. UV-induced mutations in p53 tumour suppressor genes. Such biomarkers might constitute a person's own "built in" UV risk monitoring device.

For some people, artificial sources of UV represents a significant component of their exposure. Occupational exposures and elective exposures such as from cosmetic sunbeds are important in this respect. Measurement studies are required in these areas.

Standardized monitoring of exposure to the sun in at risk populations, particularly children, should be evaluated as a guide to public health action to control melanoma.

15.4 Terrestrial Plants

Particular attention must be given to the impact on food production in the developing world and to development of crop varieties resistant to higher levels of UV radiation.

Substantial research is needed to describe and evaluate the effects of enhanced UV on plants, specifically in the following areas:

1. Field validations on crop plants should be extended to determine whether UV affects yield in other agriculturally important plants.

2. Studies should be initiated to determine the impacts on ecosystems. Little is known of the effects of UV in other ecosystems such as forests, where 80% of net primary production is currently stored.

3. It is important to study natural plants because they serve in supplying new drugs, medicines and other natural products. They also act as a reservoir of genetic diversity for modern crop breeding programmes.

4. Studies are needed to elucidate how UVB effects are modified by additional factors such as carbon dioxide, temperature, water and nutrient stress, heavy metals, diseases, and pests.

5. Of increasing interest are man-made air pollutants such as sulphur dioxide and nitrogen oxides, which are known to have damaging effects on crops and forests. Attention should be focused on whether the negative effects of these air pollutants may be aggravated by UV radiation.

6. The manner and magnitude of adaptation to increased UV, especially UVB, such as by increased screening pigments or enhanced DNA damage repair capacity, need to be investigated both as adaption capacity of individual plants and as genetically based changes in plant populations. The latter also provides a basis for plant breeding interventions for agricultural and tree species.

15.5 Aquatic Ecosystems

Current data suggest that predicted increases in UV, especially UVB radiation could have important negative effects in the marine environment. However, uncertainties regarding the magnitude of these effects remain large, including problems of extrapolating laboratory findings to the open sea, and the almost complete absence of data on long-term effects on ecosystems. Additional information is needed in several areas before more reliable assessments of risk are possible. Research is needed to:

1. Determine accurate and appropriate biological action spectra for selected endpoints of key marine species.

2. Produce dose-response data on a greater variety of ecologically important primary producers than is now available, as well as data for key higher organisms within the food web.

3. Determine long-term effects for embryos or larvae exposed to UVB radiation. Is the survival of the adult population (or their offspring) affected?

4. Determine effects of enhanced UV on major ecosystems, including the Antarctic ecosystems.

5. Obtain data on the mechanisms of damage and ranges of possible adaptation or genetic selection in response to increased UVB radiation.

6. Relate UVB penetration into the water column and through ice both in laboratory and field research to determine effects on phytoplankton and zooplankton.

7. Develop biomarkers to monitor current levels of UV damage in phytoplankton and zooplankton.

15.6 Human Health

15.6.1 *Skin*

To a substantial degree, answers are still required to the following questions regarding the relationship between sun exposure and both melanoma and non-melanocytic skin cancer. Research is needed to determine:

1. The quantitative relationship between radiant exposure and incidence of these cancers; and in particular the shape of the exposure-response relationship.

2. How the effect of sun exposure is modified by: age at exposure, time since last exposure and pattern of exposure, particularly whether a particular dose is received intermittently or more-or-less continuously.

3. Biomarkers of UV exposure or early effects in the skin, e.g. UV-induced mutations for UV exposure and skin cancer risk.

4. The importance of UVA in causing skin cancers, both relative to UVB and comparatively between melanoma and non-melanocytic cancer.

5. The importance of indirect (e.g. oxidative) as opposed to direct UV damage in causing these cancers.

6. The contribution of sun exposure to the aetiology of these cancers in dark-skinned populations and how, in general, cutaneous sensitivity modifies both quantitatively and qualitatively the relationship between sun exposure and skin cancer.

7. If the associations of red hair and freckling with skin cancer are explained by effects of skin pigmentation or sensitivity to the sun or mediated by other susceptibility mechanisms.

8. If pigmentary characteristics or cutaneous sun sensitivity explain most of the ethnic variation in skin cancer incidence or are there other ethnically related susceptibility characteristics.

9. Whether the relationships between sun exposure and BCC and SCC are the same.

10. The role of UV-induced mutations of critical genes in causing melanoma.

11. The role of sun exposure in causing cancer of the lip. An epidemiological study is required with adequate control of potential confounding with alcohol and tobacco use.

12. The relationship between use of sunlamps and sunbeds (artificial tanning) and both melanoma and non-melanocytic skin cancer. Adequate control of likely confounding with sun exposure is required.

13. The effects of the interaction between UVB and the rest of the solar spectrum in relation to DNA repair, malignant transformation, and skin tumour development.

14. Additional animal models, particularly for the study of the experimental induction of malignant melanoma. Further, an action spectrum for induction of melanoma should be developed in *M.*

domestica to see if the apparent response of UVA exposure observed in hybrid fish can be confirmed.

15.6.2 Immune System

Suppression of immune functions results from UV exposure of humans. The following studies are needed to adequately assess the consequent risk to human health.

1. Studies to determine whether systemic effects occur in humans as a result of UV exposure.

2. Establish immunological biomarkers that could identify persons who are susceptible to specific long-term UV-induced immune suppression, e.g. to infectious agents.

3. Human and rodent studies are needed to determine the relationship between UV exposure and susceptibility to infection and vaccine effectiveness, and quantitative comparison of the relative sensitivities of mice and humans.

4. Studies of the effects of UVB on immune function in human skin of all types to determine if all skin types show the same quality and quantity of effects.

5. Studies to examine whether currently available sunscreens provide adequate protection and whether dietary supplements are protective. Specifically:

    a) Protective effects for immunosuppression;
    b) Systemic toxicity based on penetration of organic chemicals in sunscreens;
    c) Carcinogenicity assays.

6. Studies of the spectral effectiveness of UV in producing immune function defects and enhanced susceptibility to disease.

7. Research to determine the role of UVB exposure in immediate-type hypersensitivity (allergic) reactions as well as specific antibody responses, particularly as it relates to impact on incidence and severity of asthma.

8. Research on the effects of UV on the development of autoimmune disease and on underlying mechanisms.

9. Studies on systemic effects caused by release of cytokines within the epidermis and blood stream.

15.6.3 Eye

Two issues underscore the need for undertaking studies of health risks of UV exposure of the eye on a priority basis. First, there is evidence of the depletion of the ozone layer and the reported consequent increase in ambient UV which will impact on many eye diseases. Second, the overall ageing of the population worldwide would further compound the magnitude of the cataract and other eye problems.

1. There is a need for well-conducted epidemiological studies to be undertaken to define the strength of the association between UVA and UVB exposure with cataract and other eye conditions, including climatic droplet keratopathy and pterygium, at both the individual and community levels. Ideally, this should be undertaken in a variety of locations. Careful attention needs to be given to quantifying, for each study participant, ocular exposure to UV and exposure to other possible risk factors that may confound observed associations.

2. Techniques need to be refined for measuring the proportion of UV of different wavelengths incident upon the human cornea and lens, and how these are affected by the behavioural response to avoid direct exposure to bright sunlight, and by different ground surfaces.

3. Studies should be conducted to provide data on the quantitative relationship between exposure to UV and cataract and other lesions of the anterior eye. In relation to this there is an urgent need to establish an internationally agreed system for grading the type and severity of cataract.

4. Investigations of the role of personal solar exposure in causing ocular melanoma, including the protective effect of ocular devices.

5. The relationship between sunlamp or sunbed exposure and malignant melanoma of the eye needs to be evaluated.

6. The relative efficacy of different protective devices, headwear and eye wear needs to be determined.

7. Techniques need to be defined for measuring the proportion of UV of different wavelengths penetrating the human cornea and lens in the intact eye, in view of possible retinal effects.

8. The action spectra for chronic exposure leading to ocular damage needs to be determined in primates and other animals. This includes action spectra for cataract formation, pterygium, climatic droplet keratopathy, and macular changes in aphakic animals.

9. Risks to aphakic people and those with intraocular lens implants for retinal changes, mainly from UVA and short wavelengths in the visible part of the spectrum, need to be determined.

15.7 Laboratory Studies

Little is known about the mechanisms of interaction of UV and environmental chemical agents on biological systems. Many widely distributed natural or artificial chemicals (pesticides, halocarbons, etc.) can be altered by UV, resulting in photoproducts that may be less or more biologically effective than the parent compound. Furthermore, many chemicals can be activated by UV *in situ* in biological systems and this activation may elicit a biological effect which neither the chemical nor the radiation alone exhibits (Psoralens). An international registry of agents that interact with light to cause adverse health effects would speed identification of such agents.

Much of the information on the chemical and biological effects of UV comes from experiments using UVC (particularly 254 nm) radiation not found in sunlight reaching the earth's surface. There are studies showing direct and indirect effects on cells and cellular constituents of UVB, UVA, and visible light that differ considerably from those of UVC. Thus, the chemical and biological effects of the wavelengths of UV found in sunlight should be studied. There is evidence that visible light can, under different conditions, either help cells to repair UV-induced damage or can potentiate the detrimental effects of UV. Thus, to better understand the effects of sunlight on humans and the environment, experiments should be performed using natural sunlight or artificial lamps with well-known continuous spectra.

Cellular and molecular studies needed include:

1. Extension of relevant biological action spectra to the UVA/visible wavelengths, as well as interactions between UVA and UVB radiation. Crucial spectra required include:

- pre-mutagenic lesions
- gene activation
- activation of viruses specially HIV (activation of DNA binding, promoter activity, viral replication)

2. Determination of the free radical/oxidative component of UVB and UVA radiation effects. Determine the reactive intermediates involved.

3. Determination of adaptation responses in human cells.

4. Determination of endogenous cellular antioxidant defences in eye tissue and skin.

5. Elucidation of DNA repair pathways in humans using the advanced technology available for analyses of gene and function.

6. Identification of key endogenous and exogenous sensitizers.

7. Studies to examine the effect of UV on the balance between Th1 and Th2 cells.

15.8 Education

It is essential to educate the general population and workers concerning the profound importance of sunlight and the possibilities of either UV deprivation or of acute and chronic UV injury. It is also important to overcome the lack of respect for the possible adverse effects on health from overexposure to sunlight, simply because sunlight is ubiquitous, and the concept that, if something is natural, it must be totally beneficial and safe. In this context there is a need to standardize a UV exposure index that can be used as part of health information/education campaigns.

15.9 Administration

An international panel composed of key national experts, with its secretariat at WHO, should be formed with the following terms of reference:

(i) to identify gaps in knowledge and set research priorities needed for a better health risk assessment of exposure to UV

(ii) to evaluate and monitor progress of research

(iii) to establish mechanisms for funding research and initiate projects where crucial gaps in knowledge have been identified

(iii) to facilitate international cooperation on UV monitoring efforts, including instrumentation intercomparisons, calibration standardization and uniform analysis of data, and

(iv) to facilitate international cooperation in measurement of human UV exposure, monitoring of trends in occurrence of UV health effects, and epidemiological studies of the relationship between UV exposure and health effects

(v) to provide a database of research projects to facilitate cooperation between researchers and institutions involved in research.

16. PREVIOUS EVALUATIONS BY INTERNATIONAL BODIES

16.1 United Nations Environment Programme

UNEP has undertaken a number of reviews on the environmental effects of increased UV intensities resulting from ozone depletion (1989, 1991, 1992). Their findings on each issue are summarized below:

16.1.1 Ozone

Significant global scale decreases in total ozone have occurred over the past ten years. All other factors being constant, there is no scientific doubt that decreases in total ozone will increase UVB radiation at ground level. Tropospheric ozone and aerosols may have masked the consequences of stratospheric ozone depletion for UVB in some industrialized regions. There are no reliable estimates of the direction or magnitude of effects of any cloud cover trends on UVB. Efforts to improve local and regional air quality may bring to light the increases in UVB associated with the depletion of stratospheric ozone.

16.1.2 Human health

The induction of immunosuppression by UVB has now been demonstrated in humans, not only those of light pigmentation, but also deeply pigmented individuals. This places all of the world's populations at risk of the potential adverse impacts of UVB on the immune system, including possible increases in the incidence or severity of infectious disease.

An increased number of adverse ocular effects have been associated with exposure to UV. These include age-related nearsightedness, deformation of the lens capsule, and nuclear cataract (a form of cataract which previous information excluded from consideration). These effects appear to be independent of pigmentation. Estimates of risk would increase slightly if one were to include nuclear cataract among the forms of cataract increasing with ozone depletion. It is now predicted that, all other things being equal, a sustained 10% decrease in ozone will be associated with between 1.6 and 1.75 million additional cases of cataract per year world-wide.

Recent information on the relationship of nonmelanoma skin cancer to UV exposures confirms previous findings and has allowed refinement of the carcinogenic action spectrum. Incorporation of this new information into the risk estimation process has led to slightly lower predictions. It is now predicted that a sustained 10% decrease in ozone will be associated with 26% increase in non-melanoma skin cancer. All other things remaining constant, this would mean an increase in excess of 300,000 cases per year world-wide.

16.2 International Agency for Research on Cancer

The carcinogenicity of ultraviolet has been evaluated by IARC (1992, 1993). IARC concluded that "There is sufficient evidence in humans for the carcinogenicity of solar radiation. Solar radiation causes cutaneous melanoma and nonmelanocytic skin cancer". With respect to other potential sources of UV, IARC has concluded that there is limited evidence for the carcinogenicity of exposure to fluorescent lighting and there is inadequate evidence for the carcinogenicity of other artificial sources of UV. Readers are referred to these excellent monographs for more details - much of which has been incorporated in this text.

16.3 World Health Organization

WHO and its Regional Office for Europe have completed reviews on the health effects of ultraviolet (WHO, 1979, 1989). They concluded that all people are exposed to UV from sunlight, and the risk to health varies with geographical, genetic and other factors. Similar risks are involved in the increasing exposure of people to UV from artificial sources, such as those used for suntanning, in phototherapy and in industrial processes. The biological effects of a single exposure differ significantly from the effects of repeated and cumulative exposures. Both types of risk increase markedly with excessive exposure.

Most observed biological effects of UVB are extremely detrimental to living organisms. Much less is known about the biological effects of UVA. It can augment the biological effects of UVB, and doses of UVA, which alone do not show any biological effects, can in the presence of certain chemical agents, result in injury to tissues (phototoxicity, photoallergy, enhancement of photocarcinogenesis).

All those who work out of doors are potentially at risk of overexposure, the consequences of which may be both acute and long-term effects. The fashion of exposing a large part of the body to sunlight has during recent years increased the exposure of the skin, resulting in quite high UV doses. This is true not only for outdoor work but is now also normal during leisure periods, as exemplified by the holiday exodus of a large part of the population of the northern European countries to the Mediterranean coast.

16.4 International Commission on Non-Ionizing Radiation Protection

Through its predecessor committee IRPA/INIRC the ICNIRP was involved in the publication of the original review of the health effects of UV (WHO/UNEP/IRPA, 1979). It has recommended international guidelines on limits (IRPA/INIRC, 1991) as shown in Chapter 13. It has also recommended against the use of sunlamps for cosmetic purposes (IRPA/INIRC, 1991a). A review of the studies on fluorescent lighting with reference to UV levels has suggested that they do not seem to be associated with an increased risk of malignant melanoma (IRPA/INIRC, 1991).

REFERENCES

Abrahams PJ, Huitema BA, & van der Eb AJ (1984) Enhanced reactivation and enhanced mutagenesis of herpes simplex virus in normal human and xeroderma pigmentosum cells. Mol Cell Biol, **4**: 2341-2346.

ACGIH (1993) Threshold limit values for chemical substances and physical agents and biological exposure indices. Cincinnati, Ohio, The American Conference of Governmental Industrial Hygienists.

Adam SA, Sheaves JK, Wright NH, Mosser G, Harris RW, & Vessey MP (1981) A case-control study of the possible association between oral contraceptives and malignant melanoma. Br J Cancer, **44**: 45-50.

Adams JS, Clemens TL, Parrish JA, (1982) Vitamin D synthesis and metabolism after UV irradiation of normal and vitamin D deficient subjects. N Engl J Med, **306**: 722-725.

Ainsleigh HG (1993) Beneficial effects of sun exposure on cancer mortality. Prev Med, **22**: 132-140.

Akslen LA & Mørkve O (1992) Expression of p53 protein in cutaneous melanoma. Int J Cancer, **52**: 13-16.

Albino AP, Nanus DM, Davis ML, & McNutt NS (1991) Lack of evidence of Ki-*ras* codon 12 mutations in melanocytic lesions. J Cutan Pathol, **18**: 273-278.

Alcalay J, Freeman SE, Goldberg LH, & Wolf JE (1990) Excision repair of pyrimidine dimers induced by simulated solar radiation in the skin of patients with basal cell carcinoma. J Invest Dermatol, **95**: 506-509.

Anderson RR & Parrish JA (1981) The optics of human skin. J Invest Dermatol, **77**: 13-19.

Andley UP (1987) Photodamage to the eye. Yearly review. Photochem Photobiol, **46**: 1057-1066.

Angel P, Poting A, Mallick U, Rahmsdorf HJ, Schorpp M, & Herrlich P (1986) Induction of metallothionein and other mRNA species by carcinogens and tumour promoters in primary human skin fibroblasts. Mol Cell Biol, **6**: 1760-1766.

Ansel JC, Mountz J, Steinberg AD, DeFabo E, & Green Ira (1985) Effects if UV radiation on autoimmune strains of mice: Increased mortality and accelerated autoimmunity in BXSB male mice. J Invest Dermatol, **85**: 181-186.

Araneo BA, Dowell T, Moon HB, & Daynes RA (1989) Regulation of murine lymphokine production *in vivo*. Ultraviolet radiation exposure depresses Il-2 and enhances IL-4 production by T cells through an Il-1 dependent mechanism. J Immunol, **143**: 1737-1744.

Arlett CF & Harcourt SA (1983) Variation in response to mutagens amongst normal and repair-defective human cells. In: Lawrence CW ed. Induced mutagenesis: Molecular mechanisms and their implications for environmental protection. New York, London, Plenum Press, pp 249-267.

Arlett CF, Harcourt SA, Cole J, Green MH, & Anstey AV (1992) A comparison of the response of unstimulated and stimulated T-lymphocytes and fibroblasts from normal, Xeroderma pigmentosum and trichothiodystrophy donors to the lethal action of UVC. Mutat Res, **273**: 127-135.

Armstrong BK (1984) Melanoma of the skin. Br Med Bull, **40**: 346-350.

Armstrong BK (1988) Epidemiology of malignant melanoma: intermittent or total accumulated exposure to the sun? J Dermatol Surg Oncol, **14**: 835-849.

Armstrong BK (1993) Implications of increased solar UVB for cancer incidence. In: Chanin ML ed. The role of the stratosphere in global change. Berlin, Heidelberg, New York, Springer-Verlag, pp 517-540.

Armstrong BK & English DR (1988) The epidemiology of acquired melanocytic naevi and their relationship to malignant melanoma. Pigment Cell, **9**: 27-47.

Armstrong BK, Woodings TL, Stenhouse NS, & McCall MG (1983) Mortality from cancer in migrants to Australia 1962 to 1971. Perth, University of Western Australia.

Armstrong BK, de Klerk NH, & Holman CDJ (1986) Etiology of common acquired melanocytic nevi: constitutional variables, sun exposure and diet. J Natl Cancer Inst, **77**: 329-335.

Atkin M, Fenning J, Heady JA, Kennaway EL, & Kennaway NM (1949) The mortality from cancer of the skin and lip in certain occupations. Br J Cancer, **3**: 1-15.

Aubry F & MacGibbon B (1985) Risk factors of squamous cell carcinoma of the skin. A case-control study in the Montreal region. Cancer, **55**: 907-911.

Auerbach H (1961) Geographic variation in incidence of skin cancer in the United States. Public Health Rep, **76**: 345-348.

Augustsson A, Stierner U, Rosdahl I, & Suurküla M (1990) Melanocytic naevi in sun-exposed and protected skin in melanoma patients and controls. Acta Dermato-Venereol, **71**: 512-517.

Azizi E, Lusky A, Kushelevsky AP, & Schewach-Millet N (1988) Skin type, hair colour and freckles are predictors of decreased minimal erythema ultraviolet radiation dose. J Am Acad Dermatol, **19**: 32-38.

Azizova AO, Islomov AI, Roshchupkin DI, Predvoditelev DA, Remizov AN, & Vladimir YA (1980) Free radicals formed on ultraviolet irradiation of the lipids of biological membrane. Biophysics, **24**: 407-414.

Baadsgaard O, Wulf HC, Wantzin GL, & Cooper KD (1987) UVB and UVC, but not UVA, potently induce the appearance of T6-DR+ antigen-presenting cells in human epidermis. J Invest Dermatol, **89**: 113-118.

Baadsgaard O, Lisby S, Wulf HC, Wantzin GL, & Cooper KD (1989) Rapid recovery of Langerhans cell alloreactivity, without induction of autoreactivity, after *in vivo* ultraviolet A, but not ultraviolet B exposure of human skin. J Immunol, **142**: 4213-4218.

Baadsgaard O, Salvo B, Mannie A, Dass B, Fox DA, & Cooper KD (1990) *In vivo* ultraviolet-exposed human epidermal cells activate T suppressor cell pathways that involve CD4+CD45RA+ suppressor-inducer T cells. J Immunol, **145**: 2854-2861.

Baasanhu J, Johnson GJ, Burendei G, & Minassian DC (in press) Prevalence and causes of blindness and visual impairment in Mongolia: A survey of populations aged 40 and older. Bull. World Health Organ.

Bachem A (1956) Ophthalmic ultraviolet action spectra. Am J Ophthalmol, **41**: 969-975.

Baird EA, McHenry PM, & MacKie RM (1992) Effect of maintenance chemotherapy in childhood on numbers of melanocytic naevi. Br Med J, **305**: 799-801.

Baker KS & Smith RC (1982) Spectral irradiance penetration in natural waters. In: Calkins J ed. The role of solar ultraviolet radiation in marine ecosystems. New York, London, Plenum Press, pp 223-246.

Barbareschi M, Girlando S, Cristofolini P, Cristofolini M, Togni R, & Boi S (1992) p53 Protein expression in basal cell carcinoma. Histopathology, **21**: 579-581.

Barker & Brainard (1993) Personal communication.

Barker JNWN & MacDonald DM (1988) Eruptive dysplastic naevi following renal transplantation. Clin Exp Dermatol, **13**: 123-125.

Barnes PW, Jordan PW, Gold WG, Flint SD, & Caldwell MM (1988) Competition, morphology and canopy structure in wheat (Triticum aestivum L.) and wild oat (Avena fatua L.) exposed to enhanced ultraviolet-B radiation. Funct Ecol, **2**: 319-330.

Barnes PW, Flint SD, & Caldwell MM (1990) Morphological responses of crop and weed species of different growth forms to ultraviolet-B radiation. Am J Bot, **77**: 1354-1360.

Barrett SF, Robbins JH, Tarone RE, & Kraemer KH (1991) Evidence for defective repair of cyclobutane pyrimidine dimers with normal repair and other DNA photoproducts in a transcriptionally active gene transfected into Cockayne syndrome cells. Mutat Res, **255**: 281-291.

Basu-Modak S & Tyrrell RM (1993) Singlet oxygen. A primary effector in the UVA/near visible light induction of the human heme oxygenase gene. Cancer Res. **53**: 4505-4510.

Bech-Thomsen N, Wulf HC, Poulsen T, & Lundgren K (1988a) Pretreatment with long-wave ultraviolet light inhibits ultraviolet-induced skin tumor development in hairless mice. Arch Dermatol, **124**: 1215-1218.

Bech-Thomsen N, Wulf HC, & Lundgren K (1988b) Pre-treatment with UVA influences broad-spectrum UV photocarcinogenesis in hairless mice (Abstract). In: Rikles E ed. Proceedings of the 10th International Congress on Photobiology, Jerusalem. Jerusalem, Israel, International Association of Biology, p 34.

Beer JZ & Smudzka BZ (1991) Activation of human immunodeficiency virus by radiation. In: Seymour CB & Murhersill C ed. New developments in fundamental and applied radiology. London, Taylor and Francis, pp 113-123.

Beitner H, Norell SE, Ringborg U, Wennersten G, & Mattson B (1990) Malignant melanoma: aetiological importance of individual pigmentation and sun exposure. Br J Dermatol, **122**: 43-51.

Beral V & Robinson N (1981) The relationship of malignant melanoma, basal and squamous skin cancers to indoor and outdoor work. Br J Cancer, **44**: 886-891.

Beral V, Evans S, Shaw H, & Milton G (1982) Malignant melanoma and exposure to fluorescent lighting at work. Lancet, **ii**: 290-293.

Berger DS & Urbach F (1982) A climatology of sunburning ultraviolet radiation. Photochem Photobiol, **35**: 187-192.

Bergmanson JP, Pitts DG, & Chu LW (1988) Protection from harmful UV radiation by contact lens. J Am Optom Assoc, **59**:,178-182.

Bergmanson JP, Pitts DG, & Chu LW (1987) The efficacy of a UV-blocking soft contact lens in protecting cornea against UV radiation. Acta Opthtalmol, **65**: 279-286.

Beukers R & Berends W (1960) Isolation and identification of the irradiation product of thymine. Biochim Biophys Acta, **41**: 550-551.

Bhatnagar R, West KP, Vitale S, Sommer A, Joshi S, & Venkataswamy G (1991) Risk of cataract and history of severe diarrhoeal disease in Southern India. Arch Ophthalmol, **109**: 696-699.

Bhuyan, K.C. and Bhuyan, D.K. (1983) Molecular mechanism of caractogenesis I reactive species of oxygen as triggering agents II. Evidence of lipid peroxidation and membrane damage. In Oxy Radicals, their scavenger syst. Proc. Int. Conf. Superoxide Dismutase 3rd, vol. 2 (Ed. G. Cohen and R.A. Greenwald), pp 343-356, Elsevier, New York.

Bidigare RR (1989) Potential effects of UVB radiation on marine organisms of the Southern Ocean: distributions of phytoplankton and krill during Austral spring. Photochem Photobiol, **50**: 469-477.

Birch-Hirschfeld A (1914) The pathological effect of radiant energy on the eye. 1. Blinding by sunlight. Ergebn Allg Path des Menschen und der Tiere **16,** 619-634.

Bishop L (1992) Statistical considerations in network design and data analysis. Presentation to UVB Workshop: A review of the science and status of measuring and monitoring programs. Washington, DC, Science and Policy Associates, Inc.

Bissett DL, Hannon DP, & Orr TV (1989) Wavelength dependence of histological, physical and visible changes in chronically UV-irradiated hairless mouse skin. Photochem Photobiol, **50**: 763-769.

Bittersmann E, Holzwarth AR, Agel G, & Nultsch W (1988) Picosecond time-resolved emission spectra of photoinhibited and photobleached Anabaena variabilis. Photochem Photobiol, **47**: 101-105.

Black HS (1987a) Photocarcinogenesis and diet. Fed Proc, **46**: 1901-1905.

Black HS (1987b) Potential involvement of free radical reactions in ultraviolet light mediated cutaneous damage. Photochem Photobiol, **46**: 213-221.

Black HS & Chan JT (1975) Suppression of ultraviolet light-induced tumor formation by dietary antioxidants. J Invest Dermatol, **65**: 412-412.

Black HS, Thornby JI, Gerguis J, & Lenger, W (1992) Influence of dietary omega-6,-3 fatty acid sources on the initiation and promotion stages of photocarcinognesis. Photochem Photobiol, **56**: 195-199.

Blum, HF (1948) Sunlight as a causal factor in cancer of the skin of man. J Natl Inst Cancer, **9**: 247-258.

Blum HF, Butler EG, Dailey TH, Daube JR, Mawe RC, & Soffen GA (1959) Irradiation of mouse skin with single doses of ultraviolet light. J Natl Cancer Inst, **22**: 979-993.

Blumthaler M, Ambach W, & Daxecker F (1987) On the threshold radiant exposure for keratitis solaris. Invest Opthalmol Vis Sci, **28**: 1713-1716.

Blyth WA, Hill TJ, Field HJ, & Harbour DA (1976) Reactivation of herpes simples virus infection by ultraviolet light and possible involvement of prostaglandins. J Gen Virol, **33**: 547-550.

Bochow TW, West SK, Azar A, Munoz B, Sommer A, & Taylor HR (1989) Ultraviolet light exposure and risk of posterior subcapsular cataracts. Arch Ophthalmol, **107**: 369-372.

Boettner EA & Wolter JR (1962) Transmission of the ocular media. Invest Ophthalmol Vis Sci, **1**: 776-783.

Boiteux S, O'Connor TR, & Laval J (1987) Formamido pyrimidine-DNA glycosylase of Escherichia coli: cloning and sequencing of the fpg structural gene and overproduction of the protein. EMBO J, **6**: 3177-3183.

Booth F (1985) Heredity in one hundred patients admitted for excision of pterygia. Aust N Z J Ophthalmol, **13**: 59-61.

Bornman JF & Vogelmann TC (1991) Effect of UV-B radiation on leaf optical properties measured with fibre optics. J Exp Vot, **42**: 547-554.

Bose B, Agarwal S & Chafterjee SN (1989) UV-A induced lipid peroxidation in liposomal membrane. Radiat. Environ. Biophys. **28** 59-65.

Bose SN & Davies RJH (1984) The photoreactivity of T-A sequences in oligodeoxyribonucleotides and DNA. Nucl Acids Res, **12**: 7903-7913.

Bouwes-Bavinck JN (1992) Risk of skin cancer in renal-transplant recipients. Leiden, The Netherlands (Thesis).

Boyle J, Mackie RM, Briggs JD, Junor BJR, & Aitchison TC (1984) Cancer, warts, and sunshine in renal transplant patients: A case-control study. Lancet, **1**: 702-705.

Bradley MO, Hsu IC, & Harris CC (1979) Relationships between sister chromatid exchange and mutagenicity, toxicity and DNA damage. Nature (Lond), **282**: 318-320.

Brash DE & Haseltine WA (1982) UV-induced hotspots occur at DNA damage hotspots. Nature (Lond), **298**: 189-192.

Brash DE, Rudolph JA, Simon JA, Lin A, McKenna GJ, Baden HP, Halperin AJ, & Pontén J (1991) A role for sunlight in skin cancer: UV-induced p53 mutations in squamous cell carcinoma. Proc Natl Acad Sci (USA), **88**: 10124-10128.

Braun J (1991) The protective function of phenolic compounds of rye- and oat seedlings against UV-B radiation and their biosynthetic regulation, (Thesis) pp. 1-237 in Karlsr Beitr Entw Okophysiol **9**, M. Tevini (ed.), Bot Inst II, Karlsruhe.

Braun J & Tevini M (1991) Regulation of UV-Protective pigment synthesis in the epidermal layer of rye seedlings (*Secale cereale L. cv. Kustro*). Photochem Photobiol, **37**: 318-321.

Bridges BA (1990) Sunlight, DNA damage and skin cancer: a new perspective. Jpn J Cancer Res, **81**: 105-107.

Brilliant LB, Grasset NC, Pokhrel RP, Kolstad A, Lepkowski JM, Brilliant GE, Hawks WN, & Pararajasegaram R (1983) Associations among cataract prevalence, sunlight hours, and altitude in the Himalayas. Am J Epidemiol, **118**: 250-264.

Brodkin RH, Kopf AW, & Andrade R (1969) Basal-cell epithelioma and elastosis: a comparison of distribution. In: Urbach F ed. Biologic effects of ultraviolet radiation. Oxford, New York, Pergamon Press, pp 581-618.

Brühl C & Crutzen PJ (1989) On the disproportionate role of tropospheric ozone as a filter against solar UV radiation. Geophys Res Lett, **16**: 703-706.

Bruls WAG, Slaper H, Van der Leun JC, & Berrens L (1984) Transmission of human epidermis and stratum corneum as a function of thickness in the ultraviolet and visible wavelengths. Photochem Photobiol, **40**(4): 485-494.

Bhuyan KC & Bhuyan DK (1983) Molecular mechanism of cataractogenesis, I. Reactive species of oxygen as triggering agents, II. Evidence of lipid peroxidation and membrane damage. In (ed. Cohen G & Greenwald RA) Oxy Radicals, their scavenger syst. Proc. Int. Conf. Superoxide Dismutase 3rd, vol 2, Elsevier, New York, pp 343-356.

Cadet J, Ravanat JC, Buchko GW, Yeo HC, & Ames BN (in press) Singlet oxygen DNA damage: chromatographic and mass spectrometry analysis of damage products. Methods Enzymol.

Caldwell MM (1976) The effect of solar UV-B radiation (280-315 nm) on higher plants: implications of stratosphere ozone reduction. In: Castellani A ed. Research in photobiology. New York, London, Plenum Press, pp 597-607.

Caldwell MM, Termura AH, & Tevini M (1989) The changing solar ultraviolet climate and the ecological consequences for higher plants. Trends Ecol Evol, **4**: 363-366.

Cameron ME (1965) Pterygium throughout the world. Springfield, Illinois, Charles C. Thomas.

Campbell CC, Quinn AG, & Rees JL (1993) Codon 12 Harvey-*ras* mutations are rare events in non-melanoma human skin cancer. Br J Dermatol, **128**: 111-114.

Carretto JJ, Carignana MO, Daleo G, & de Marco SG (1990) Occurrence of mycosporine-like amino acids in the red tide dinoflagellate Alexandrium excavarum, UV-photoprotective compounds. J Plankton Res, **12**: 909-921.

Cartwright LE & Walter JF (1983) Psoralen-containing sunscreen is tumorigenic in hairless mice. J Am Acad Dermatol, **8**: 830-836.

Cerutti PA & Netrawali M (1979) Formation and repair of DNA damage induced by indirect action of ultraviolet light in normal and xeroderma pigmentosum skin fibroblasts. Radiat Res, **Suppl**: 423-432.

Cervenka J, Witkop CJ, Okoro AN, & King RA (1979) Chromosome breaks and sister chromatid exchanges in albinos in Nigeria. Clin Genet, **15**: 17-21.

Césarini JP & Muel B (1989) Erythema induced by quartz-halogen sources. Photodermatology, **6**: 222-227.

Challoner AVJ, Corless D, & Davis A (1976) Personnel monitoring of exposure to ultraviolet radiation. Clin Exp Dermatol, **1**: 175-179.

Chamberlain J & Moss SH (1987) Lipid peroxidation and other membrane damage produced in Escherichia coli K1060 by near-UV radiation and deuterium oxide. Photochem Photobiol, **45**: 625-630.

Chamberlin GJ & Chamberlin DG (1980) Colour: It's measurement, computation and application. London, Heyden & Son, p 46.

Chan GL, Peak MJ, Peak JG, & Haseltine WA (1986) Action spectrum for the formation of endonuclease-sensitive sites and (6-4) photoproducts induced in a DNA fragment by ultraviolet radiation. Int J Radiat Biol, **50**: 641-648.

Chatterjee A, Milton RC, & Thyle S (1982) Prevalence and aetiology of cataract in Punjab. Br J Ophthalmol, **66**: 35-42.

Christman MF, Morgan RW, Jacobson FS, & Ames BN (1985) Positive control of a regulon for defences against oxidative stress and some heat shock proteins in Salmonella typhimurium. Cell, **41**: 753-762.

Chu G & Chang E (1988) Xeroderma pigmentosum group E cells lack a nuclear factor that binds to damaged DNA. Science, **242**: 564-567.

CIE (1987) International lighting vocabulary published jointly by the International Electrotechnical Commission (IEC) and the International Commission on Illumination (CIE). Geneva, International Electrotechnical Commission (ISBN 2-8273-0006-0).

CIE (1990) Report on photosensitising chemicals - Updated in 1993. Vienna, International Commission on Illumination.

CIE (1991) Sunscreen testing (UVB). Vienna, Commission on Illumination (CIE Technical report - Publication No. CIE 90).

Cleaver JE (1973) Xeroderma pigmentosum - progress and regress. J Invest Dermatol, **60**: 374-380.

Clemmesen J (1965) Statistical studies in the aetiology of malignant neoplasms. I. Review and results. Copenhagen, Munksgaard, p 409.

Coffman RL, Seymour WP, Lebman DA, Hirakkki DD, Christiansen JA, Shrader B, Cherwinski HM, Savelkoul HF, Finkelman FD, Bond MW, & Mosmann TR (1988) The role of helper T cell products in mouse B cell differentiation and isotype regulation. Immunol Rev, **102**: 5-28.

Cogan DG & Kinsey VE (1946) Action spectrum for keratitis produced by ultraviolet radiation. Arch Ophthalmol, **35**: 670-677.

Cole CA, Forbes PD, & Davies RE (1986) An action spectrum for UV photocarcinogenesis. Photobiology, **43**: 275.

Colin J, Bonissent JF, & Resnikoff S (1985) Epidemiology of the exfoliation syndrome. Proceedings of the 17th Congress of the European Society of Ophthalmolology, Helsinki, pp 230-231.

Collmann GW, Shore DL, Shy CM, Checkoway H, & Luria AS (1988) Sunlight and other risk factors for cataract: an epidemiological study. Am J Public Health, **78**: 1459-1462.

Colston K, Berger U, & Coombes RC (1989) Possible role for vitamin D in controlling breast cancer cell proliferation. Lancet, **1**: 188-191.

Connor MJ & Wheeler LA (1987) Depletion off cutaneous glutathione by ultraviolet radiation. Photochem Photobiol, **46**: 239-245.

Cooke KR & Fraser J (1985) Migration and death from malignant melanoma. Int J Cancer, **36**: 175-178.

Coombs BD, Sharples KJ, Cooke KR, Skegg DCG, & Elwood JM (1992) Variation and covariates of the number of benign nevi in adolescents. Am J Epidemiol, **136**: 344-355.

Cooper KD (1993) Human studies in photo immunology. Photochem Photobiol, **57**: 745.

Cooper KD, Neises GR, & Katz SI (1986) Antigen-presenting OKM5+ melanophages appear in human epidermis after ultraviolet radiation. J Invest Dermatol, **861**: 363-370.

Cooper KD, Oberhelman BS, Hamilton MS, Baadsgaard O, Terhune M, LeVee G, Anderson T, & Koren H (1992) UV exposure reduces immunization rates and promotes tolerance to epicutaneous antigens in humans; relationship to dose, $CD1a^-$ DR^+ epidermal macrophage induction and Langerhans cell depletion. Proc Natl Acad Sci (USA), **89**: 8497-8501.

Corominas M, Kamino H, Leon J & Pellicer A (1991) Oncogene activitation in human benign tumors of the skin (keratoacanthomas): Is H-ras involved in differentiation as well as proliferation? Proc Natl Acad Sci (USA), **86**: 6372-6376.

Coronel VP, Dai QJ, Vergara BS, & Teramura AH (1990) Preliminary study on response of rice seedlings to enhanced UV-B radiation. Int Rice Res Newsl, **15**: 37.

Coroneo MT (1993) Pterygium as an early indicator of ultraviolet insolation: a hypothesis. Br J Ophthalmol, **77**: 734-739.

Correll DL, Clark CO, Goldberg B, Goodrich VR, Hayes DR, Klein WH, & Schecher WD (1992) Spectral ultraviolet-B radiation fluxes at the earth's surface: long-term variations at 39°N, 77°W. J Geogr Res, **97**: 7579-7591.

Cox CWJ (1987) Ultraviolet irradiance levels in welding processes. In: Passachier WF & Bosnjakovic BFM ed. Human exposure to ultraviolet radiation: Risks and regulations. Amsterdam, Oxford, New York, Elsevier Science Publishers, pp 383-386.

Cristofolini M, Franceschi S, Tasin L, Zumiani G, Piscioli F, Talamini R, & La Vecchia C (1987) Risk factors for cutaneous malignant melanoma in a northern Italian population. Int J Cancer, **39**: 150-154.

Crombie IK (1981) Distribution of malignant melanoma on the body surface. Br J Cancer, **43**: 842-849.

Cruickshanks KJ, Klein R, & Klein BE (1993) Sunlight and age-related macular degeneration: the Beaver Dam Eye Study. Arch Ophthalmol, **111**: 514-518.

Cunningham ML, Johnson JS, Giovanazzi SM, & Peak MJ (1985) Photosensitized production of superoxide anion by monochromatic (290-405 nm) ultraviolet irradiation of NADH and NADPH coenzymes. Photochem Photobiol, **42**: 125-128.

Cyrlin MN, Pedris-Leftick A, & Sugar J (1980) Cataract formation in association with ultraviolet photosensitivity. Ann Ophthalmol, **12**: 786-790.

Czochralska B, Bartosz W, & Shugar D (1984) Oxidation of excited-state NADH and NAD dimer in aqueous medium - involvement of O2- as a mediator in the presence of oxygen. Biochim Biophys Acta, **801**: 403-409.

Danielle RP (1988) Pathophysiology of the asthmatic syndromes. In: Danielle RP ed. Immunologic diseases of the lung. Boston, Blackwell Scientific Publishers, pp 503-516.

Dardanoni L, Gafá L, Paterno R, & Pavone G (1984) A case-control study on lip cancer risk factors in Ragusa (Sicily). Int J Cancer, **34**: 335-337.

Dargent JL, Lespagnard L, Heenan M, & Verhest A (1992) Malignant melanoma occurring in a case of oculocutaneous albinism. Histopathology, **21**: 74-76.

Darrell RW & Bachrach CA (1963) Pterygium among veterans. Arch Ophthalmol, **70**: 158-169.

Davies DM (1985) Calcium metabolism in healthy men deprived of sunlight. Ann N Y Acad Sci, **453**: 21-27.

Daynes RA & Spellman CW (1977) Evidence for the generation of suppressor cells by UV radiation. Cell Immunol, **31**: 182-187.

Daynes RA, Spellman CW, Woodward JG, & Stewart DA (1977) Studies into the transplantation biology of ultraviolet light-induced tumours. Transplantation, **23**: 343-348.

De Fabo EC & Kripke ML (1979) Dose-response characteristics of immunologic unresponsiveness to UV-induced tumors produced by UV irradiation of mice. Photochem Photobiol, **30**: 385-390.

De Fabo EC & Noonan FP (1983) Mechanism of immune suppression by ultraviolet irradiation *in vivo*. J Exp Med, **157**: 84-98.

de Gruijl FR & van der Leun JC (1980) A dose-response model for skin cancer induction by chronic UV exposure of a human population. J Theor Biol, **83**: 487-504.

de Gruijl FR & van der Leun JC (1982) Systemic influence of pre-irradiation of a limited skin area on UV-tumorigenesis. Photochem Photobiol, **35**: 379-383.

de Gruijl FR & van der Leun JC (1983) Follow up on systemic influence of partial pre-irradiation on UV-tumorigenesis. Photochem Photobiol, **38**: 381-383.

de Gruijl FR & van der Leun JC (1991) Action spectra for carcinogenesis. In: Urbach F ed. Biological responses to UVA. Overland Park, Kansas, Valdemar Publishing Company, p 91.

de Gruijl FR, van der Meer JB, & van der Leun JC (1983) Dose-time dependency of tumor formation by chronic UV exposure. Photochem Photobiol, **37**: 53-62.

de Gruijl FR, Sterenborg HJCM, Forbes PD, Davies RE, Cole C, Kelfkens G, van Weelden H, Slaper H, & van der Leun JC (1993) Wavelength dependence of skin cancer induction by ultraviolet radiation of albino hairless mice. Cancer Res, **53**: 53-60.

Denkins Y, Fidler IJ, & Kripke ML (1989) Exposure of mice to UV-B radiation suppresses delayed hypersensitivity to Candida albicans. Photochem Photobiol, **49**: 615-619.

Desai ID, Sawant PL, & Tappel AL (1964) Peroxidative and radiation damage to isolated lysosomes. Biochim Biophys Acta, **86**: 277-285.

Detels R & Dhir SP (1967) Pterygium: a geographical study. Arch Ophthalmol, **78**: 485-491.

Devary Y, Gottlieb RA, Smeal T & Karin M (1992) The mammalian ultraviolet response is triggered by activation of Src tyrosine kinases. Cell **71**: 1081-1091.

Devary Y, Rosette C, Di Donato JA, & Karin M (1993) NFkB activation by ultraviolet light not dependent on a nuclear signal. Science, **261**: 1442-1445.

Dhir SP, Detels R, & Alexander ER (1967) The role of environmental factors in cataract, pterygium and trachoma. Am J Ophthalmol, **64**: 128-135.

Diffey BL (1977) The calculation of the spectral distribution of natural ultraviolet radiation under clear sky conditions, Phys Med Biol, **22**: 309-316.

Diffey BL (1986) Use of UVA sunbeds for cosmetic tanning. Br J Dermatol, **225**: 67-76.

Diffey BL (1987) Analysis of the risk of skin cancer from sunlight and solaria in subjects living in northern Europe. Photodermatology, **4**: 118-126.

Diffey BL (1988) The risk of skin cancer from occupational exposure to ultraviolet radiation in hospitals. Phys Med Biol, **33**(10): 1187-1193.

Diffey BL (1989) Ultraviolet radiation and skin cancer: Are physiotherapists at risk? Physiotherapy, **75**(10): 615-616.

Diffey BL (1989a) Ultraviolet radiation dosimetry with polysulphone film. In: Diffey BL ed. Radiation measurement in photobiology. New York, London, San Francisco, Academic Press, pp 135-159.

Diffey BL (1990) Human exposure to ultraviolet radiation. Semin Dermatol, **9**: 2-10.

Diffey BL (1993) A photobiological evaluation of lamps used in the phototherapy of seasonal affective disorder. J Photochem Photobiol, **B17**: 203-207.

Diffey BL (1993a) Personal communication.

Diffey BL & Cheeseman J (1992) Sun protection with hats. Br J Dermatol, **127**: 10-12.

Diffey BL & McKinlay AF (1983) The UVB content of 'UVA fluorescent lamps' and its erythemal effectiveness in human skin. Phys Med Biol, **28**: 351-358.

Diffey BL & Robson J (1992) The influence of pigmentation and illumination on the perception of erythema. Photodermatol Photoimmunol Photomed, **9**: 45-47.

Diffey BL, Tate TJ, & Davis A (1979) Solar dosimetry of the face: the relationship of natural ultraviolet exposure to basal cell carcinoma localisation. Phys Med Biol, **24**: 931-939.

Diffey BL, Challoner AVJ, & Key PJ (1980) A survey of the ultraviolet radiation emissions of photochemotherapy units. Br J Dermatol, **102**: 301-306.

Diffey BL, Larko O, & Swanbeck G (1982) UVB doses received during different outdoor activities and UVB treatment of psoriasis. Br J Dermatol, **106**: 33-41.

Dillon J, Wang RH, & Atherton S (1990) Photochemical and photophysical studies on human lens constituent. Photochem Photobiol, **52**: 849-854.

Dion M & Hammelin C (1987) Relationship between enhanced reactivation and mutagenesis of UV-irradiated human cytomegalovirus in normal human cells. EMBO J, **6**: 397-399.

Djavuheri-Mergny M, Maziére JC, Santus R, Mora L, Maziére C, Auclair M & Dubertet C (1993) Exposure to long wavelength ultraviolet radiation decreases processing of low density lipoprotein by cultured human fibroblasts. Photochem Photobiol **57**: 302-305.

Döhler G (1990) Effect of UVB (290-320nm) radiation on uptake of 15N-nitrate by marine diatoms. Berlin, Heidelberg, New York, Springer-Verlag, pp 354-359.

Döhler G & Alt MR (1989) Assimilation of ^{15}N-ammonia during irradiance with ultraviolet-B and monochromatic light by Thalassiosira rotula, C R Acad Sci Paris, **D308**, 513-518.

Dolezal JM, Perkins ES, & Wallace RB (1989) Sunlight, skin sensitivity, and senile cataract. Am J Epidemiol, **129**: 559-568.

Doll R (1991) Urban and rural factors in the aetiology of cancer. Int J Cancer, **47**: 803-810.

Doll R, Muir C, & Waterhouse J ed. (1970) Cancer incidence in five continents, Volume II. Berlin, Heidelberg, New York, Springer-Verlag.

Doniger J, Jacobson ED, Krell K, & DiPaolo JA (1981) Ultraviolet light action spectra for neoplastic transformation and lethality of syrian hamster embryo cells correlate with spectrum for pyrimidine dimer formation in cellular DNA. Proc Natl Acad Sci (USA), **78**: 2378-2383.

Dorn HF (1944b) Illness from cancer in the United States: IV. Illness from cancer of specific sites classed in broad groups. Public Health Rep, **59**: 65-77.

Dorn HF (1944a) Illness from cancer in the United States. Public Health Rep, **59**: 33-48.

Dorn CR, Taylor DON, & Schneider R (1971) Sunlight exposure and risk of developing cutaneous and oral squamous cell carcinomas.in white cats. J Natl Cancer Inst, **46**: 1073-1078.

Doughty MJ & Cullen A (1990) Long-term effects of a single dose of ultraviolet B on albino rabbit cornea. II. Deturgescence and fluid pump assessed *in vitro*. Photochem Photobiol, **54**: 439-449.

Driscoll CMH (1992) Solar UV trends and distributions. Natl Radiat Prot Board Bull, **137**: 7-13.

Dubin N, Moseson M, & Pasternack BS (1986) Epidemiology of malignant melanoma: pigmentary traits, ultraviolet radiation, and the identification of high-risk populations. Recent Results Cancer Res, **102**: 56-75.

Duke-Elder WS (1926) The pathological action of light upon the eye. I. Action on the outer eye: Photophthalmia. Lancet, **1**: 1137-1141.

Duvic M, Lowe L, Rapini RP, Rodriguez S, & Levy ML (1989) Eruptive dysplastic nevi associated with human immunodeficiency virus infection. Arch Dermatol, **125**: 397-401.

Dyall-Smith D & Varigos G (1985) The malignant potential of papillomavirus. Aust J Dermatol, **26**: 102-107.

Eggersdorfer B & Häder DP (1991) Phototaxis, gravitaxis and vertical migration in the marine dinoflaggelates. Acta Protozool **30**(2): 63-71.

Eisenstark A & Perrot G (1987) Catalase has only a minor role in protection against ultraviolet radiation damage in bacteria. Mol Gen Genet **207**: 68-72.

Eisman JA, MacIntyre I, Martin TJ, Frampton RJ, & King RJB (1980) Normal and malignant breast tissue is a target organ for 1,25-$(OH)_2$ vitamin D_3. Clin Endocrinol, **13**: 267-272.

Elliott R (1961) The aetiology of pterygium. Trans Ophthalmol Soc N Z, **13**: 22-41.

Ellison MJ & Childs JD (1981) Pyrimidine dimers induced in Escherichia coli DNA by ultraviolet radiation present in sunlight. Photochem Photobiol, **34**: 465-469.

Elmets CA, Bergstresser PR, Tigelaar RE, Wood PJ, & Streilein JW (1983) Analysis of the mechanism of unresponsiveness produced by haptens painted on skin exposed to low dose ultraviolet radiation. J Exp Med, **158**: 781-794.

Elwood, JM & Gallagher RP (1983) Site distribution of malignant melanoma. Can Med Assoc J, **128**: 1400-1404.

Elwood JM, Gallagher RP, Hill GB, Spinelli JJ, Pearson JCG, & Threlfall W (1984) Pigmentation and skin reaction to sun as risk factors for cutaneous melanoma: Western Canada melanoma study. Br Med J, **288**: 99-102.

Elwood JM, Gallagher RP, Davison J, & Hill GB (1985a) Sunburn, suntan and the risk of cutaneous malignant melanoma: the Western Canada melanoma study. Br J Cancer, **51**: 543-549.

Elwood JM, Gallagher RP, Hill GB, & Pearson JCG (1985b) Cutaneous melanoma in relation to intermittent and constant sun exposure: the Western Canada melanoma study. Int J Cancer, **35**: 427-433.

Elwood JM, Williamson C, & Stapleton PJ (1986) Malignant melanoma in relation to moles, pigmentation, and exposure to fluorescent and other lighting sources. Br J Cancer, **53**: 65-74.

Elwood JM, Whitehead SM, Davison J, Stewart M, & Galt M (1990) Malignant melanoma in England: risk associated with naevi, freckles, social class, hair colour, and sunburn. Int J Epidemiol, **19**: 801-810.

Emmett EA (1973) Ultraviolet radiation as a cause of skin tumors. Crit Rev Toxicol, **2**, 211-255.

Engel A, Johnson M, & Haynes S (1988) Health effects of sunlight exposure in the United States. Arch Dermatol, **124**: 72-79.

English DR & Armstrong BK (in press) Cutaneous malignant melanoma. In: Schottenfeld, D Fraumeni. J eds, Cancer epidemiology and prevention, New York, Oxford University Press.

Enninga IC, Groenendijk RTL, Filon AR, van Zeeland AA, & Simons JWIM (1986) The wavelength dependence of UV-induced pyrimidine dimer formation, cell killing and mutation induction in human diploid skin fibroblasts. Carcinogenesis, **7**: 1829-1836.

Epe B, Pflaum M, & Boiteux S (1993) DNA damage induced by photosensitisers in cellular and cell-free systems. Mutat Res **299**: 135-145.

Epstein JH (1965) Comparison of the carcinogenic and cocarcinogenic effects of ultraviolet light on hairless mice. J Natl Cancer Inst, **34**: 741-745.

Epstein JH (1985) Animal models for studying photocarcinogenesis. In: Maibach H & Lowe N ed. Models in Dermatology. Basel, Karger, vol 2, pp 303-312.

Epstein JH (1988) Photocarcinogenesis promotion studies with benzoyl peroxide (BPO) and croton oil. J Invest Dermatol, **91**: 114-116.

Epstein JH & Epstein WL (1962) Cocarcinogenic effect of ultraviolet light on DMBA tumor initiation in albino mice. J Invest Dermatol, **39**: 455-460.

Epstein JH & Roth HL (1968) Experimental ultraviolet light carcinogenesis. A study of croton oil promoting effects. J Invest Dermatol, **50**: 387-389.

Epstein JH, Tuffanelli DL, & Dubois EL (1965) Light sensitivity and lupus erythematosus. Arch Dermatol, **91**: 483-485.

Epstein JH, Epstein WL, & Nakai T (1967) Production of melanomas from DMBA-induced 'blue nevi' in hairless mice with ultraviolet light. J Natl Cancer Inst, **38**: 19-30.

Eriksen P (1987) Occupational applications of ultraviolet radiation: risk evaluation and protection techniques. In: Passchier WF & Bosnjakovic BFM ed. Human exposure to ultraviolet radiation: Risks and regulations. Amsterdam, Oxford, New York, Elsevier Science Publishers, pp 317-331.

Everett MA, Olsen RL, & Sayer RM (1965) Ultraviolet erythema. Arch Dermatol, **92**: 713-719.

Farr PM, Marks JM, Diffey BL, & Ince P (1988) Skin fragility and blistering due to the use of sunbeds. Br Med J, **296**: 1708-1709.

FDA (1988) Quality control guide for sunlamp products, Washington, DC, US Dept. Health and Human Services, (HHS Publication FDA No. 88-8234).

FDA (1992) Medications that increase sensitivity to light (prepared by Levine JI). Rockville, Maryland, Food and Drug Administration, Center of Devices and Radiological Health.

Findlay GM (1928) Ultra-violet light and skin cancer. Lancet, **ii**: 1070-1073.

Finsen NR (1901) The treatment of lupus vulgaris by concentrated chemical rays. In: Phototherapy. London, Edward Armold, pp 73-75.

Fisher GJ & Johns HE (1976) Pyrimidine photohydrates. In: (Ed. Wang, S.) Photochemistry and Photobiology of Nucleic Acids, vol. 1, New York, Academic Press, pp 169-224.

Fisher MS & Kripke ML (1977) Systemic alteration induced in mice by ultraviolet light irradiation and its relationship to ultraviolet carcinogenesis. Proc Natl Acad Sci (USA), **74**: 1688-1692.

Fisher MS, Menter JM, & Willis I (1989) Ultraviolet radiation-induced suppression of contact hypersensitivity in relation to padimate O and oxybenzone. J Invest Dermatol, **92**: 337-341

Fitzpatrick TB & Sober AJ (1985) Sunlight and skin cancer. N Engl J Med, **313**: 818-820.

Fitzpatrick TB, Pathak MA, Magnus IA, & Curwen WL (1963) Abnormal reactions of man to light. Annu Rev Med, **14**: 195-214.

Fitzpatrick TB, Pathak MA, Harber LC, Seiji M, & Kukita A (1974) Sunlight and man. Tokyo, University of Tokyo Press.

Fleming ID, Barnawell JR, Burlison PE, (1975) Skin cancer in black patients. Cancer, **35**: 600-605.

Forbes PD, Davies RE, Sambuco CP, & Urbach F (1989) Topical urocanic acid enhances UV-induced skin tumors in hairless mice by topical application of the sunscreen 2-ethylhexyl-p-methoxycinnamate. J Toxicol Cutan Ocul Toxicol, **8**: 209-226.

Forbes PD, Blum HF, & Davies RE (1981) Photocarcinogenesis in hairless mice: dose-response and the influence of dose-delivery. Photochem Photobiol, **34**: 361-365.

Forbes PD, Davies RE, Urbach F, Berger D, & Cole C (1982) Simulated stratospheric ozone depletion and increased ultraviolet radiation: effects on photocarcinogenesis in hairless mice. Cancer Res, **42**: 2796-2803.

Forbes PD, Davies RE, & Urbach F (1978) Experimental ultraviolet photocarcinogenesis: wavelength interactions and time-dose relationships. Natl Cancer Inst Monogr, **50**: 31-38.

Forsius H (1988) Exfoliation syndrome in various ethnic populations. Acta Ophthalmol, **68**(Suppl 184): 71-85.

Foster HM & Webb SJ (1988) Skin cancer in the North Solomons. Aust N Z J Surg, **58**: 397-401.

Fragu P, Lemarchand-Venencie F, Benhamou S, Francois P, Jeannel D, Benhamou E, Sezary-Lartigau I, & Avril MF (1991) Long-term effects in skin and thyroid after radiotherapy for skin angiomas - A French retrospective cohort study. Eur J Cancer, **27**: 1215-1222.

Franklin WA, Lo KM, & Haseltine WA (1982) Alkaline lability of fluorescent photoproducts produced in ultraviolet light-irradiated DNA. J Biol Chem, **157**: 13535-13543.

Frederick JE, Snell HE, & Haywoood EK (1989) Solar ultraviolet radiation at the earth's surface. Photochem Photobiol, **51**: 443-450.

Freeman RG (1975) Data on the action spectrum for ultraviolet carcinogenesis. J Natl Cancer Inst, **55**: 1119-1122.

Freeman SE, Hacham H, Gange RW, Maytum DJ, Sutherland JC, & Sutherland BM (1989) Wavelength dependence of pyrimidine dimer formation in DNA of human skin irradiated in situ with ultraviolet light. Proc Natl Acad Sci (USA), **86**: 5605-5609.

Friedberg EC (1984) DNA repair. New York, Freeman and Company.

Friedmann PS, White SI, Parker S, Moss C, & Matthews JNS (1989) Antigenic stimulation during ultraviolet therapy in man does not result in immunological tolerance. Clin Exp Immunol, **76**: 68-72.

Fuchs J & Packer L (1991) Photooxidative stress in the skin. In: Sies H Ed. Oxidative stress: oxidants and antioxidants. New York, London, San Francisco, Academic Press, pp 554-584.

Fuchs J, Huflejt M, Rothfuss L, Carcamero G, & Packer L (1989) Impairment of enzymic and nonenzymic antioxidants in skin by UVB irradiation. J Invest Dermatol **93**, 769-773.

Fuller CJ, Faulkner H, Bendich A, Parker RS, & Roe DA (1992) Effect of β-carotene supplementation on photosuppression of delayed-type hypersensitivity in normal young men. Am J Clin Nutr, **56**: 684-690.

Funnell SGP & Keast D (1985) The effect of ultraviolet radiation on the generation of plaque-forming cells and on T-suppressor cell activity to sheep erythrocytes. Photodermatology, **3**: 64-72.

Gaboriau F, Morlière P, Marquis I, Maysan A, Gèze M, & Dubertret L (1993) Membrane damage induced in cultured human skin fibroblasts by UVA irradiation. Photochem Photobiol, **58**: 515-520.

Gafa L, Filippazzo MG, Tumino R, Dardanoni G, Lanzarone F, & Dardanoni L (1991) Risk factors of nonmelanoma skin cancer in Ragusa, Sicily: a case-control study. Cancer Causes Control, **2**: 395-399.

Gallagher, RP (1988) Ocular melanoma in farmers (Letter to the Editor). Am J Ind Med, **13**: 523-525.

Gallagher PE & Duker NJ (1986) Detection of UV purine photoproduct in a defined sequence of human DNA. Mol Cell Biol, **6**: 707-709.

Gallagher RP, Elwood JM, & Hill GB (1986) Risk factors for cutaneous malignant melanoma: the Western Canadian melanoma study, Rec Res Cancer Res, **102**: 38-55.

Gallagher RP, Threlfall WJ, Jeffries E, Band PR, Spinelli J, & Coldman AJ (1984) Cancer and aplastic anemia in British Columbia farmers. J Natl Cancer Inst, **72**: 1311-1315.

Gallagher CH, Greenoak GE, Reeve VE, Canfield PJ, Baker RSU, & Bonin AM (1984a) Ultraviolet carcinogenesis in the hairless mouse skin - influence of the sunscreen 2-ethylhexyl-p-methoxycinnamate. Aust J Exp Biol Med Sci, **62**: 577-588.

Gallagher RP, Elwood JM, Rootman J, Spinelli JJ, Hill GB, Threlfall WJ, & Birdsell JM (1985) Risk factors for ocular melanoma: Western Canada melanoma study. J Natl Cancer Inst, **74**: 775-778.

Gallagher PE, Weiss RB, Brent TP, & Duker NJ (1989) Wavelength dependence of DNA incision by a human ultraviolet endonuclease. Photochem Photobiol, **49**: 363-367.

Gallagher RP, Ma B, McLean DI, Yang CP, Ho V, Carruthers JA, & Warshawski LM (1990a) Trends in basal cell carcinoma, squamous cell carcinoma, and melanoma of the skin from 1973 through 1987. J Am Acad Dermatol, **23**: 413-421.

Gallagher RP, McLean DI, Yang CP, Coldman AJ, Silver HKB, Spinelli JJ, & Beagrie M (1990b) Anatomic distribution of acquired melanocytic nevi in white children. A comparison with melanoma: the Vancouver mole study. Arch Dermatol, **126**: 466-471

Gallagher RP, McLean DI, Yang CP, Coldman AJ, Silver HKB, Spinelli JJ, & Beagrie M (1990c) Suntan, sunburn and pigmentation factors and the frequency of acquired melanocytic nevi in children. Similarities to melanoma: the Vancouver mole study. Arch Dermatol, **126**: 770-776

Gallagher RP, Rivers JK, Yang CP, (1991) Melanocytic nevus density in Asian, Indo-Pakistani, and white children: The Vancouver mole study. J Am Acad Dermatol, **25**: 507-12.

Gange RW, Blackett AD, Matzinger EA, Sutherland BM, & Kochevar IE (1985) Comparative protection efficiency of UVA- and UVB-induced tans against erythema and formation of endonuclease-sensitive sites in DNA by UVB in human skin. J Invest Dermatol, **85**: 362-364.

Garbe C, Krüger S, Stadler R, Guggenmoos-Holzmann I, & Orfanos CE (1989) Markers and relative risk in a German population for developing malignant melanoma. Int J Dermatol, **28**: 517-523.

Garcia-Pichel F & Castenholz RW (1991) Characterization and biological implications of scytonemin, a cyanobacterial sheath pigment, J Phycol, **27**: 395-409.

Garland C & Garland F (1980) Do sunlight and vitamin D reduce the likelihood of colon cancer? Int J Epidemiol, **9**: 227-231.

Garland CF, Comstock GW, Garland FC, Felsing K, Shaw EK, & Gorham ED (1989) Serum 25-hydroxyvitamin D and colon cancer: 8-year prospective study. Lancet, **2**: 1176-1178.

Garland FC, Garland CF, Gorham ED, & Young JF (1990) Geographic variation in breast cancer mortality in the United States: A hypothesis involving exposure to solar radiation. Prev Med, **19**: 614-622.

Garland CF Garland FC, & Gorham ED (1992) Could sunscreens increase melanoma risk? (Letter) Am J Public Health, **82**(4): 614-615.

Garner A (1989) The pathology of tumours at the limbus. Eye, **3**: 210-217.

Garsen J, Goettsch W, de Gruy F, & van Loveren H (1993) UVB suppresses immunity and resistance against systemic infections in the rat. Photochem Photobiol, **57**: 755.

Gasparro F & Fresco J (1986) Ultraviolet-induced 8,8-adenine dehydromimers in oligo- and polynucleotides. Nucl Acids Res, **14**: 4239-4251.

Gellin GA, Kopf AW, & Garfinkel L (1965) Basal cell epithelioma. A controlled study of associated factors. Arch Dermatol, **91**: 38-45.

Gensler HL (1988) Enhancement of chemical carcinogenesis in mice by systemic effects of ultraviolet radiation. Cancer Res, **48**: 620-623.

Gensler HL (1989) Reduction of immunosuppression in UV-irradiated mice by dietary retinyl palmitate plus canthaxanthin. Carcinogenesis, **10**: 203-207.

Gensler HL & Bowden GT (1987) UVB-Induced modulation of mouse skin tumor induction by benzo[a]pyrene (Abstract no. 546). Proc Am Assoc Cancer Res, **28**: 137.

Gensler HL & Welch K (1992) Prevalence of tumor prevention rather than tumor enhancement when repetitive UV radiation treatments precede initiation and promotion. Carcinogenesis, **13**: 9-13.

Gerrish KE & Gensler HL (1993) Prevention of photocarcinogenesis by dietary vitamin E. Nutr Cancer, **19**: 125-133.

Giannini SH (1986a) Suppression of pathogenesis in cutaneous leishmaniasis by UV irradiation. Infect Immun, **51**: 838-843.

Giannini SH (1986b) Effects of UV-B on infectious disease. In: Titus JG ed. Effects of changes in stratospheric ozone and global climate. Washington, DC, US Environmental Protection Agency, vol 2, pp 101-112.

Giannini SH (1987) Abrogation of skin lesions in cutaneous leishmaniasis by ultraviolet irradiation. In: Hart DT ed. Leishmaniasis: The first centenary (1885-1985) new strategies for control. New York, London, Plenum Press, pp 677-684 (NATO ASI Series A: Life Sciences).

Giannini SH (1992) Effects of ultraviolet B irradiation on cutaneous leishmaniasis. Parasitology Today, **8**: 44-48.

Gibbs NK (1993) Is ultraviolet immunosuppression initiated by photosomerisation of urocanic acid. In: de Gruijl FR ed. The dark side of sunlight. Utrecht, The Netherlands, Utrecht University.

Gies HP & Roy CR (1990) Bilirubin phototherapy and potential UVR hazards. Health Phys, **58**: 313-320.

Gies HP, Roy CR, & Elliott G (1986) Artificial suntanning: Spectral irradiance and hazard evaluation of ultraviolet sources. Health Phys, **50**(6): 691-703.

Gies HP, Roy CR, & Elliot G (1990) A proposed UVR protection factor for sunglasses. Clin Exp Optom, **73**: 183-189.

Gies HP, Roy CR, & Elliott G (1992) Ultraviolet radiation protection factors for personal protection in both occupational and recreational situations. Radiat Prot Aust, **10**(3): 59-66.

Gies HP, Roy CR, Herlihy E, & Rivers J (1992a) Personal dosimetry of solar UVB using polysulphone film Congress Proceedings (IRPA 8) vol 1, p 791, Montreal, May 1992, International Radiation Protection Association.

Gilchrest BA (1990) Actinic injury. Annu Rev Med, **41**: 199-210.

Gilchrest BA, Soter NA, Stoff JS, & Mihm MC Jr (1981) The human sunburn reaction: histologic and biochemical studies. J Am Acad Dermatol, **5**: 411-422.

Giles GG, Marks R, & Foley P (1988) Incidence of non-melanocytic skin cancer treated in Australia. Br Med J, **296**: 13-17.

Glass AG & Hoover RN (1989) The emerging epidemic of melanoma and squamous cell skin cancer. J Am Med Assoc, **262**: 2097-2100.

Goldberg LH & Altman A (1984) Benign skin changes associated with chronic sunlight exposure. Cutis, **34**: 33-39.

Goodman GJ, Marks R, Selwood TS, Ponsford MW, & Pakes W (1984) Non-melanocytic skin cancer and solar keratoses in Victoria - clinical studies II. Aust J Dermatol, **25**: 103-106.

Gorham ED, Garland CF, & Garland FC (1989) Acid haze air pollution and breast and colon cancer mortality in 20 Canadian cities. Can J Public Health, **80**: 96-100.

Gorham ED, Garland FC, & Garland CF (1990) Sunlight and breast cancer incidence in the USSR. Int J Epidemiol, **19**: 820-824.

Graham S, Marshall J, Haughey B, Stoll H, Zielezny M, Brasure J, & West D (1985) An inquiry into the epidemiology of melanoma. Am J Epidemiol, **122**: 606-619.

Gray RH, Johnson GJ, & Freedman A (1992) Climatic droplet keratopathy. Surv Ophthalmol, **36**: 241-253.

Greaves MW, Hensby CN, Black AK, Plummer NA, Fincham N, Warin AP, & Camp R (1978) Inflammatory reactions induced by ultraviolet irradiation. Bull. Cancer, **65**: 299-304.

Green AC (1984) Sun exposure and the risk of melanoma. Aust J Dermatol, **25**: 99-102.

Green AC (1991) Premature ageing of the skin in a Queensland population. Med J Aust, **155**: 473-478.

Green AC & Battistutta D (1990) Incidence and determinants of skin cancer in a high-risk Australian population. Int J Cancer, **46**: 356-361.

Green A & O'Rourke MGE (1985) Cutaneous malignant melanoma in association with other skin cancers. J Natl Cancer Inst, **74**: 977-980.

Green A & Siskind V (1983) Geographical distribution of cutaneous melanoma in Queensland. Med J Aust, **1**: 407-410.

Green AES, Sawada T, & Shettle EP (1974) The middle ultraviolet reaching the ground. Photochem Photobiol, **19**: 251.

Green AC, Siskind V, Bain C, & Alexander J (1985) Sunburn and malignant melanoma. Br J Cancer, **51**: 393-397.

Green AC, Beardmore G, Hart V, Leslie D, Marks R, & Staines D (1988a) Skin cancer in a Queensland population. J Am Acad Dermatol, **19**: 1045-1052.

Green AC, Sorahan T, Pope D, Siskind V, Hansen M, Hanson L, Leech P, Ball PM, & Grimley RP (1988b) Moles in Australian and British schoolchildren (Letter to the Editor). Lancet, **ii**: 1497.

Green C, Diffey BL, & Hawk JLM (1992) Ultraviolet radiation in the treatment of skin disease. Phys Med Biol, **37**(1): 1-20.

Green A, Smith P, McWhirter W, Oregan P, Battistutta D, Yarker ME, & Lape K (1993a) Melanocytic naevi and melanoma in survivors of childhood cancer. Br J Cancer, **67**: 1053-1057.

Green A, MacLennan R, Youll P, & Martin N (1993b) Site distribution of cutaneous melanoma in Queensland. Int J Cancer, **53**: 232-236.

Greenberg JT, Monach PA, Chou JH, Josephy PD, & Demple B (1990) Positive control of a global antioxidant defence regulon activated by superoxide-generating agents in Escherichia coli. Proc Natl Acad Sci (USA), **87**: 6181-6185.

Greene MH & Wilson J (1985) Second cancer following lymphatic and hematopoietic cancers in Connecticut, 1935-82. Natl Cancer Inst Monogr, **68**: 191-217.

Greene MH, Young TI, & Clark WH Jr (1981) Malignant melanoma in renal transplant recipients. Lancet, **May 30**: 1196-1199.

Grob JJ, Gouvernet J, Aymar D, Mostaque A, Romano MH, Collet AM, Noe MC, Diconstanzo MP, & Bonerandi JJ (1990) Count of benign melanocytic nevi as a major indicator of risk for nonfamilial nodular and superficial spreading melanoma. Cancer, **66**: 387-395.

Guerry RK, Ham WT, & Mueller HA (1985) Light toxicity in the posterior segment. In: Duane TD & Jaeger EA ed. Clinical ophthalmology. Philadelphia, Pennsylvania, Harper and Row, pp 1-17.

Guex-Crosier Y & Herbort CP (1993) Presumed corneal intraepithelial neoplasia associated with contact lens wear and intense ultraviolet light exposure. Br J Ophthalmol, **77**: 191-192.

Gupta AK, Cardella CJ, & Haberman HF (1986) Cutaneous malignant neoplasms in patients with renal transplants. Arch Dermatol, **122**: 1288-1293.

Gupta AK, Stern RS, Swanson NA, Anderson TF, & Arbor A (1988) Cutaneous melanomas in patients treated with psoralens plus ultraviolet A. J Am Acad Dermatol, **19**: 67-76.

Gutteridge JMC (1985) Superoxide dismutase inhibits the superoxide-driven Fenton reaction at two different levels. FEBS Lett, **185**: 19-23.

Häder DP & Worrest RC (1991) Effects of enhanced solar radiation on aquatic ecosystems. Photochem Photobiol, **53**: 717-725.

Häder DP & Lui SM (1991) Mobility and gravitactic orientation of the flagellate, Euglena gracilis, impaired by artificial and solar UVB radiation. Curr Microbiol, **21**: 161-168.

Haenszel W (1963) Variations in skin cancer incidence within the United States. Natl Cancer Inst Monogr, **10**: 225-243.

Halprin KM, Comerford M, Presser SE, & Taylor JR (1981) Ultraviolet light treatment delays contact sensitization to nitrogen mustard. Br J Dermatol, 105: 71-76.

Ham WT, Mueller HA, Ruffolo JJ, Millen JE, Cleary SF, & Guerry RK (1984) Basic mechanisms underlying the production of photochemical lesions in the mammalian retina. Curr Eye Res, 3: 165-174.

Hanchette CL & Schwartz GC (1992) Geographic patterns of prostatecancer mortality. Evidence for a protective effect of ultraviolet radiation. Cancer, **70**: 2861-2869.

Hardie IR, Strong RW, Hartley LCJ, Woodruff PWH, & Clunie GJA (1980) Skin cancer in Caucasian renal allograft recipients living in a subtropical climate. Surgery, **87**: 177-183.

Hartevelt MM, Bouwes Bavinck JN, Kootte AMM, Vermeer BJ, & Vandenbroucke JP (1990) Incidence of skin cancer after renal transplantation in the Netherlands. Transplantation, **49**: 506-509.

Hawk, JLM (1984) Photosensitising agents used in the United Kingdom. Clin Expl Dermatol, **9**: 300-302.

Hayashi Y & Aurelian L (1986) Immunity to herpes simplex virus type 2: Viral antigen-presenting capacity of epidermal cells and its impairment by ultraviolet irradiation. J Immunol, **136**: 1087-1092.

Haynes RH (1966) The interpretation of microbiol inactivation and recovery phenomena. Radiat Res, **Suppl 6**: 1-29.

Health Council of the Netherlands (1986) UV radiation: Human exposure to ultraviolet radiation. The Hague, Health Council of the Netherlands (Report 1986/93).

Hedblom EE (1961) Snowscape eye protection. Arch Environ Health, **2**; 685-704.

Hefferren JJ, Cooley RO, Hall JB, Olsen NH, & Lyon HW (1971) Use of ultraviolet illumination in diagnosis. J Am Dent Assoc, **82**: 1353-1360.

Herity B, O'Loughlin G, Moriarty MJ, & Conroy R (1989) Risk factors for non-melanoma skin cancer. Ir Med J, 82: 151-152.

Hersey P, Hasic E, Edwards A, Bradley M, Maran G, & McCarthy WH (1983a) Immunological effects of solarium exposure. Lancet, **1**: 545-548.

Hersey P, Haran G, Hasic E, & Edwards A (1983b) Alteration of T cell subsets and induction of suppressor T cell activity in normal subjects after exposure to sunlight. J Immunol, **31**: 171-174.

Hersey P, MacDonald M, Burns C, Schibeci S, Matthews H, & Wilkinson FJ (1987) Analysis of the effect of sunscreen agent on the suppression of natural killer cell activity induced in human subjects by radiation from solarium lamps. J Invest Dermatol, **88**: 271-276.

Hersey P, MacDonald M, Henderson C, Schibeci S, D'Alessandro G, Pryor M, & Wilkinson FJ (1988) Suppression of natural killer cell activity in humans by radiation from solarium lamps depleted of UVB. J Invest Dermatol, **90**: 305-310.

Hess C (1907) Experiments on the effect of ultraviolet light on the lens. Arch f Augenheilk **57** 185-196.

Higginson J & Oettlé AG (1959) Cancer incidence in the Bantu and "Cape Colored" races of South Africa: Report of a cancer survey in the Transvaal (1953-55). J Natl Cancer Inst, **24**: 589-671.

Hill D, White V, Marks R, Theobald T, Borland R, & Roy C (1992) Melanoma prevention: behavioural and nonbehavioural factors in sunburn among an Australian urban population. Prev Med, **21**: 654-669.

Hiller R, Sperduto RD, & Ederer F (1977a) Epidemiological associations with cataract in the 1971-72 national health and nutrition examination survey. Am J Epidemiol, **105**: 450-459.

Hiller R, Giacometti L, & Yuen K (1977b) Sunlight and cataract: an epidemiologic investigation. Am J Epidemiol, **105**: 450-459.

Hiller R, Sperduto RD, & Ederer F (1983) Epidemiologic associations with cataract in the 1971-1972 national health and nutrition examination survey. Am J Epidemiol, **118**: 239-249.

Hiller R, Sperduto RD, & Ederer F (1986) Epidemiologic associations with nuclear, cortical, and posterior subcapsular cataracts. Am J Epidemiol, **124**: 916-925.

Hirschfeld S, Levine AS, Ozato K, & Protic M (1990) A constitutive damage-specific DNA binding protein is synthesized at higher levels in UV-irradiated primate cells. Mol Cell Biol, **10**: 2041-2048.

Hoeijmakers JHJ & Bootsma D (1990) Molecular genetics of eucaryotic DNA excision repair. Cancer Cells, **2**: 311-320.

Hoffman JS (1987) Ultraviolet radiation and melanoma (with a special focus on assessing the risks of stratospheric ozone depletion). Washington, DC, US Environmental Protection Agency, Office of Air and Radiation (EPA 400/1-87-001D).

Hogan DJ, To T, Gran L, Wong D, & Lane PR (1991) Risk factors for basal cell carcinoma. Int J Dermatol, **28**: 591-594.

Holick MF (1985) The photobiology of vitamin D and its consequences for human. Ann N Y Acad Sci, **453**: 1-3.

Hollows F & Moran D (1981) Cataract - the ultraviolet risk factor. Lancet, **2**: 1249-1250.

Holly EA, Kelly JW, Shpall SN, & Chiu S-H (1987) Number of melanocytic nevi as a major risk factor for malignant melanoma. J Am Acad Dermatol, **17**: 459-468.

Holly EA, Aston DA, Char DH, Kristiansen JJ, & Ahn DK (1990) Uveal melanoma in relation to ultraviolet light exposure and host factors. Cancer Res, **50**: 5773-5777.

Holly EA, Aston DA, Ahn DK, Kristiansen JJ, & Char DH (1991) No excess prior cancer in patients with uveal melanoma. Ophthalmology, **98**: 608-611.

Holm-Hansen O (1990) UV radiation in Arctic waters: Effects on rates of primary production (Appendix G). La Jolla, CA, USA, Scripps Institution of Oceanography, pp 1-17.

Holman CDJ & Armstrong BK (1984) Pigmentary traits, ethnic origin, benign nevi, and family history as risk factors for cutaneous malignant melanoma. J Natl Cancer Inst, **72**: 257-266.

Holman CDJ, Gibson IM, Stephenson M. & Armstrong BK (1983) Ultraviolet irradiation of human body sites in relation to occupation and outdoor activity: field studies using personal UVR dosimeters. Clin Exp Dermatol, **8**: 269-277.

Holman CDJ, Armstrong BK, Evans PR, Lumsden GJ, Dallimore KJ, Meehan CJ, Beagley J, & Gibson IM (1984a) Relationship of solar keratosis and history of skin cancer to objective measures of actinic skin damage. Br J Dermatol, **110**: 129-138.

Holman CD, Evans PR, Lumsden GJ, & Armstrong BK (1984b) The determinants of actinic skin damage: problems of confounding among environmental and constitutional variables. Am J Epidemiol, **120**: 414-422.

Holman CDJ, Armstrong BK, & Heenan PJ (1986) Relationship of cutaneous malignant melanoma to individual sunlight-exposure habits. J Natl Cancer Inst, **76**: 403-414.

Hoover R (1977) Effects of Rugs - Immunosuppression. In: Hiatt HH, Watson JD, & Winsten JA ed. Origins of human cancer. Book A: Incidence of cancer in humans. Proceedings of the Cold Spring Harbor Conferences on Cell Proliferation. Cold Spring Harbor, New York, Cold Spring Harbor Laboratory, vol 4.

Hoppeler Th, Hendrickson Ph, Dietrich C, & Reme (1988) Morphology and time-course of defined photochemical lesions in the rabbit retina. Curr Eye Res, **7(9):** 849-860.

Howie S, Norval M, & Maingay J (1986) Exposure to low-dose ultraviolet radiation suppresses delayed-type hypersensitivity to herpes simplex virus in mice. J Invest Dermatol, **86:** 125-128.

Howie SEM, Ross JA, Norval M, & Maingay JP (1986) In vivo*In vivo* modulation of antigen presentation generates Ts rather than TDH in HSV-1 infection. Immunology, **60**: 419-423.

Hsu J, Forbes PD, Harber LC, & Lakow E (1975) Induction of skin tumors in hairless mice by a single exposure to UV radiation. Photochem Photobiol, **21:** 185-188.

Hughes BR, Cunliffe WJ, & Bailey CC (1989) Excess benign melanocytic naevi after chemotherapy for malignancy in childhood. Br Med J, **299:** 88-91.

Hunter DJ, Colditz GA, Stampfer MJ, Rosner B, Willett WC, & Speizer FE (1990) Risk factors for basal cell carcinoma in a prospective cohort of women. Ann Epidemiol, **1**: 13-23.

Hunter DJ, Colditz GA, Stampfer MJ, Rosner B, Willett WC, & Speizer FE (1992) Diet and risk of basal cell carcinoma of the skin in a prospective cohort of women. Ann Epidemiol, **2**: 231-239.

Husain Z, Yang Q, & Biswas DK (1990) cHa-ras Proto oncogene. Amplification and overexpression in UVB-induced mouse skin papillomas and carcinomas. Arch Dermatol, **126:** 324-330.

Husain Z, Pathak MA, Flotte T, & Wick MM (1991) Role of ultraviolet radiation in the induction of melanocytic tumors in hairless mice following 7,12-dimethylbenz(a)anthracene application and ultraviolet irradiation. Cancer Res, **51:** 4964-4970.

Hyman LG, Lilienfeld AM, Ferris FL, & Fine SL (1983) Senile macular degeneration: a case-control study. Am J Epidemiol, **118:** 213-227.

IARC (1993) In: Kricker A, Armstrong BK, Jones ME & Burton RD ed. Health, solar UV radiation and environmental change. Lyon, International Agency for Research on Cancer (IARC Technical Report No. 13).

IARC (1992) Solar and ultraviolet radiation. Lyon, International Agency for Research on Cancer (Monographs on the Evaluation of Carcinogenic Risks to Humans, Volume 55).

IARC (1980) International Agency for Research on Cancer, Monographs on the Evaluation of the Carcinogenic Risk of Chemicals to Humans, Vol 24, Some Pharmaceutical Drugs, Lyon, 101-124.

Ignatiades L (1990) Photosynthetic capacity of the surface microlayer during the mixing period. J Planktonic Res, **12:** 851-860.

Imlay JA, Chir SM, & Linn S (1988) Science, **240:** 640-642.

IRPA/INIRC (1985) International Radiation Protection Association/ International Non-Ionizing Radiation Committee. Concepts, units and terminology for NIR protection. Health Phys, **49(6)**: 1329-1362.

IRPA/INIRC (1991a) International Radiation Protection Association/ International Non-Ionizing Radiation Committee. Health issues of ultraviolet A sunbeds used for cosmetic purposes. Health Phys, **61(2)**: 285-288.

IRPA/INIRC (1991b) International Radiation Protection Association/ International Non-Ionizing Radiation Committee. In: Duchêne AS, Lakey JRA, & Repacholi MH ed. IRPA guidelines on protection against non-ionizing radiation., New York, McGraw-Hill.

Isaacson C, Selzer G, Kaye V, Greenberg M, Woodruff JD, Davies J, Ninin D, Vetten D, & Andrew, M (1978) Cancer in the urban blacks of South Africa. S Afr Cancer Bull, **22**: 49-84.

Ishizaki K, Tsujimura T, Nakai M, Nishigori C, Sato K, Katayama S, Kurimura O, Yoshikawa K, Imamura S, & Ikenaga M (1992) Infrequent mutation of the *ras* genes in skin tumors of Xeroderma Pigmentosum patients in Japan. Int J Cancer, **50:** 382-385.

Italian-American Cataract Study Group (1991) Risk factors for age-related cortical, nuclear, and posterior subcapsular cataracts. Am J Epidemiol, **133:** 541-553.

Ito A & Ito T (1983) Possible involvement of membrane damage in the inactivation by broad-band near-UV radiation in Saccharomyces cerevisiae cells. Photochem Photobiol **37**: 395-401.

Iversen OH (1988) Skin tumorigenesis and carcinogenesis studies with 7,12-dimethylbenz[a]anthracene, ultraviolet light, benzoyl peroxide (Panoxyl gel 5%) and ointment gel. Carcinogenesis, **9:** 803-809.

Jagger J (1985) Solar-UV actions on living cells. New York, Praeger.

Jeevan A & Kripke ML (1990) Alteration of the immune response to Mycobacterium bovis BCG in mice exposed chonically to low doses of UV radiation. Cell Immunol, **130:** 32-41.

Jeevan A, Evans R, Brown EL, & Kripke ML (1992a) Effect of local ultraviolet irradiation on infections of mice with Candida albicans, Mycobacterium bovis BCG, and Schistosoma mansoni. J Invest Dermatol, **99:** 59-64.

Jeevan A, Gilliam K, Heard H, & Kripke ML (1992b) Effects of ultraviolet radiation on the pathogenesis of Mycobacterium lepraemurium infection in mice. Exp Dermatol, **1:** 152-160.

Jeevan A, Ullrich SE, Dizon V, & Kripke ML (1992c) Supernantants from ultraviolet-irradiated keratinocytes decrease the resistance and delayed-type hypersensitivity response to Mycobacterium bovis bacillus Calmette-Guerin in mice and impair the phagocytic ability of macrophages. Photodermatol Photoimmunol Photomed, **9:** 255-263.

Jeffery SW & Humphrey GH (1975) New spectrophotometric equations for determining chlorophylls a, b, c_1 and C_2 in higher plants, algae, and natural phytoplankton. Biochem Physiol Pflanz, **167:** 191-194.

Jensen OM & Bolander (1980) Trends in malignant melanoma of the skin, WHO Stat Q, **33:** 2-26.

Johnson GJ (1981) Aetiology of spheroidal degeneration of the cornea in Labrador. Br J Ophthalmol, **65**: 270-283.

Johnson GJ & Overall M (1978) Histology of spheroidal degeneration of the cornea in Labrador. Br J Ophthalmol, **62:** 53-61.

Johnson GJ, Paterson GD, Green JS, & Perkins ES (1981) Ocular conditions in a labrador community In: Harvald B & Hansen JP ed. Circumpolar health 81. Copenhagen, Nordic Council for Arctic Medical Research.

Johnson GJ, Minassian DC, & Franken S (1989) Alterations of the anterior lens capsule associated with climatic keratopathy. Br J Ophthalmol, **73:** 229-234

Jones CA, Huberman E, Cunningham ML, & Peak MJ (1987a) Mutagenesis and cytotoxicity in human epithelial cells by far- and near-ultraviolet radiations : action spectra. Radiat Res, **110:** 244-254.

Jones SK, Moseley H, & Mackie RM (1987b) UVA-induced melanocytic lesions. Br J Dermatol, **117:** 111-115.

Jones ME, Shugg D, Dwyer T, Young B, & Bonett A (1992) Interstate differences in incidence and mortality from melanoma: a re-examination of the latitudinal gradient. Med J Aust, **157:** 373-377.

Jose JG (1986) Posterior cataract induction by UVB radiation in albino mice. Exp Eye Res, **42:** 11-20.

Jose JG & Pitts DG (1985) Wavelength dependency of cataracts in albino mice following chronic exposure. Exp Eye Res, **41:** 545-563.

Kalimo K, Loulu L, & Jansen CT (1983) Effect of a single UVB or PUVA exposure on immediate and delayed skin hypersensitivity reactions in humans. Correlation to erythemal response and Langerhans cell depletion. Arch Dermatol Res, **275:** 374-378.

Karai I & Horiguchi S (1984) Pterygium in welders. Br J Ophthalmol, **68:** 347-349.

Karentz D & Lutze LH (1990) Evaluation of biologically harmful ultraviolet radiation in Antarctica with a biological dosimeter designed for aquatic environments. Limnol Oceanogr, **35:** 549-561.

Karentz D, Mc Euen FS, Land MC, & Dunlap WC (1991) Survey of microsporine-like amino acid compounds in Antarctic marine organisms: potential protection from ultraviolet exposure. Mar Biol, **108:** 157-166.

Karjalainen S, Salo H, & Teppo L (1989) Basal cell and squamous cell carcinoma of the skin in Finland Int J Dermatol, **28:** 445-450.

Kataoka H & Fujiwara Y (1991) UV damage specific protein in xeroderma pigmentosum complementation group E. Biochem Biophys Res Commun, **175:** 1139-1143.

Katz L, Ben-Tuvia S, & Steinitz R (1982) Malignant melanoma of the skin in Israel: effect of migration. In: Magnus K ed Trends in cancer incidence: Causes and practical implication. Washington, New York, Hemisphere, pp 419-426.

Kelfkens G, van Weelden H, de Gruijl FR, & van der Leun JC (1991) Influence of dose rate in ultraviolet tumorigenesis. J Photochem Photobiol, **B10**: 41-50.

Kelfkens G & van der Leun JC (1989) Skin temperature changes after irradiation with UVB or UVC: Implications for the mechanism underlying ultraviolet erythema. Phys Med Biol, **34**: 599-608.

Keller, AZ (1970) Cellular types, survival, race, nativity, occupations, habits and associated diseases in the pathogenesis of lip cancers. Am J Epidemiol, **91**, 486-499.

Kelly, GE, Meikle, WD, & Moore, DE (1989) Enhancement of UV-induced skin carcinogenesis by azathioprine: role of photochemical sensitisation. Photochem Photobiol, **49**, 59-65.

Kelly GE, Meikle WD, & Sheil AGR (1987) Effects of immunosuppressive therapy on the induction of skin tumors by ultraviolet irradiation in hairless mice. Transplantation, **44**, 429-434.

Kennedy JC, Poltier RH, & Pross DC (1990) Photodynamic therapy with endogenous protoporphyrin. IX. Basic principles and present clinical experience. J Photochem Photobiol, **6:** 143-148.

Keyse SM (1993) The induction of gene expression in mammalian cells by radiation. Sem Cancer Biol, **4:** 119-128.

Keyse SM & Tyrrell RM (1989) Heme oxygenase is the major 32-kDa stress protein induced in human skin fibroblasts by UVA radiation, hydrogen peroxide and sodium arsenite. Proc Natl Acad Sci (USA), **86**: 99-103.

Khlat M, Vail A, Parkin M, & Green A (1992) Mortality from melanoma in migrants to Australia: variation by age at arrival and duration of stay. Am J Epidemiol, **135:** 1103-1113.

Kim TY, Kripke ML, & Ullrich SE (1990) Immunosuppression by factors released from UV-irradiated epidermal cells: Selective effects on the generation of contact and delayed hypersensitivity after exposure to UVA or UVB radiation. J Invest Dermatol, **94:** 26-32.

Kinlen LJ, Sheil AGR, Peto J, & Doll R (1979) Collaborative United Kingdom-Australasian study of cancer in patients treated with immunosuppressive drugs. Br Med J, **2:** 1461-1466.

Klamen DK & Tuveson RW (1982) The effect of membrane fatty acid compositions on the near-UV (300-400 nm) sensitivity of Escherichia coli K1060. Photochem Photobiol, **35:** 167-173.

Klepp O & Magnus K (1979) Some environmental and bodily characteristics of melanoma patients. A case-control study. Int J Cancer, **23:** 482-486.

Kligman LH, Kaidbey KH, Hitchens VM, & Miller SA (1987) Long wavelength (>340 nm) ultraviolet-A induced damage in hairless mice is dose dependent. In: Passchier W & Bosnjakovi, BFM ed., Human exposure to ultraviolet radiation: Risks and regulations. Amsterdam, Oxford, New York, Elsevier Science Publishers, pp 77-81.

Knekt P, Aromaa A, Maatela J, Alfthan G, Aaran RK, Nikkari T, Hakama M, Hakulinen T, & Teppo, L (1991) Serum micronutrients and risk of cancers of low incidence in Finland. Am J Epidemiol, **134**: 356-361.

Kollias, N, Sayre RM, Zeise L, & Cehedekel MR (1991) Photoprotection by melanin, J Photochem Photobiol, **9**: 135-160

Kopecky KE, Pugh GW Jr, Hughes DE, Booth GD, & Cheville, NF (1979) Biological effect of ultraviolet radiation on cattle: bovine ocular squamous cell carcinoma. Am J Vet Res, **40:** 1783-1788.

Kopf AW, Lazar M, Bart RS, Dubin N, & Bromberg J (1978) Prevalence of nevocytic nevi on lateral and medial aspects of arms. J Dermatol Surg Oncol, **4:** 153-158.

Kopf AW, Lindsay AC, Rogers GS, Friedman RJ, Rigel DS, & Levenstein M (1985) Relationship of nevocytic nevi to sun exposure in dysplastic nevus syndrome. J Am Acad Dermatol, **12:** 656-662.

Kraemer KH, Lee MM, & Scotto J (1987) Xeroderma Pigmentosum Arch Dermatol, **123:** 241-50.

Kraemer KH, Seetharam S, Protic-Sabljic M, Brash DE, Bredberg A, & Seidman MM (1988) Defective DNA repair and mutagenesis by dimer and non-dimer photoproducts in xeroderma pigmentosum measured with plasmid vectors. In: Freidberg EC & Hanawalt PC ed. Mechanisms and consequences of DNA damage processing. New York, Alan R. Liss, pp 325-335.

Kramer GF & Ames BN (1987) Oxidative mechanisms of toxicity of low-intensity near-UV light in Salmonella typhimurium. J Bacteriol, **164:** 2259-2266.

Kremers JJM & van Norren D (1988) Two classes of photochemical damage to the retina. In. Lasers and light in ophthalmology. Amsterdam, Berkeley, Milano, Klugler Publications, vpl 2, pp 41-52.

Kress S, Sutter C, Strickland PT, Mukhtar H, Schweizer J, & Schwarz M (1992) Carcinogen-specific mutational pattern in the p53 gene in ultraviolet B radiation-induced squamous cell carcinomas of mouse skin. Cancer Res, **52:** 6400-6403.

Kricker A, Armstrong BK, English DR, & Heenan PJ (1991a) Pigmentary and cutaneous risk factors for non-melanocytic skin cancer - a case-control study. Int J Cancer, **48**: 650-662.

Kricker A, Armstrong BK, English D, Heenan PJ, & Randell PL (1991b) A case-control study of non-melanocytic skin cancer and sun exposure in Western Australia (Abstract No. III, P2). Cancer Res Clin Oncol, **117**(Suppl II): S75.

Kricker A, English DR, Randell PL, Heenan PJ, Clay CD, Delaney TA, & Armstrong BK (1990) Skin cancer in Geraldton, Western Australia: a survey of incidence and prevalence. Med J Aust, **152**: 399-407.

Kricker A, Armstrong BK, Jones ME, & Burton RC (1993) Health, solar UV radiation and environmental change. IARC Technical Report No 13. Lyon, International Agency for Research on Cancer.

Kripke ML (1974) Antigenicity of murine skin tumors induced by ultraviolet light. J Natl Cancer Inst, **53:** 1333-1336.

Kripke Ml & Fidler IJ (1980) Enhanced experimental metastasis of ultraviolet light-induced fibrosarcomas in ultraviolet light-iradiated syngeneic mice. Cancer Res, **40**: 625-629.

Kripke ML & Fisher MS (1976) Immunologic parameters of ultraviolet carcinogenesis. J Natl Cancer Inst, **57:** 211-215.

Kripke ML & Sass ER ed. (1978) International Conference on Ultraviolet Carcinogenesis. Natl Cancer Inst Monogr, **50**: 16-17.

Kripke ML, Lofgreen JS, Beard J, Jessup JM, & Fisher MS (1977) *In vivo* immune responses of mice during carcinogenesis by ultraviolet irradiation. J Natl Cancer Inst, **59**: 1227-1230.

Kromberg JG & Jenkins T (1982) Prevalence of albinism in the South African Negro. S Afr Med J, **61:** 383-386.

Kromberg JGR, Castle D, Zwane EM, & Jenkins T (1989) Albinism and skin cancer in southern Africa. Clin Genet, **36**: 43-52.

Kulandaivelu G, Neducheshian N & Annamalainathan K (1993) Ultraviolet-B (280-320) radiation induced changes in photochemical activities and polypeptide components of C_3 and C_4 chloroplasts. Photosynthetica, **25**:12-14.

Kune GA, Bannerman S, Field B, Watson LF, Clelan H, Merenstein D, & Vitetta L (1992) Diet, alcohol, smoking, serum β-carotene, and vitamin A in male nonmelanocytic skin cancer patients and controls. Nutr Cancer, **18**: 237-244.

Lancaster HO & Nelson J (1957) Sunlight as a cause of melanoma: a clinical survey. Med J Aust, **1**: 452-456.

Langer B & Wellmann E (1990) Phytochrome induction of photoreactivation in Phaseolus vulgaris L. seedlings. Photochem Photobiol, **52**: 861-864.

Larko O & Diffey BL (1983) Natural UVB radiation received by people with outdoor, indoor and mixed occupations and UVB treatment of psoriasis. Clin Exp Dermatol, **8**: 279-285.

Lassam NJ, From L, & Kahn HJ (1993) Overexpression of p53 is a late event in the development of malignant melanoma. Cancer Res, **53**: 2235-2238.

Laycock KA, Lee SF, Brady RH, & Pepose JS (1991) Characterization of a murine model of recurrent herpes simples viral keratitis induced by ultraviolet B radiation. Invest Ophthalmol Vis Sci, **32**: 2741-2746.

Lê, MG, Cabanes, PA, Desvignes, V, Chanteau, MF, Mlika, N, & Avril, MF (1992) Oral contraceptive use and risk of cutatneous malignant melanoma in a case-control study in French women. Cancer Causes Control, **3**, 199-205.

Leach, JF, McLeod, VE, Pingstone, AR, Davis, A and Deane, GHW (1978) Measurement of the ultraviolet doses received by office workers. Clinical and Experimental Dermatology, **3**,77-79.

Leclerc, JE, Borden, A and Lawrence, CW (1991) The thymine-thymine pyrimidine-pyrimidine (6-4) ultraviolet light photoproduct is highly mutagenic and specifically induces 3'-thymine-to-cytosine transition in Escherichia coli Proc Natl Acad Sci USA, **88**: 9685-9689.

Lee JAM (1989) The relationship between malignant melanoma of the skin and exposure to sunlight. Photochem Photobiol, **50**: 493-496.

Lee GA & Hirst LW (1992) Incidence of ocular surface epithelial dysplasia in metropolitan Brisbane: a 10-year survey. Arch Ophthalmol, **110**: 525-527.

Lerman S (1980) Human ultraviolet radiation cataracts. Ophthalmic Res, **12**: 303-314.

Leske MC, Chylack LT, Wu S, & The Lens Opacities Case-Control Study Group (1991) The lens opacities case-control study: risk factors for cataract. Arch Ophthalmol, **109**: 244-251.

Levi F, La Vecchia C, Te V-C, & Mezzanotte G (1988) Descriptive epidemiology of skin cancer in the Swiss canton of Vaud. Int J Cancer, **42**: 811-816.

Levine EA, Ronan SG, Shirali SS, & Das Gupta TK (1992) Malignant melanoma in a child with oculocutaneous ablinism. J Surg Oncol, **51**: 138-142.

Lew RA, Sober AJ, Cook N, Marvell R, & Fitzpatrick TB (1983) Sun exposure habits in patients with cutaneous melanoma: a case control study. J Dermatol Surg Oncol, **9**: 981-986.

Lewis MG (1967) Malignant melanoma in Uganda (The relationship between pigmentation and malignant melanoma on the soles of the feet). Br J Cancer, **21**: 483-495.

Ley RD (1993) Photoreactivation in humans. Proc Natl Acad Sci (USA), **90**: 4337.

Ley RD Peak MJ, & Lyon LL (1983) Induction of pyrimidine dimers in epidermal DNA of hairless mice by UVB: an action spectrum. J Invest Dermatol, **80**: 188-191.

Ley RD (1985) Photoreactivation of UV-Induced pyrimidine dimers and erythema in the marsupial Monodelphis domestica. Proc Natl Acad Sci (USA), **82**: 2409-2411.

Ley RD, Applegate LA, Stuart TD, & Fry RJM (1987) UV radiation-induced skin tumors in Monodelphis domestica. Photodermatology, **4**: 144-147.

Ley RD, Applegate LA, Padilla RS, & Stuart TD (1989) Ultraviolet radiation-induced malignant melanoma in Monodelphis domestica. Photochem Photobiol, **50**: 1-5.

Ley RD, Applegate LA, Fry RJM, & Sanchez AB (1991) Photoreactivation of ultraviolet radiation-induced skin and eye tumors of Monodelphis domestica. Cancer Res, **51**: 6539-6542.

Li YF, Kim ST, & Sancer A (1993) Evidence for lack of DNA photoreactivity enzyme in humans. Proc Natl Acad Sci (USA), **90**: 4389-4393.

Lieu F-M, Yamanishi K, Jonishi K, Kishimoto S, & Yasuno, H (1991) Low incidence of Ha-*ras* oncogene mutations in human epidermal tumors. Cancer Lett, **59**: 231-235.

Lill PH (1983) Latent period and antigenicity of murine tumors induced in C3H mice by short-wavelength ultraviolet radiation. J Invest Dermatol, **81**: 342-346.

Lindberg JG (1917) Clinical study on iris depigmentation and on transparency of iris in cataract and in normal eyes among elderly persons. Dissertation, Helsinki, Finland (in Swedish).

Lindelöf B, Sigurgeirsson B, Tegner E, Larkö O, Johannesson A, Berne B, Christensen OB, Andersson T, Törngren M, Molin L, Nylander-Lundqvist E, & Emtestam L (1991) PUVA and cancer; a large-scale epidemiological study. Lancet, **338**: 91-93.

Lindqvist C (1979) Risk factors in lip cancer: a questionnaire survey. Am J Epidemiol, **109**: 521-530.

Lippke JA, Gordon LK, Brash D, & Haseltine WA (1981) Distribution of UV light-induced damage in a defined sequence of human DNA: Detection of alkaline-sensitive lesions at pyrimidine nucleoside-cytidine sequences. Proc Natl Acad Sci (USA), **78**: 3388-3392.

Lischko AM, Seddon JM, Gragoudas ES, Egan KM, & Glynn RJ (1989) Evaluation of prior primary malignancy as a determinant of uveal melanoma. A case-control study. Ophtalmology, **96**: 1716-1721.

Logani MK, Sambuco CP, Forbes PD, & Davies RE (1984) Skin-tumour promoting activity of methyl ethyl ketone peroxide - a potent lipid-peroxidizing agent. Food chem Toxicol, **22**: 879-882.

Luande J, Henschke CI, & Mohammed N (1985) The Tanzanian human albino skin. Cancer, **55**: 1823-1828.

Lubin D, Frederick JE, Booth CR, Lucas T, & Neuschuler D (1989) Measurements of enhanced springtime ultraviolet radiation at Palmer Station, Antarctica. Geophys Res Lett, **16**: 783-785.

Lynch DH & Daynes RA (1983) Evaluation of naturally occurring cell-mediated cytotoxic activity in normal and UV-irradiated mice. Transplantation, **35**: 216-223.

Lynge E & Thygesen L (1990) Occupational cancer in Denmark. Cancer incidence in the 1970 census population. Scand J Work Environ Health, **16**(Suppl 2): 1-35.

Lytle CD, Miller SA, Jacobs ME, Cyr WH, James RH, Kaczmarek RG, Beer JZ, Landry RJ, Sharkness CM, Gaylor D, & De Gruijl FR (1993) An estimation of squamous cell carcinoma risk from ultraviolet radiation emitted by fluorescent lamps. In : Proceedings of the 1993 Meeting of the American Society for Photobiology, Chicago, 26-30 June 1993.

McCormick JP, Fisher JR, Pachlatko JP, & Eisenstark A (1976) Characterization of a cell lethal product from the photooxidation of tryptophan: hydrogen peroxide. Science, **198**: 468-469.

McCredie M & Coates MS (1989) Cancer incidence in migrants to New South Wales; 1972 to 1984, New South Wales Central Cancer Registry. Woolloomooloo, New South Wales Cancer Council, pp 22-23, 62-63.

MacDonald EJ (1948) Malignant melanoma in Connecticut. In: The biology of melanomas. New York, Academy of Sciences, pp 71-81 (Special publication of the Academy of Sciences No. 4).

McGregor JM, Barker JNWN, & MacDonald DM (1992) The development of excess numbers of melanocytic naevi in an immunosuppressed identical twin. Clin Exp Dermatol, **16**: 131-132.

Mack TM, & Floderus B (1991) Malignant melanoma risk by nativity, place of residence at diagnosis, and age at migration. Cancer Causes Control, **2**: 401-411.

Mackenzie FD, Hirst LW, Battistutta D, & Green A (1992) Risk analysis in the development of pterygia. Ophthalmol, **99**: 1056-1061.

MacKie RM & Aitchison T (1982) Severe sunburn and subsequent risk of primary cutaneous malignant melanoma in Scotland. Br J Cancer, **40**: 55-960.

MacKie RM, Freudenberger T, & Aitchison TC (1989) Personal risk-factor chart for cutaneous melanoma. Lancet, **ii**: 487-490.

McKinlay AF (1992) Artificial sources of UVA radiation. Loss and emission characteristics. In: Urbach F ed Biological responses to UVA radiation. Vandermor Pub Corp Kansas.

McKinlay AF & Diffey BL (1987) A reference action spectrum for ultraviolet induced erythema in human skin. CIE J, **6:** 17-22

McKinlay AF & Whillock MJ (1987) Measurements of ultraviolet radiation from fluorescent lamps used for general lighting and other purposes in the UK. In: Passchhier WF & Bosnjakovic BFM ed. Human exposure to ultraviolet radiation: Risks and regulations., Amsterdam, Oxford, New York, Elsevier Science Pubishers, pp 253-258.

McKinlay AF, Whillock MJ, & Meulemans CCE (1989) Ultraviolet radiation and blue-light emissions from spotlights incorporating tungsten halogen lamps. London, National Radiological Protection Board (Report NRPB No. R228).

McKinlay AF, Harlen F, & Whillock MJ (1988) Hazards of optical radiation: A guide to sources, uses and safety. Bristol, Philadelphia, Adam Hilger.

Madewell BR, Conroy JD, & Hodgkins EM (1981) Sunlight-skin cancer association in the dog: a report of three cases. J Cutan Pathol, **8**: 434-443.

Magnus K (1977) Incidence of malignant melanoma of the skin in 5 Nordic countries: significance of solar radiation. Int J Cancer, **20**: 477.

Magnus K (1986) Malignant melanoma in Norway. Tidsskr Nor Lacgeforen, **106**: 2309-2313.

Magnus K (1991) The Nordic profile of skin cancer incidence. A comparative epidemiological study of the three main types of skin cancer. Int J Cancer, **47**: 12-19.

Mandal TK & Chatterjee SN (1980) Ultraviolet- and sunlight-induced lipid peroxidation in liposomal membrane. Radiat Res, **83**: 290-302.

Mao W & Hu T (1982) An epidemiologic survey of senile cataract in China. Chin Med J, **95**: 813-818.

Marks R & Hill D ed. (1992) The public health approach to melanoma control: Prevention and early detection. Geneva, International Union Against Cancer (UICC Publication).

Marks R, Ponsford MW, Selwood TS, Goodman G, & Mason G (1983) Non-melanocytic skin cancer and solar keratoses in Victoria. Med J Aust, **2**: 619-622.

Marks R, Jolley D, Dorevitch AP, & Selwood TS (1989) The incidence of non-melanocytic skin cancers in an Australian population: results of a five-year prospective study. Med J Aust, **150**: 475-478.

Marks R, Staples M, & Giles GG (1993) Trends in non melanocytic skin cancer treated in Australia: the second national survey. Int J Cancer, **53**: 585-590.

Martin EK (1912) The effects of ultra-violet rays upon the eye. Proc of the Soc Ser B, **85**: 319-334.

Mathews-Roth MM & Krinsky NI (1987) Carotenoids affect development of UV-B induced skin cancer. Photochem Photobiol, **46**: 507-509.

Matsunaga T, Hieda K, & Nikaido O (1991) Wavelength dependent formation of thymine dimers and (6-4) photoproducts in DNA by monochromatic ultraviolet light ranging from 150 to 365 nm. Photochem Photobiol, **54**: 403-410.

Matsuoka LY, Wortsman J, Hanifan N, & Holick MF (1988) Chronic sunscreen use decreases circulating concentration of 25-hydroxy vitamin D. A preliminary study. Arch Dermatol, **124**: 1802-1804.

Mayne LV, Mullenders LHF, & vasn Zeeland AA (1988) Cockayne syndrome: a UV sensitive disorder with a defect in the repair of tanscribing DNA but normal overall excision repair. In: Friedberg EC & Hanawalt PC ed. Mechanisms and consequences of DNA damage processing. New York, Alan R. Liss, pp 349-353.

Menzies, SW, Greenoak, GE, Reeve, VE, & Gallagher, CH (1991) Ultraviolet radiation-induced murine tumors produced in the absence of ultraviolet radiation-induced systemic tumor immunosuppression. Cancer Res, **51**: 2773-2779.

Miguel AG & Tyrrell RM (1983) Induction of oxygen-dependent lethal damage by monochromatic UVB (313 nm) radiation: strand breakage, repair and cell death. Carcinogenesis **4**, 375-380.

Milham S Jr (1983) Occupational mortality in Washington State 1950-1979. Cincinnati, Ohio, National Institute for Occupational Safety and Health (DHSS (NIOSH) Publication No. 83-116).

Minassian DC, Mehra V, & Johnson GJ (1992) Mortality and cataract: findings from a population-based longitudinal study. Bull World Health Organ, **70**: 219-223.

Miskin R & Ben-Ishai R (1981) Induction of placmenogen activator by UV light in normal and Xeroderma pigmentosum fibroblasts. Proc Natl Acad Sci (USA), **78**: 6236-6240.

Mitchell DL, Pfeifer GP, Taylor JS, Zdienicka MZ, & Nikaido O (1993) Biological role of (6-4) photoproducts and cyclobutane dimers. In: Shima A, Ichihashi M, Fujiwara Y, & Takebe H ed. Frontiers of photobiology. Amsterdam, Oxford, New York, Elsevier Science Publishers, pp 337-344.

Mitchell DL & Rosenstein BS (1987) The use of specific radioimmunoassays to determine action spectra for the photolysis of (6-4) photoproducts. Photochem Photobiol, **45**: 781-786.

Mitchell RL & Andersen IC (1965) Catalase Photoinactivation. Science **150**: 74.

Moan J & Dahlback A (1992) The relationship between skin cancers, solar radiation and ozone depletion. Br J Cancer, **65**: 916-921.

Modan B, Alfandary E, Shapiro D, Lusky A, Chetrit A, Shewach-Millet M, & Moushovitz M (1993) Factors affecting the development of skin cancer after scalp irradiation. Radiat Res, **134**: 125-128.

Mohan M, Sperduto RD, Angra SK, Milton RC, Mathur RL, Underwood BA, Jaffery N, Pandya CB, Chhabra VK, Vajpayee RB, Kalra VK, Sharma YR, & The Indian-US Case-Control Study Group (1989) India-US case-control study of age-related cataracts. Arch Ophthalmol, **107**: 670-676.

Moan J, Dahlbach A, Henriksen T, & Magnus K (1989) Biological amplification factor for sunlight-induced nonmelanoma skin cancer at high latitudes. Cancer Res, **49**: 5207-5212.

Molès J-P, Moyret C, Guillot B, Jeanteur P, Guilhou J-J, Theillet C, & Basset-Sèguin N (1993) p53 Mutations in human epithelial skin cancers. Oncogene, **8**: 583-588.

Molesworth EH (1927) Rodent ulcer. Med J Aust, **1**: 878-899.

Møller H, Mellemgaard A, Jacobsen GK, Pedersen D, & Storm HH (1993) Incidence of second primary cancer following testicular cancer. Eur J Cancer, **29A**: 672-676.

Mooy CM, Van der Helm MJ, Van der Kwast ThH, De Jong PTVM, Ruiter DJ, & Zwarthoff EC (1991) No N-*ras* mutations in human uveal melanoma: the role of ultraviolet light revisited. Br J Cancer, **64**: 411-413.

Moran DJ & Hollows FC (1984) Pterygium and ultraviolet radiation: a positive correlation. Br J Ophthalmol, **68**: 343-346.

Morimoto S & Kunihiko Y (1989) Psoriasis and vitamin D: A review of our experience. Arch Dermatol, **125**: 231-234.

Morin RJ, Hu B, Peng S-K, & Sevanian A (1991) Cholesterol oxides and carcinogenesis. J Clin Lab Anal, **5**: 219-225.

Morison WL (1984) The effect of a sunscreen containing para-aminobenzoic acid on the systemic immunologic alterations induced in mice by exposure to UVB radiation. J Invest Dermatol, **83**: 405-408.

Morlière P, Mayson A, Santus R, Huppe G, Mazière JP, & Dubertet L (1991) UVA-induced lipid peroxidation in cultured human fibroblasts. Biochem Biophys Acta, **1084(3)**: 261-268.

Morlière P, Moysan A, Gaboriou F, Santus R, Mazière JC, & Dubertret L (1992) Ultraviolet A et la peau: implications d'espèces activées de l'oxygène, tendances actuelles et résultats récents. Pathol Biol, **40**: 160-168.

Moseley H (1988) Hospital Physicists' Association - Non-ionizing radiation, medical physics handbook 18. Bristol, Philadelphia, Adam Hilger Publishers.

Mountin JW & Dor H(1939) Some peculiarities in the geography of cancer. J Am Med Assoc, **113**: 2405-2410.

Muir C, Waterhouse J, Mack T, Powell J, & Whelan S ed. (1987) Cancer incidence in five continents, Vol V (IARC Scientific Publications No 88), Lyon, International Agency for Research on Cancer.

Munkata N (1993) Biological effective dose of solar ultraviolet radiation estimated by spore dosimetry in Tokyo since 1989. Photochem Photobiol, **58**(3): 386-392.

Munch-Petersen B, Frentz G, Squire B, Wallevik K, Horn CC, Reymann F, & Faber M (1985) Abnormal lymphocyte response to uv radiation in multiple skin cancer. Carcinogenesis, **6**: 843-845.

Murali NS & Teramura AH (1987) Insensitivity of soyabean photosynthesis to UVB radiation under phosphorus deficiency. J Plant Nutr, **10**: 501-515.

Murphy GF, Walsh Lj, Kaidby K, & Lavker RM (1991) UV and sunbeds (Abstract) Clin. Res. **39**,195.

Murphy GM, Wright J, Nicholls DSH, McKee PH, Messenger AG, Hawk JLM, & Levene GM (1989) Sunbed induced pseudoporphyria. Br J Dermatol, **120**: 555-562.

NSF (1993) National Science Foundation, Div Polar Programs, Report to P Penhale (NSF) & CR Booth (Biospherical Instruments), Antarctic Support Assoc US.

Nachtwey DB & Rundel RD (1981) A photobiological evaluation of tanning booths. Science, **211**: 405-407.

Nakazawa H, English D, Randell PL, Nakazawa K, Martel N, Armstrong BK, & Yamasaki H (in press) UV and skin cancer; specific p53 gene mutation in normal skin as a biologically relevant exposure measurement. Proc Natl Acad Sci (USA).

Naumann GOH & Apple D (1986) Pathology of the eye. Berlin, Heidelberg, New York, Springer-Verlag.

Nelemans PJ, Groenendal H, Kiemeney LALM, Rampen FHJ, Ruiter DJ, & Verbeek ALM (1993) Effect of intermittent exposure to sunlight on melanoma risk among indoor workers and sun sensitive individuals. Environ Health Perspect, **101**(3): 252-255.

Nelson EW, Eichwald EJ, & Shelby J (1987) Increased ultraviolet radiation-induced skin cancers in cyclosporine-treated mice. Transpl Proc, **19**: 526-527.

NIH (1991) Executive summary: Guidelines for the diagnosis and management of asthma. Bethesda, Maryland, National Institutes of Health, US Department of Health and Human Services (Publication No. 91-3042A).

Noell WK, Walker VS, & Kang BS (1966) Retinal damage by light in rats. Invest Ophthalmol Vis Sci, **5**: 450-473.

Noonan FP & De Fabo EC (1990) Ultraviolet-B-dose-response curves for local and systemic immunosuppression are identical. Photochem Photobiol, **52**, 801-810.

Noonan FP, Kripke ML, Pedersen GM, & Green MI (1981a) Suppression of contact hypersensitivity in mice by ultraviolet irradiation is associated with defective antigen presentation. Immunology, **43**: 527-533.

Noonan FP, De Fabo EC, & Kripke ML (1981b) Suppression of contact hypersensitivity by UV radiation and its relationship to UV-induced suppression of tumor immunity. Photochem Photobiol, **34**: 683-689.

Noonan FP, De Fabo EC, & Morrison H (1988) Cis-urocanic acid, a product formed by ultraviolet B irradiation of the skin, initiates an antigen presentation defect in splenic dendritic cells *in vivo*. J Invest Dermatol, **90**: 92-99.

Norbury KC, Kripke ML, & Budmen M (1977) *In vitro* reactvity of macrophages and lymphocytes from ultraviolet-irradiated mice. J Natl Cancer Inst, **59**: 1231-1235.

Norn MS (1982) Spheroid degeneration, pinguecula, and pterygium among Arabs in the Red Sea Territory, Jordan. Acta Ophthalmol, **60**: 949-954.

Norval M, Howie SE, Ross JA, & Maingay JP (1987) A murine model of herpes simplex virus recrudescence. J Gen Virol, **68**: 2693-2698.

Nultsch W, Pfan J, & Huppertz K (1990) Photoinhibition of photosynthetic oxygen production and its recovery in the subtidal red data Polyneura hilliae, Bot. Acta, **103**: 62-67.

O'Beirn SF, Judge P, Urbach F, MacCon CF, & Martin F (1970) Skin cancer in County Galway, Ireland. Proc Natl Cancer Conf, **6**: 489-500.

Oberhelman L, Koren H, & Cooper KD (1992) Depressed capacity to contact sensitiza women at the onset of menses; elevated contact sensitization capacity during mid cycle can be inhibited by UV. Clin Res, **40**: 542A.

O'Dell BL, Jessen RT, Becker LE, Jackson RT, & Smith EB (1980) Diminished immune response in sun-damaged skin. Arch Dermatol, **116**: 559-561.

Oettlé,AG (1963) Skin cancer in Africa. Natl Cancer Inst Monogr, **10**: 197-214.

Office of Population, Censuses and Surveys (1986) Occupational mortality: the registrar general's decennial, supplement for Great Britain 1979-80, 1982-83. London, Office of Population Censuses and Surveys, Her Majesty's Stationary Office (Report Series DS No. 6).

Oldenburg JB, Gritz DC, & McDonnell PJ (1990) Topical ultraviolet light-absorbing chromophore protects against experimental photokeratitis. Arch Ophthalmol, **108**: 1142-1144.

O'Loughlin C, Moriarty MJ, Herity B, & Daly, L (1985) A re-appraisal of risk factors for skin carcinoma in Ireland: a case control study. Ir J Med Sci, **154**: 61-65.

Olsen JH & Jensen OM (1987) Occupation and risk of cancer in Denmark. An analysis of 93 810 cancer cases, 1970-1979. Scand J Work Environ Health, **13**(Suppl 1): 1-91.

Oluwasanmi JO, Williams AO, & Alli AF (1969) Superficial cancer in Nigeria. Br J Cancer, **23**: 714-728.

Omdahl JR, Garry TJ, & Hunsaker A (1982) Nutritional status in the healthy elderly population: vitamin D. Am J Clin Nutr, **6**: 1225-1233.

Organisciak DT & Winkler BS (1993) Retinal light damage: Practical and theoretical considerations. In: Osborne N & Chader G ed. Progress in retinal research. Oxford, New York, Seoul, Tokyo, Pergamon Press.

Orth AB, Teramura AH, & Sisler HD (1990) Effects of UV-B radiation on fungal disease development in Cucumis sativus. Am J Bot, **77**: 1188-1192.

Ostendfeld-Åkerblom A (1988) Pseudoexfoliation in Eskimos (Inuit) in Greenland. Acta Ophthalmol, **66**: 467-468.

Østerlind A (1987) Trends in incidence of ocular malignant melanoma in Denmark 1943-1982. Int J Cancer, **40**: 161-164.

Østerlind A, Olsen JH, Lynge E, & Ewertz M (1985) Second cancer following cutaneous melanoma and cancers of the brain, thyroid, connective tissue, bone, and eye in Denmark, 1943-80. Natl Cancer Inst Monogr, **68**: 361-388.

Østerlind A, Hou-Jensen K, & Jensen OM (1988a) Incidence of cutaneous malignant melanoma in Denmark 1978-1982. Anatomic site distribution, histologic types, and comparison with non-melanoma skin cancer. Br J Cancer, **58**: 385-391.

Østerlind A, Tucker MA, Stone BJ, & Jensen OM (1988b) The Danish case-control study of cutaneous malignant melanoma. II. Importance of UV-light exposure. Int J Cancer, **42**: 319-324.

Otani T & Mori R (1987) The effects of UV irradiation of the skin on herpes simplex virus infection: Alteration in immune function mediated by epidermal cells and in the course of infection. Arch Virol, **96**(1-2): 1-15.

Oxholm A, Oxholm P, Staberg B, & Bendtzen K (1988) Immunohistological detection of interleukin-like molecule and tumor necrosis factor in human epidermis before and after UVB-irradiation *in vivo*. Br J Dermatol, **118**: 369-376.

Paffenbarger RS Jr, Wing AL, & Hyde RT (1978) Characteristics in youth predictive of adult-onset malignant lymphomas, melanomas, and leukemias: brief communication. J Natl Cancer Inst, **60**: 89-92.

Paksoy N, Bouchardy C, & Parkin DM (1991) Cancer incidence in Western Samoa. Int J Epidemiol, **20**: 634-641.

Pang Q & Hays JB (1991) UV-B inducible and temperature-sensitive photoreactivation of cyclobutane pyrimidine dimers in Arabidopsis thaliana. Plant Physiol, **95**: 536-543.

Parkin DM, Muir CS, Whelan SL, Gao Y-T, Ferlay J, & Powell J ed. (1992) Cancer incidence in five continents, Vol VI (IARC Scientific Publications No. 120), Lyon, International Agency for Research on Cancer.

Parrish JA, Jaenicke KF, & Anderson RR (1982) Erythema and melanogenesis action spectra of normal human skin. Photochem Photobiol, **36**: 187-191.

Patrick MH (1977) Studies on thymine-derived UV photoproducts in DNA - I. Formation and biological role of pyrimidine adducts in DNA. Photochem Photobiol, **25**: 357-372.

Peak MJ & Peak JG (1982) Single-strand breaks induced in *Bacillus subtilis* DNA by ultraviolet light: action spectrum and properties. Photochem Photobiol, **35**: 675-680.

Peak JG & Peak MJ (1990) Ultraviolet light induces double-strand breaks in DNA of cultured human P3 cells as measured by neutral filter elution. Photochem Photobiol, **52**: 387-393.

Peak JG & Peak MJ (1991) Comparison of initial yields of DNA-to-protein crosslinks and single-strand breaks induced in cultured human cells by far-and near-ultraviolet light, blue light and x-rays, Mutat Res, **246**: 187-191.

Peak MJ, Peak JG, Moehring MP, & Webb RB (1984) Ultrviolet action spectrum for DNA dimer induction, lethality, and mutagenesis in *Escherichia coli* with emphasis on the UVB region. Photochem Photobiol, **40**: 613-620.

Peak MJ, Peak JG, Sikorski RS, & Jones CA (1985a) Induction of DNA-protein crosslinks in human cells by ultraviolet and visible radiations: action spectrum. Photochem Photobiol, **41**: 295-302.

Peak MJ, Peak JG, & Jones CA (1985b) Different (direct and indirect) mechanisms for induction of DNA-protein crosslinks in human cells by far- and near-ultraviolet radiation (290 and 405 nm). Photochem Photobiol, **42**: 141-146.

Peak MJ, Peak JG, & Carnes BA (1987) Induction of direct and indirect single-strand breaks in human cell DNA by far and near-ultraviolet radiations: action spectrum and mechanisms. Photochem Photobiol, **45**: 381-387.

Perna JJ, Mannix ML, Ronney JF, Notkins AL, & Straus SE (1987) Reactivation of latent herpes simplex virus infection by ultraviolet light: A human model. J Am Acad Dermatol, **17**(3): 473-478.

Philips (1983) Lighting, comprehensive handbook including technical section. Croydon, Philips Lighting.

Pierceall WE, Mukhopadhyay T, Goldberg LH, & Ananthasswamy HN (1991) Mutations in the P53 tumor suppressor gene in human cutaneous squamous cell carcinomas. Mol Carcinog, **4**: 445-449.

Piltingsrud HV, Fong CW, & Odland LT (1978) An evaluation of ultraviolet radiation personnel hazards from selected 400-watt high intensity discharge lamps. Am Ind Hyg Assoc J, **39**: 406-413.

Pincus MW, Rollings PK, Craft AB, & Green A (1991) Sunscreen use on Queensland beaches, Australia. J Dermatol, **32**: 21.

Pitcher H & Longtreth J (1991) Melanoma mortality and exposure to ultraviolet radiation: An empirical relationship. Environ Int, **17**: 7-21.

Pitts DG (1974) The human ultraviolet action spectrum. Am J Optom Arch Am Acad Optom, **51**: 946-960.

Pitts DG (1978) The ocular effects of ultraviolet radiation. Am J Optom Phys Optics, **55**: 19-35.

Pitts DG, Cullen AP, & Hacker PD (1977) Ocular effects of ultraviolet radiation from 295 to 365nm. Invest Ophthalmol Vis Sci, **16**: 932-939.

Pound AW (1970) Induced cell proliferation and the initiation of skin tumour formation in mice by ultraviolet light. Pathology, **2**: 269-275.

Prystowsky JH (1988) Photoprotection and the vitamin D status of the elderly. Arch Dermatol, **124**: 1844-1848.

Punnonen K, Puntela A, & Ahotupa M (1991) Effects of ultraviolet A and B irradiation on lipid peroxidation and activity of the antioxidant enzymes in keratinocytes in culture. Photochem Photoimmunol Photomed, **8**: 3-6.

Putvinsky AV, Sokolov AI, Roshchupkin DI, & Vladimirov Ya (1979) Electric breakdown of bilayer phospholipid membranes under ultraviolet irradiation-induced lipid peroxidation. FEBS Lett, **106**: 53-55.

Quan MB & Moy RL (1991) The role of human papillomavirus in carcinoma. J Am Acad Dermatol, **25**: 698-705.

Quintern LE, Horneck G, Eischweiler V, & Büker H (1992) A biofilm used as ultraviolet dosimeter. Photochem Photobiol, **55**: 389-395.

Rady P, Scinicariello F, Wagner RF, & Tyring SK (1992) p53 Mutations in basal cell carcinomas. Cancer Res, **52**: 3804-3806.

Rapp LM & Smith SC (1992) Morphorlogical comparisons between rhodopsin-mediated and short wavelength classes of retinal light damage. Invest Ophthalmol Vis Sci, **33**: 3367-3377.

Rasanen L, Reunala T, Lehto M, Jansen C, Rantala I, & Leinikki P (1989) Immediate decrease in antigen-presenting function and delayed enhancement of interleukin-1 production in human epidermal cells after *in vivo* UVB irradiation. Br J Dermatol, **120**: 589-596.

Rathbun WB (1989) In: Dolphin D, Poulson R, & Avramoric O ed. Coenzymes and cofactors - Volume III, Glutathione. New York, John Wiley and Sons, Inc., pp 467-509.

Raven JA, (1991) Responses of aquatic photosynthetic organisms to increased solar UVB. J Photochem Photobiol, **B9**: 239-244.

Reeve VE, Greenoak GE, Gallagher CH, Canfield PJ, & Wilkinson FJ (1985) Effect of immunosuppressive agents and sunscreens on UV carcinogenesis in the hairless mouse. Aust J Exp Biol Med Sci, **63**: 655-665.

Reeve VE, Matheson M, Greenoak GE, Canfield PJ, Boehm-Wilcox C, & Gallagher CH (1988) Effect of dietary lipid on UV light carcinogenesis in the hairless mouse. Photochem Photobiol, **48**: 689-696.

Reeve VE, Greenoak GE, Canfield PJ, Boehm-Wilcox C, & Gallagher CH (1989) Topical urocanic acid enhances UV-induced tumour yield and malignancy in hairless mouse. Photochem Photobiol, **49**: 459-464.

Reeve VE, Bosnic M, & Boehm-Wilcox C (1990) Effect of ultraviolet (UV) radiation and UVB-absorbing sunscreen ingredients on 7,12-dimethyllbenz(a)anthracene-initiated skin tumorigenesis in hairless mice. Photodermatol Photoimmunol Photomed, **7**: 222-227.

Reeve VE, Bosnic M, Boehm-Wilcos C, & Ley RD (1991) Differential protection by two sunscreens from UV radiation-induced immunosuppression. J Invest Dermatol, **97**: 624-628.

Reeve VE, Bosnic M, & Rozinova E (1993) Carnosine (beta-alanylhistidine) protects from the suppression of contact hypersensitivity by ultraviolet B (280-320 nm) radiation or by cis urocanic acid. Immunology, **78**: 99-104.

Remé CH, Braschler U, Roberts J, & Dillon J (1991) Light damage in the rat retina: effect of a radioprotective agent (WR-77913) on acute rod outer segment disk disruption. Photochem Photobiol, **54**: 137-142.

Reynolds P, Saunders LD, Layefsky ME, & Lemp GF (1993) The spectrum of acquired immunodeficiency syndrome (AIDS)-associated malignancies in San Francisco, 1980-1987. Am J Epidemiol, **137**: 19-30.

Rhodes AR, Albert LS, Barnhill RL, & Weinstock MA (1991) Sun-induced freckles in children and young adults: A correlation of clinical and histopathologic features. Cancer, **67**: 1990-2001.

Rigel DS, Friedman RJ, Levenstein MJ, & Greenwald DI (1983) Relationship of fluorescent lights to malignant melanoma: another view. J Dermatol Surg Oncol, **9**: 836-838.

Ringvold A & Davangar M (1985) Changes in the rabbit corneal stroma caused by UV irradiation. Acta Ophthalmol, **63**: 601-606.

Ringvold A, Davander M, & Olsen EG (1982) Changes of the cornea epithelium after ultraviolet radiation. Acta Ophthalmol, **60**: 41-52.

Rippey J & Schmaman A (1972) Skin tumours of Africans. In: Marshall J ed. Essays on tropical dermatology. Amsterdam, Excerpta Medica, vol 2, pp 98-115.

Rivas JM & Ullrich SE (1992) Systemic suppression of delayed-type hypersensitivity by supenatants from UV-irradiated keratinocytes. An essential role for keratinocyte-derived Il-10. J Immunol, **149**: 3865-3871.

Rivers JK, Norris PG, Murphy GM, Chu AC, Midgley G, Morris J, Morris RW, Young AR, & Hawk JLM (1989) Tanning, photoprotection, acute adverse effects and immunological changes. Br J Dermatol, **120**: 767-777.

Ro YS, Cooper PN, Lee JA, Quinn AG, Harrison D, Lane D, Horne CHW Rees JL, & Angus B (1993) p53 Protein expression in benign and malignant skin tumours. Br J Dermatol, **128**: 237-241.

Roberts DL (1990) Incidence of non-melanoma skin cancer in West Glamorgan, South Wales. Br J Dermatol, **122**: 399-403.

Roberts LK & Daynes RA (1980) Modification of the immunogenic properties of chemically induced tumors arising in hosts treated concomitantly with ultraviolet light. J Immunol, **125**: 438-447.

Roberts JE, Kinley J, Young A, Jenkins G, Atherton S, & Dillon J (1991) *In vivo* and photophysical studies on photooxidative damage to lens proteins and their protection by radioprotectors. Photochem Photobiol, **53**: 33-38.

Robinson JK & Rademaker AW (1992) Relative importance of prior basal cell carcinomas, continuing sun exposure, and circulating T-Lymphocytes on the development of basal cell carcinoma. J Invest Dermatol, **99**: 227-231.

Roffo AH (1934) Cancer et soleil: carcinomes et sarcomes provoqués par l'action du soleil in toto. Bull Assoc Fr Étude Cancer, **23:** 590-616.

Roff AH (1939) Physico-chemical etiology of cancer (with special emphasis on the association with solar radiation). Strahlentherapie, **66**: 328-350 (in German).

Ros J (1990) On the effect of UV-radiation on elongation growth of sunflower seedlings (Helianthus annuus L.)(Thesis), pp. 1-157 in Karlst. Beitr. Entw Okophysiol **8**, M Tevini (ed), Bot Inst II, Karlsruhe.

Roschupkin DJ, Pelenitsyn AB, Potapenko AY, Talitsky VV & Vladimirov YA (1975) Study of the effects of ultraviolet light on biomembranes - IV. The effect of oxygen on UV-induced hemolysis and lipid photoperoxidation in rat erythrocytes and liposomes. Photochem. Photobiol. **21**: 63-69.

Rose EF (1973) Pigment variation in relation to protection and susceptibility to cancer. Pigment Cell, **1**:, 236-45.

Rosen ES (1986) Filtration of non-ionizing radiation by the ocular media. In: Cronley-Dillon J, Rosen ES, & Marshall J ed. Hazards of light: myths and realities of eye and skin. Oxford, New York, Pergamon Press, pp 145-152.

Rosenstein BS & Ducore JM (1983) Induction of DNA strand breaks in normal human fibroblasts exposed to monochromatic ultraviolet and visible wavelengths in the 240-546 nm range. Photochem Photobiol, **38**: 51-55.

Rosenthal F, Phoon C, Bakalian A, & Taylor H (1988) The ocular dose of ultraviolet radiation to outdoor workers. Invest Ophthalmol Vis Sci, **29**: 649-656.

Rosenthal F, Safran M, & Taylor H (1985) The ocular dose of ultraviolet radiation from sunlight exposure. Photochem Photobiol, **42**: 163-171.

Roshchupkin DI, Pelenitsyn AB, Potapenko AY, Talitsky VV, & Vladimirov YA (1975) Study of the effects of ultraviolet light on biomembranes. IV. The effect of oxygen on UV-induced hemolysis and lipid photoperoxidation in rat erythrocytes and liposomes. Photochem Photobiol, **21**: 63-69.

Ross JA, Howie SE, Norval M, Maingay J, & Simpson TJ (1986) Ultraviolet-irradiated urocanic acid suppresses delayed-type hypersensitivity to herpes simplex virus in mice. J Invest Dermatol, **87**: 630-633.

Roth M, Müller J, & Boyle JM (1987) Immunochemical determination of an initial step in thymine dimer excision repair in xeroderma pigmentosum variant fibroblasts and biopsy material from the normal population and patients with basal cell carcinoma and melanoma. Carcinogenesis, **8**: 1301-1307.

Roy CR & Gies HP (1993) Personal protection against solar ultraviolet radiation. In: Proceedings of the International Symposium on UV, Munich 4-6 May 1993. German Ministry of the Environment, Munich, Germany, pp 47-52.

Roy CR, Gies HP, & Elliot G (1988) Solar ultraviolet radiation: personel exposure and protection. J Occup Health Safety (Aust N Z), **4**: 133.

Roza L, Baan RA, Van Der Leun JC, Kligman L, & Young AR (1989) UVA hazards in skin associated with the use of tanning equipment. J Photochem Photobiol, **B3**: 281-287.

Russell WO, Wynne ES, Loquvam GS, & Mehl DA (1956) Studies on bovine ocular squamous carcinoma ('cancer eye'). I. Pathological anatomy and historical review. Cancer, **9**: 1-52.

Ryel RJ, Barnes PW, Beyschlag W, Caldwell MM, & Flint SD (1990) Plant competition for light analyzed with a multispecies canopy model. I Model development and influence of enhanced UV-B conditions on photosynthesis in mixed wheat and wild oat canopies. Oecologia, **82**: 304-310.

Sadamori N, Mine M, & Honda T (1991) Incidence of skin cancer among Nagasaki atomic bomb survivors. J Radiation Res, **32, Suppl 2**: 217-225.

Saftlas AF, Blair A, Cantor KP, Hanrahan L, & Anderson HA (1987) Cancer and other causes of death among Wisconsin farmers. Am J Ind Med, **11:** 119-129.

Schaeffer L, Ray R, Humbert S, Moncollin V, Vermeulen W, Hoeijmakers JHJ, Chambon P, & Egly JM (1993) The basic transcription factor BTF2/TFIIH contains a helicase involved in both transcription and DNA repair. Science, Apr 2; 206(5104):37-38.

Scharffetter K, Wlaschek M, Hogg A, Bolsen K, Schothorst A, Goerz G, Krieg T, & Plewig G (1991) Arch Dermatol Res, **283**: 506-511.

Schmitt C, Schmitt J, Wegener A, & Hockwin O (1988) Effect of an aldose reductase inhibitor, AL-1576, on the development of UV-B and X-Ray cataract. Graefe's Arch Clin Exp Ophthlamol, **226**: 455-460.

Schothorst AA, Slaper H, Schouten R, & Suurmond D (1985) UVB dose in maintenance psoriasis phototherapy versus solar UVB exposure. Photodermatology, **3**: 213-220.

Schwartz GG & Hulka BS (1990) Is vitamin D deficiency a risk factor for prostate cancer? Anticancer Res, **10**: 1307-1311.

Schwartz SM & Weiss NS (1988) Place of birth and incidence of ocular melanoma in the United States. Int J Cancer, **41**: 174-177.

SCOPE/UNEP (1993) Effects of increased ultraviolet radiation on global ecosystems (Workshop proceedings). Paris, Scientific Committee on Problems of the Environment, United Nations Environment Programme.

Scotto J, Kopf AW, & Urbach F (1974) Non-melanoma skin cancer among Caucasians in four areas of the United States. Cancer, **34**: 1333-1338.

Scotto J & Fears TR (1987) The association of solar ultraviolet and skin melanoma incidence among Caucasians in the United States. Cancer Invest, **5**: 275-283.

Scotto J, Fears TR, & Fraumeni JF Jr (1982) Solar radiation. In: Schottenfeld D & Fraumeni JF Jr ed. Cancer epidemiology and prevention. Philadelphia, Pennsylvania, W.B. Saunders Company, pp 254-276.

Scotto J, Fears TR, & Fraumeni JF Jr (1983) Incidence of nonmelanoma skin cancer in the United States. Bethesda, Maryland, National Cancer Institute (NIH Publication No. 83-2433).

Scotto J, Cotton G, Urbach F, Berger D, & Fears T (1988) Biologically effective ultraviolet radiation: surface measurements in the US 1974-1985. Science, **235**: 762-764.

Seddon JM, Gragoudas ES, Glynn RJ, Egan KM, Albert DM, & Blitzer PH (1990) Host factors, UV radiation and risk of uveal melanoma. A case-control study. Arch Ophthalmol, **108**: 1274-1280.

Serrano H, Scotto J, Shornick G, Fears TR, & Greenberg ER (1991) Incidence of nonmelanoma skin cancer in New Hampshire and Vermont. J Am Acad Dermatol, **24**: 574-579.

Servilla KS, Burnham DK, & Daynes RA (1987) Ability of cyclosporine to promote the growth of transplanted ultraviolet radiation-induced tumors in mice. Transplantation, **44**; 291-295.

Setlow RB, Grist E, Thompson K, & Woodhead AD (1993) Wavelengths effective in induction of malignant melanoma. Proc Natl Acad Sci (USA), **90**: 6666-6670.

Setlow RB, Woodhead AD, & Grist E (1989) Animal model for ultraviolet radiation-induced melanoma: platyfish-swordtail hybrid. Proc Natl Acad Sci (USA), **86**: 8922-8926.

Shea CR, McNutt NS, Volkenandt M, Lugo J, Prioleau PG, & Albino AP (1992) Overexpression of p53 protein in basal cell carcinoma of human skin. Am J Pathol, **141**: 25-20.

Shearer GM & Clerici M (1992) T-helper cell immune dysfunction in asymptomatic HIV-1 seropositive individuals: The role of TH1-TH2 cross regulation. In: Coffman RL ed. Regulation and functional significance of T-cell subsets. Prog Chem Immunol, **54**, 21-43

Shetlar MD (1980) Cross-linking of proteins to nucleic acids by ultraviolet light. Photochem Photobiol Rev, **5**: 105-197.

Shibata T, Katoh N, Hatano T, & Sasaki K. Population based case-control study of cortical cataract in the Noto area, Japan, Ophthalmic Res. (1993, in press).

Shore RE (1990) Overview of radiation-induced skin cancer in humans. Int J Radiat Biol, **57**: 809-827.

Shore RE, Albert RE, Reed M, Harley N, & Pasternack BS (1984) Skin cancer incidence among children irradiated for ringworm of the scalp. Radiat Res, **100**: 192-204.

Shukla VK, Hughes DC, Hughes LE, McCormick F, & Padua RA (1989) *ras* mutations in human melanotic lesions: K-*ras* activation is a frequent and early event in melanoma development. Oncogene Res, **5**: 121-127.

Siemiatycki J (1991) Risk factors for cancer in the workplace. Boca Raton, Florida, CRC Press.

Simon JC, Cruz PD, Bergstresser PR, & Tigelaar RE (1990) Low dose ultraviolet B-irradiated Langerhans cells preferentially activate $CD4^+$ cells of the T helper 2 subset. J Immunol, **145**: 2087-2091.

Simon JC, Tigelaar RE, Bergstresser PR, Edelbaum D, & Cruz PD (1991) Ultraviolet B radiation converts Langerhans cells from immunogenic to tolerogenic antigen-presenting cells. J Immunol, **146**: 485-491.

Sjovall P, Christensen OB, & Moller H (1985) Single exposure to ultraviolet irradiation and elicitation of human allergic contact dermatitis. Acta Derm Venereol, **65**: 93-96.

Slaper H (1987) Skin cancer and UV exposure: Investigations on the estimation of risks. University of Utrecht, The Netherlands (PhD Thesis).

Slaper H, Schothorst AA, & Van der Leun JC (1986) Risk evaluation of UVB-therapy for psoriasis: comparison of calculated risk for UVB-therapy and observed risk in PUVA-treated patients. Photodermatology, **3**: 271-283.

Sliney, DH (1983) Eye protective techniques for bright light. Ophthalmology **90(8)**, 937-944.

Sliney D (1986) Physical factors in cataractogenesis: ambient ultraviolet radiation and temperature. Invest Ophthalmol Vis Sci, **27**(5):, 781-790.

Sliney DH (1987) Estimating the solar ultraviolet radiation exposure to an intraocular lens implant, J Cataract Refract Surg, **13**(5),296-301.

Sliney DH & Wolbarsht ML (1980) Safety with lasers and other optical sources -A comprehensive handbook. New York, London, Plenum Press.

Smith KC (1976) The radiation-induced addition of proteins and other molecules to nucleic acids. In: Wang SY ed. Photochemistry and photobiology of nucleic acids. New York, London, San Francisco, Academic Press, vol 2, pp 187-218.

Smith GJ & Ryan KG (1993) The effect of changes on differences in Robertson-Berger radiometer responsitivity on solar ultraviolet-B measurement. Photochem Photobiol, **58**(4): 512-514.

Smith RC, Baker KS, Holm-Hansen O, & Olson R (1980) Photoinhibition of photosynthesis in natural waters. Photochem Photobiol, **31**: 585-592.

Smith EL, Walworth NC, & Holick MF (1986) Effects of 2 alpha-25-dihydrxy vitamin D3 on the morphologic and biological differentiation of cultured human epidermal keratinocytes grown in serum-free conditions. J Invest Dermatol, **86**: 709-714.

Söderberg PG (1989) Mass alteration in the lens after exposure to ultraviolet radiation, 300nm. Acta Ophthalmol, **67**: 633-644.

Söderberg PG (1991) Na and K in the lens after exposure to radiation in the 300 nm wavelength region. J Photochem Photobiol, **8**: 279-294.

Soparker CN, O'Brien JM, & Albert DM (1993) Investigation of the role of the *ras* protooncogene point mutation in human uveal melanomas. Invest Ophthalmol Vis Sci, **34**: 2203-2209.

Sorahan T & Grimley RP (1985) The aetiological significance of sunlight and fluorescent lighting in malignant melanoma: a case-control study. Br J Cancer, **52**; 765-769.

Spector A (1991) In: Sies H ed. The lens and oxidative stress. Endogenous antioxidant defences in human blood plasma in oxidative stress: Oxidants and antioxidants. New York, London, San Francisco, Academic Press.

Spellman CW & Daynes RA (1978) Properties of ultraviolet light-induced suppressor lymphocytes within a syngeneic tunour system. Cell Immunol, **36**: 383-387.

Spellman CW, Woodward JG, & Daynes RA (1977) Modification of immunological potential by ultrviolet radiation. I Immune status of short-term UV-irradiated mice. Transplantation, **24**: 112-119.

Spitzer WO, Hill GB, Chambers LW, Helliwell BE, & Murphy HB (1975) The occupation of fishing as a risk factor in cancer of the lip. N Engl J Med, **293**: 419-424.

Spruance SL (1985) Pathogenesis of herpes simplex labialis: Experimental induction of lesions with UV light. J Clin Microbiol, **22**: 366-368.

Staberg B, Wulf HC, Poulsen T, Klemp P, & Brodthagen H (1983) Carcinogenic effect of sequential artificial sunlight and UVA irradiation in hairless mice. Consequences for solarium 'therapy'. Arch Dermatol, **119**: 641-643.

Stadtman ER (1990) Metal ion catalysed oxidation of protein-biochemical mechanism and biological consequences. Free Radic Biol Med, **9**: 315-325

Stamnes K, Tsay SC, Wiscombe WJ, & Jayaweera K (1988) Numerically stable algorithm for discreet-ordinate method radiative transfer in multiple scattering and emitting media. Appl Optics, **27**: 2502-2509.

Stein B, Rahmsdorf HJ, Steffen A, Liffin M, & Herrlich P (1989) UV-induced damage is an intermediate step in UV-induced expression of human immunodeficiency virus type 1, collagenase, c-fos and metallothionein. Mol Cell Biol, **9**: 5169-5181.

Steinitz R, Parkin DM, Young JL, Bieber CA, & Katz L ed. (1989) Cancer incidence in Jewish migrants to Israel, 1961-1981 (IARC Scientific Publications No 98), Lyon, International Agency for Research on Cancer, 114-115, 134-135.

Stenbäck F (1975a) Species-specific neoplastic progression by ultraviolet light on the skin of rats, guinea pigs, hamsters and mice. Oncology, **31**: 209-225.

Stenbäck F (1975b) Ultraviolet light irradiation as initiating agent in skin tumor formation by the two-stage method. Eur J Cancer, **11**: 241-246.

Stephenson TJ, Royds J, Silcocks PB, & Bleehen SS (1992) Mutant p53 oncogene expression in keratoacanthoma and squamous cell carcinoma. Br J Dermatol, **127**: 566-570.

Sterenborg HJCM & van der Leun JC (1990) Tumorigenesis by a long wavelength UVA source. Photochem Photobiol, **51**: 325-330.

Sterenborg HJCM, van der Putte SCJ, & van der Leun JC (1988) The dose-response relationship of tumorigenesis by ultraviolet radiation of 254 nm. Photochem Photobiol, **47**: 245-253.

Stern RS & Docken W (1986) An exacerbation of SLE after visiting a tanning salon. J Am Med Assoc, **255**: 3120.

Stern RS & Lange R (1988) Non-melanoma skin cancer occurring in patients treated with PUVA five to ten years after the first treatment. J Invest Dermatol, **91**: 120-124.

Stern RS, Thibodeau LA, & Kleinerman RA (1979) Risk of cutaneous carcinoma in patients treated with oral methoxsalen photochemotherapy. N Engl J Med, **300**: 809-813.

Stocker R & Frei B (1991) In Sies H ed. Endogenous antioxidant defences in human blood plasma in oxidative stress: Oxidants and antioxidants.New York, London, San Francisco, Adacemic Press.

Stretch JR, Gatter KC, Ralfkiaer E, Lane DP, & Harris, AL (1991) Expression of mutant p53 in melanoma. Cancer Res, **51**: 5976-5979.

Strickland PT, Burns FJ, & Albert, RE (1979) Induction of skin tumors in the rat by single exposure to ultraviolet radiation. Photochem Photobiol, **30**: 683-688.

Strickland PT, Creasia D, & Kripke ML (1985) Enhancement of two-stage skin carcinogenesis by exposure of distant skin to UV radiation. J Natl Cancer Inst, **74**: 1129-1134.

Strickland PT, Vitasa BC, West SK, Rosenthal FS, Emmett EA, & Taylor HR (1989) Quantitative carcinogenesis in man: solar ultraviolet B dose dependence of skin cancer in Maryland watermen. J Natl Cancer Inst, **81**: 1910-1913.

Stryker WS, Stampfer MJ, Stein EA, Kaplan L, Louis TA, Sober A, & Willett WC (1990) Diet, plasma levels of beta-carotene and alpha-tocopherol, and risk of malignant melanoma. Am J Epidemiol, **131**: 597-611.

Sullivan JH & Teramura AH (1991) The effects of UV-B radiation on loblolly pine. 2 Growth of field-grown seedlings, Trees (Berl) **6**(3):115-120.

Sutherland JC & Griffin K (1981) Absorption spectrum of DNA for wavelengths greater than 300nm. Radiat Res, **86**: 399-410.

Swerdlow AJ, English JSC, MacKie RM, O'Doherty CJ, Hunter JAA, Clark J, & Hole DJ (1988) Fluorescent lights, ultraviolet lamps, and risk of cutaneous melanoma. Br Med J, **297**: 647-650.

Sydenham MM, Wong CF, Hirst LW, & Collins MJ (1991) Cular UVB dosimetry made possible for the first time using a CR-39 contact lens. In: Proceedings of 22nd Session of CIE, Melbourne. Vienna, International Commission of illumination, vol 1, part 2, pp 27-28.

Talbot G (1948) Pterygium. Trans Ophthalmol Soc N Z, **2**: 42-45.

Taylor HR (1979) Pseudoexfoliation, an environmental disease? Trans Ophthalmol Soc UK, **99**: 302-307.

Taylor HR (1980a) Aetiology of climatic droplet keratopathy and pterygium. Br J Ophthalmol, **64**: 154-163.

Taylor HR (1980b) The environment and the lens. Br J Ophthalmol, **64**: 303-310.

Taylor HR, West SK, Rosenthal FS, Munoz B, Newland HS, Abbey H, & Emmett EA (1988) Effect of ultraviolet radiation on cataract formation. N Engl J Med, **319**: 1429-1433.

Taylor HR, West SK, Rosenthal FS, Munoz B, Newland HS, & Emmett EA (1989) Corneal changes associated with chronic UV irradiation. Arch Ophthalmol, **107**: 1481-1484.

Taylor HR, West S, Munoz B, Rosenthal FS, Bressler SB, & Bressler NM (1992) The long-term effects of visible light on the eye. Arch Ophthalmol, **110**: 99-104.

Taylor JR, Schmieder GF, Shimizu T, & Streilein JW (1993) UVB-susceptibility is a risk factor for recurrent herpes labialis. Photochem Photobiol, **57**: 135.

Templeton AC (1967) Tumours of the eye and adnexa in Africans of Uganda. Cancer, **20**: 1689-1698.

Teppo L, Pukkala E, Hakama M, Hakulinen T, Herva A, & Saxén E (1980) Way of life and cancer incidence in Finland. A municipality-based ecological analysis. Scand J Soc Med, **Suppl 19**: 5-84.

Terman M, Reme CE, Rafferty B, Gallin PF, & Terman JS (1990) Bright light therapy for winter depression: Potential ocular effects and theoretical implications. Yearly Review. Photochem Photobiol, **51**: 781-792.

Tevini M, Braun J, & Fieser G (1991a) The protective function of the epidermal layer of rye seedlings against ultraviolet-B radiation, Photochem Photobiol, **53**: 329-333.

Tevini M, Mark U, & Saile-Mark M (1991b) Effects of enhanced solar UV-B radiation on growth and function of crop plant seedlings. In: Randall D & Blevins D ed. Current topics in plant biochemistry and physiology. Columbia, University of Missouri.

Tevini M, Mark U, Fieser G, & Saile M (1991c) Effects of enhanced solar UV-B radiation on growth and function of selected crop plan seedlings. In: Riklis, D ed. Photobiology. New York, London, Plenum Press, pp 635-649.

Tobal K, Warren W, Cooper CS, McCartney A, Hungerford J, & Lightman S (1992) Increased expression and mutation of p53 in choroidal melanoma. Br J Cancer, **66**: 900-904.

Toews GB, Bergstresser PR, & Streilein JW (1980) Epidermal langerhans cell density determines whether contact hypersensitivity or unresponsiveness follows skin painting with DNFB. J Immunol, **124**: 445-453.

Tomatis, L (1990) ed, Cancer: Causes, Occurrence and Control. Lyon, International Agency for Research on Cancer (IARC Scientific Publications No 100).

Travis, LB, Curtis, RE, Boice, JD, Hankey, BF, & Fraumeni Jr, JF (1991) Second cancers following non-Hodgkin's lymphoma. Cancer, **67**: 2002-2009.

Travis, LB, Curtis, RE, Hankey, BF, & Fraumeni Jr, JF (1992) Second cancers in patients with chronic lymphocytic leukemia. J Natl Cancer Inst, **84**: 1422-1427.

Tucker, MA, Boice, JD, Jr & Hoffman, DA (1985a) Second cancer following cutaneous melanoma and cancers of the brain, thyroid, connective tissue, bone and eye in Connecticut, 1935-82. Natl Cancer Inst Monogr, **68**: 161-189.

Tucker, MA, Misfeldt, D, Coleman, N, Clark, WH, & Rosenberg, SA (1985b) Cutaneous malignant melanoma after Hodgkin's Disease. Ann Int Med, **102**: 37-41.

Tucker, MA, Shields, JA, Hartge, P, Augsberger, J, Hoover, RN, & Fraumeni, JF, Jr (1985c) Sunlight exposure as risk factor for intraocular malignant melanoma. New Engl J Med, **313**: 789-792.

Turner, BJ, Siatkowski, RM, Augsburger, JJ, Shields, JA, Lustbader, E, & Mastrangelo, MJ (1989) Other cancers in uveal melanoma patients and their families. Am J Ophthalmol, **107**: 601-608.

Tuveson RW & Sammartano, LJ (1986) Sensitivity of HemA mutant Escherichia coli cells to inactivation by near-UV light depends on the level of supplementation with L-aminolevulinic acid. Photochem Photobiol **43**: 621-626.

Tyrrell RM (1973) Induction of pyrimidine dimers in bacterial DNA by 365 nm radiation, Photochem Photobiol **17**: 69-73.

Tyrrell RM, Ley RD & Webb RB (1974) Induction of single strand breaks (Alkali-labile bonds) in bacterial and phage DNA by near-UV (365 nm) radiation. Photochem. Photobiol. **20**: 395-398.

Tyrrell RM (1982) Cell inactivation and mutagenesis by solar ultraviolet radiation In: Hélène C, Charlier M, Montenay-Garestier Th & Laustriat G ed. Trends in Photobiology, Plenum Press, New York, pp 155-172.

Tyrrell, RM (1984) Exposure of nondividing populations of primary human fibroblasts to UV (254 nm) radiation induces a transient enhancement in capacity to repair potentially lethal cellular damage. Proc Natl Acad Sci USA **81**: 781-784.

Tyrrell, RM (1991) UVA (320-380 nm) radiation as an oxidative stress In: Sies H ed. Oxidative Stress : oxidants and antioxidants, London, Academic Press, pp 57-83.

Tyrrell, RM (1992) Inducible responses to UVA exposure. In: (ed. F. Urbach) Biological responses to ultraviolet A radiation, Valdenmar Press, Overland Park, pp. 59-64.

Tyrrell, RM and Pidoux, M (1986) Endogenous glutathione protects human skin fibroblasts against the cytotoxic action of UVB, UVA and near-visible radiations. Photochem Photobiol **44**: 561-564.

Tyrrell RM & Pidoux M (1987) Action spectra for human skin cells. Estimates of the relative cytotoxicity of the middle ultraviolet, near ultraviolet and violet regions of sunlight on epidermal keratinocytes. Cancer Res **47**: 1825-1829.

Tyrrell, RM and Pidoux, M (1988) Correlation between endogenous glutathione content and sensitivity of cultured human skin cells to radiation at defined wavelengths in the solar UV range. Photochem Photobiol **47**: 405-412.

Tyrrell, RM & Pidoux M (1989) Singlet oxygen involvement in the inactivation of cultured human fibroblasts by UVA (334 nm, 365 nm) and near-visible radiations. Photochem Photobiol **49**: 407-412.

Ullrich SE (1985) Suppression of lymphoproliferation by hapten-specific suppressor T lymphocytes from mice exposed to ultraviolet radiation. Immunology, **54**: 343-352.

Ullrich SE (1986) Suppression of the immune response to allogeneic histocompatibility antigens by a single exposure to ultraviolet radiation. Transplantation, **42**: 287-291.

Ullrich SE & Kripke ML (1984) Mechanisms in the suppression of tumor rejection produced in mice by repeated UV irradiation. J Immunol, **133**: 2786-2790.

Ullrich SE, Azizi E, Kripke ML (1986a) Suppression of the induction of delayed-type hypersensitivity reactions in mice by a single exposure to ultraviolet radiation. Photochem Photobiol, **43**: 633-638.

Ullrich SE, Yee GK, & Kripke ML (1986b) Suppressor lymphocytes induced by epicutaneous sensitization of UV-irradiated mice control multiple immunological pathways. Immunology, **58**: 185-190.

UNEP (1987) The ozone layer, United Nations Environment Programme, UNEP/GEMS Environmental Library No 2, UNEP, Nairobi.

UNEP (1989) Environmental Effects Panel Report, Van der Leun, JC, Tevini, M eds. United Nations Environment Programme , Nairobi, Kenya.

UNEP (1991) Environmental effects of ozone depletion: 1991 Update. United Nations Environment Programme, Nairobi, Kenya.

UNEP (1992) Effects of increased ultraviolet radiation on biological systems. Proceedings of meeting, Scientific Committee on Problems of the Environment (SCOPE). Budapest, United Nations Environment Programme, Nairobi, Kenya.

UNEP-WMO (1989) Scientific assessment of stratospheric ozone: 1989 WMO Global ozone research and monitoring project, United Nations Environment Programme, World Meteorological Organization, Geneva (Report No 29).

Urbach F (1987) Man and ultraviolet radiation. In: Passchier WF & Bosnjakovic BFM eds. Human exposure to ultraviolet radiation - risks and regulations. New York, Excerpta Medica.

Urbach F (1989) Testing the efficacy of sunscreens: effect of choice of source and spectral distribution of ultraviolet radiation, and choice of endpoint. Photodermatology, **6**: 177-181.

Urbach F, Davies RE, & Forbes PD (1966) Ultraviolet radiation and skin cancer in man In: Montagna W & Dobson RL eds. Advances in Biology of Skin, Oxford, Pergamon Press, Carcinogenesis, Vol VII, pp 195-214.

Urbach F, Epstein JH, & Forbes PD (1974) Ultraviolet carcinogenesis: experimental, global and genetic aspects. In: Pathak MA, Harber LC, Seiji M, & Kukita A, eds. Sunlight and Man - Normal and Abnormal Photobiological Responses, Tokyo, University of Tokyo Press, pp 259-283.

US Food and Drug Administration (1978) Sunscreen drug products for over-the-counter use. Fed Regis, **43**: 38206-28269.

US National Cancer Institute (1989) Sunscreens, Rockville, MD, Tracor Technological Resources Inc (Class Study Report; Contract No NO1-CP-71082 (7/89)).

Vågerö D, Ringbäck G, & Kiviranta H (1986) Melanoma and other tumours of the skin among office, other indoor and outdoor workers in Sweden 1961-1979. Br J Cancer, **53**: 507-512.

Vågerö D, Swerdlow AJ, & Beral V (1990) Occupation and malignant melanoma: a study based on cancer registration data in England and Wales and in Sweden. Br J Ind Med, **47**: 317-324.

Valerie K, Delers A, Bruck C, Thiriatt C, Rosenberg H, Debouck C & Rosenberg M (1988) Activation of human immmunodefficiency virus type 1 by DNA damage in human cells. Nature **333**: 78-81.

Van der Leun JC (1984) Yearly review: UV-carcinogenesis. Photochem Photobiol, **39**: 861-868.

Van der Leun JC (1987) Principles of risk reduction and protection. In: Passchier WF & Bosnjakovic BFM, eds. Human Exposure to Ultraviolet Radiation: Risks and Regulations, Amsterdam, Elsevier, pp 293-303.

Van der Leun JC (1992) Interactions of UVA and UVB in photodermatology: what was photoaugmentation? In: Urbach F ed. The Biological Responses to Ultraviolet A Radiation, Overland Park, KS Valdenmar, pp 309-319.

Van der Leun JC & de Gruijl FR (1993) Influences of ozone depletion on human and animal health. In: Tevini M ed. UV-B radiation and ozone depletion. Effects on humans, animals, plants, microorganisms, and materials. Boc Raton, Lewis Publishers, pp 95-123.

Van der Schroeff JG, Evers LM, Boot AJM & Bos JL (1990) *ras* oncogene mutations in basal cell carcinomas and squamous cell carcinomas of human skin. J Invest Dermatol, **94**: 423-425.

Van Weelden H, de Gruijl FR & van der Leun JC (1986) Carcinogenesis by UVA, with an attempt to assess the carcinogenic risks of tanning with UVA and UVB. In: Urbach F & Gange RW eds. The Biological Effects of UVA Radiation, New York, Praeger, pp 137-146.

Van Weelden H, de Gruijl FR, van der Putte SCJ, Toonstra J & van der Leun JC (1988) The carcinogenic risks of modern tanning equipment: is UVA safer than UVB? Arch Dermatol Res, **280**: 300-307.

Van't Veer LJ, Burgering BMT, Versteeg R, Boot AJM, Ruiter DJ, Osanto S, Schrier PI & Bos JL (1989) N-*ras* Mutations in human cutaneous melanoma from sun-exposed body sites. Mol Cell Biol, **9**: 3114-3116.

Varghese AJ & Wang SY (1967) Ultraviolet irradiation of DNA in vitro and in vivo produces a third thymine-derived product. Science **156**: 955-957.

Verhoeff FH, Bell L & Walker CB (1916) The pathological effects of radiant energy on the eye. Proc Am Acad Arts Sci, **510**: 1-810.

Vermeer M & Streilein JW (1990) Ultraviolet B light-induced alterations in epidermal Langerhans cells are mediated in part by tumor necrosis factor-alpha. Photodermatol Photoimmunol Photomed, **7**: 258-265.

Vermeer M, Schmieder GJ, Yoshikawa T, Van den Berg J-W, Metzman MS, Taylor JR, & Streilein JW (1991) Effects of ultraviolet B light on cutaneous immune responses of humans with deeply pigmented skin. J Invest Dermatol, **97**: 729-734.

Vile GF, Basu-Moda S, Waltner C & Tyrrell RM (1994) Haem oxygenase 1 mediates an adaptive response to oxidative stress in human skin fibroblasts. Proc Natl Acad Sci USA **91**: 2607-2610.

Vincek V, Jurimoto I, Medema JP, Prieto E, & Streilein JW (1993) Tumor necrosis factor alpha polymorphism correlates with deleterious effects of ultraviolet B light on cutaneous immunity. Cancer Res, **53**: 728-732.

Vitale S, West S, Munoz B, Schein OD, Maguire M, Bressler, N & Taylor HR (1992) Watermen Study II: mortality and baseline prevalence of nuclear opacity. Invest Ophthalmol Vi Sci, **33**: 1097.

Vitasa BC, Taylor HR, Strickland PT, Rosenthal FS, West S, Abbey H, Ng SK, Munoz B, & Emmett EA (1990) Association of nonmelanoma skin cancer and actinic keratosis with cumulative solar ultraviolet exposure in Maryland watermen. Cancer, **65**: 2811-2817.

Volkenandt M, Schlegel U, Nanus DM, & Albino AP (1991) Mutational analysis of the human p53 gene in malignant melanoma. Pigment Cell Res, **4**: 35-40.

Vuillaume M, Daya-Grosjean L, Vincens P, Pennetier JL, Tarroux P, Baret A, Calvayrac R, Taieb A & Satorin, A (1992) Striking differences in cellular catalase activity between two DNA repair-deficient diseases. Xeroderma pigmentosum and trichothiodystophy. Carcinogenesis **13**: 321-328.

Walker GC (1987) The SOS response of Escherichia coli In: Niedhardt FC, Ingraham JL, Low KB, Magasanik B, Shaechter M, Umbarger HE eds. Escherichia coli and Salmonella typhimurium. Cellular and Molecular Biology, American Society of Microbiology, Washington DC pp 1346-1357.

Walter SD, Marrett LD, From L, Hertzman C, Shannon HS, & Roy P (1990) The association of cutaneous malignant melanoma with the use of sunbeds and sunlamps. Am J Epidemiol, **131**: 232-243.

Warfel AH, Moy JA, Meola T, Sanchez M, Soter NA, & Belsito DV (1993) Effect of ultraviolet B (UVB) on the expression of human immunodeficiency virus (HIV) in mice and humans, Photochem Photobiol, **57**: 755.

Waring GO, Roth AM, & Ekins MB (1984) Clinical and pathological description of 17 cases of corneal intraepithelial neoplasia. Am J Ophthalmol, **97**: 547-559.

Waterhouse J, Muir C, Correa P, & Powell J eds (1976) Cancer Incidence in Five Continents, Lyon, International Agency for Research on Cancer, Vol III (IARC Scientific Publications No 15).

Waterhouse J, Muir C, Shanmugaratnam K, & Powell J eds (1982) Cancer Incidence in Five Continents, Lyon, International Agency for Research on Cancer, Vol IV (IARC Scientific Publications No 42).

Webb RB (1977) Lethal and mutagenic effects of near-ultraviolet radiation Photochem Photobiol Rev **2**: 169-261.

Wei Q, Matanoski GM, Farmer ER, Hedayati MA, & Grossman L (1993) DNA repair and aging in basal cell carcinoma: A molecular epidemiology study. Proc Natl Acad Sci USA, **90**: 1614-1618.

Weinstock MA, Colditz GA, Willett WC, Stampfer MJ, Bronstein BR, Mihm MC Jr, & Speizer FE (1989) Nonfamilial cutaneous melanoma incidence in women associated with sun exposure before 20 years of age. Pediatrics, **84**: 199-204.

Wellmann E, (1971) Phytochrome mediated flavone glycoside synthesis in cell suspension cultures of Petroselinum hortense after preirradiation with ultraviolet light, Planta, **101**: 283-286.

Wellmann E, (1991) Specific ultraviolet effects in plant development, J Exp Bot, (Suppl), **32:** 42.

Welsh D & Diffey B (1981) Protection against solar actinic radiation afforded by common clothing fabrics. Clinical and Experimental Dermatology **6**: 577-582.

West SK, Rosenthal FS, Bressler NM, Bressler SB, Munoz B, Fine SL, & Taylor HR (1989) Exposure to sunlight and other risk factors for age-related macular degeneration. Arch Ophthalmol, **107**: 875-879.

Wester A (1987) Ultraviolet transmission properties of sunscreens and sunglasses. In: Passchier W & Bosnjakovic B eds. Human exposure to ultraviolet radiation: risks and regulations, Elsevier, Amsterdam.

Westerveld A, Hoeijmakers JHJ, van Duin M, de Wit J, Odijk H, Pavlink A, Wood RD & Bootsma D (1984) Molecular cloning of a human DNA repair gene. Nature **310**: 425-529.

Whillock MJ, McKinlay AF, Kemmlert J & Forsgren PG (1990) Ultraviolet radiation emissions from miniature [compact] fluorescent lamps. Lighting Res Technol **22**: 125-128.

Whitaker CJ, Lee WR, & Downes JE (1979) Squamous cell skin cancer in the north-west of England, 1967-69, and its relation to occupation. Br J Ind Med, **36**: 43-51.

WHO (1948) International Statistical Classification of Diseases, Injuries and Causes of Death, Sixth Revision, Geneva.

WHO (1977) Manual of the International Statistical Classification of Diseases, Injuries, and Causes of Death. International Classification of Diseases, 1975 rev, Vol 1, Geneva, p 102.

WHO (1989) Non-ionizing radiation protection. MJ Suess & DA Benwell-Morison eds. World Health Organization Regional Office for Europe, European series No 25, WHO, Copenhagen.

WHO/UNEP/IRPA (1979) Ultraviolet Radiation, Environmental Health Criteria 14, World Health Organization, United Nations Environment Programme, WHO, Geneva.

Widmark J (1901) Ueber den Einfluss des Lichtes auf die Linse. Mitteil aus d Augenklin d Carol med chir Inst zu Stockholm **3**: 135-149.

Willis I, Menter JM, & Whyte HJ (1981) The rapid induction of cancers in the hairless mouse utilizing the principle of photoaugmentation. J Invest Dermatol, **76**: 404-408.

Wittenberg S (1986) Solar radiation and the eye: a review of knowledge relevant to eye care. Am J Optom Physiol Optics, **63**: 676-689.

WMO (1993) World Meteorological Organization Report of the second meeting of the ozone research managers of the parties to the Vienna Convention for the protection of the ozone layer. Geneva 10-12 March.

Wolf P, Donawho CK, & Kripke ML (1993a) Analysis of the protective effect of different sunscreens on ultraviolet radiation-induced local and systemic suppression of contact hypersensitivity and inflammatory responses in mice. J Invest Dermatol **100**: 254-259.

Wolf P, Yarosh DB, & Kripke ML (1993b) Effects of sunscreens and a DNA excision repair enzyme on ultraviolet radiation - induced inflammation, immune suppression and cyclobutane pyrimidine dimer formation in mice. J invest Dermatol **101**: 523-527.

Wong CF, Fleming R, & Carter SJ (1989) A new dosimeter for ultraviolet B radiation. Photochem Photobiol **50**: 611-615.

Wong L, Ho SC, Coggon D, Cruddas AM, Hwang CH, Ho CP, Robertshaw AM, & MacDonald DM (1993) Sunlight exposure, antioxidant status, and cataract in Hong Kong fishermen. J Epidemiol Comm Health, **47**: 46-49.

Wood RD, Robbins P & Lindahl T (1988) Complementation of the Xeroderma pigmentosum DNA repair defect in cell-free extracts. Cell **53**: 91-106.

Wucherpfenning V (1931) Biologie und prackische verwenbarkeit der erythemschwelle des UV. Strahlentherapie **40**: 201-244.

Yarosh D, Alas LG, Yee V, Oberyszyn A, Kibitel JT, Mitchell D, Rosenstein R, Spinowitz A, & Citron M (1992) Pyrimidine dimer removal enhanced by DNA repair liposomes reduces incidence of UV skin cancer in mice. Cancer Res, **52**: 4227-4231.

Yasumoto S, Yoshinobu H, & Aurelian L (1987) Immunity to herpes simplex virus type 2: Suppression of virus-induced responses in ultraviolet B-irradiated mice. J Immunol, **139**: 2788-2793.

Yoshida A, Ishiguro S, & Tamai M (1993) Expression of glial fibrillary acidic protein in muoller cells after lensectomy-vitrectomy. Invest. Ophthalmol. Vis. Sci. **34**: 3154-3160.

Yoshikawa T & Streilein JW (1990) On the genetic basis of the effects of ultraviolet B on cutaneous immunity. Evidence that polymorphisms at the Tnfα and Lps loci govern susceptibility. Immunogenetics, **32**: 398-405.

Yoshikawa T, Rae V, Bruins-Slot W, Van den Berg J-W, Taylor Jr, & Streilein JW (1990) Susceptibility to effects of UVB radiation on induction of contact hypersensitivity as a risk factor for skin cancer in humans. J Invest Dermatol, **95**: 530-536.

Young AR, Magnus IA, Davies AC, & Smith NP (1983) A comparison of the phototumorigenic potential of 8-MOP and 5-MOP in hairless albino mice exposed to solar simulated radiation. Br J Dermatol, **108**: 507-518.

Young AR, Walker SL, Kinley JS, Plastow SR, Averbeck D, Morlière P, & Dubertret L (1990) Phototumorigenesis studies of 5-methoxypsoralen in bergamot oil: evaluation and modification of risk of human use in an albino mouse skin model. J Photochem Photobiol B Biol, **7**: 231-250.

Young AR, Potten CS, Chadwick CA, Murphy GM, Hawk JLM & Cohen AJ (1991) Photo-protection and 5-MOP photochemoprotection from UVR-induced DNA damage in humans: the role of skin type. J Invest Dermatol, **97**: 942-948.

Yu CC, MacGregor JM, Dublin EA, Barnes DM, MacDonald DM, & Levison DA (1992) Patterns of immunostaining for p53 in benign and malignant melanocytic lesions (meeting abstract). J Pathol, **167**: (Suppl), 130A.

Zadjela E & Bisagni E (1981) 5-Methoxypsoralen, the melanogenic additive in sun-tan preparations, is tumorigenic in mice exposed to 365 nm uv radiation. Carcinogenesis, **2**: 121-127.

Zamansky G & Chou, I-N (1987) Environmental wavelength of ultraviolet light induce cytoskeletal damage. J Inv Dermatol **89**: 603-606.

Zanetti R, Rosso S, Faggiano F, Roffino R, Colonna S, & Martina G (1988) A case-control study on cutaneous malignant melanoma in the province of Torino, Italy (Fr). Rev Epidemiol Santé publ, **36**: 309-317.

Zanetti R, Franceschi S, Rosso S, Colonna S, & Bidoli E (1992) Cutaneous melanoma and sunburns in childhood in a southern European population. Eur J Cancer, **28A**: 1172-1176.

Zaridze D, Mukeria A, & Duffy SW (1992) Risk factors for skin melanoma in Moscow. Int J Cancer, **52**: 159-161.

Zaunuddin D & Sasaki K (1991) Risk factor analysis in a cataract epidemiology survey in West Samatara, Indonesia. Dev Ophthalmol, **21**: 78-86.

Ziegler A-M, Leffell DJ, Kunala S, Sharma HW, Gailani M, Simon JA, Halperin AJ, Baden HP, Shapiro PE, Bale AE, & Brash DE (1993) Mutation hotspots due to sunlight in the p53 gene of nonmelanoma skin cancers. Proc Natl Acad Sci USA, **90**: 4216-4220.

Zigman S (1993) Yearly review: ocular light damage. Photochem. Photobiol. **57**: 1060-1068.

Zigman S, Yulo T, & Schultz J (1974) Cataract induction in mice exposed to near UV light. Ophthalmol Res, **6**: 259-270.

Zigman S, Graff J, Yulo T, & Vaughen T (1975) The response of mouse ocular tissue to continuous near-UV light exposure. Invest Ophthalmol, **14**: 710-713.

Zmudzka BZ & Beer JZ (1990) Activation of human immunodeficiency virus by ultraviolet radiation. Photochem Photobiol, **52**: 1153-1162.

Zuclich JA (1989) Ultraviolet induced photochemical damage in ocular tissues. Health Physics **56**: 671-682.

Zuclich J & Kurtin W (1977) Oxygen dependence of near-ultraviolet induced corneal damage. Photochem Photobiol **25**: 133-135.

Tyrrell, RM and Pidoux, M (1986) Endogenous glutathione protects human skin fibroblasts against the cytotoxic action of UVB, UVA and near-visible radiations. Photochem Photobiol **44,** 561-564.

Ullrich SE & Kripke ML (1984) Mechanisms in the suppression of tumor rejection produced in mice by repeated UV irradiation. J Immunol, **133**, 2786-2790.

Ullrich SE, Yee GK, & Kripke ML (1986b) Suppressor lymphocytes induced by epicutaneous sensitization of UV-irradiated mice control multiple immunological pathways. Immunology, **58**, 185-190.

Ullrich SE (1985) Suppression of lymphoproliferation by hapten-specific suppressor T lymphocytes from mice exposed to ultraviolet radiation. Immunology, **54**, 343-352.

Ullrich SE (1986) Suppression of the immune response to allogeneic histocompatibility antigens by a single exposure to ultraviolet radiation. Transplantation, **42**, 287-291.

Ullrich SE, Azizi E, Kripke ML (1986a) Suppression of the induction of delayed-type hypersensitivity reactions in mice by a single exposure to ultraviolet radiation. Photochem Photobiol, **43**, 633-638.

UNEP (1993) United Nations Environment Programme. Report of the nineth meeting of the Open-Ended Working Group of the parties to the Montreal Protocol, Geneva 30 August-1 September 1993.

UNEP (1992) Effects of increased ultraviolet radiation on biological systems. Proceedings of meeting, Scientific Committee on Problems of the Environment (SCOPE). Budapest, United Nations Environment Programme, Nairobi, Kenya.

UNEP (1991) Environmental effects of ozone depletion: 1991 Update. United Nations Environment Programme, Nairobi, Kenya.

UNEP (1989) Environmental Effects Panel Report, Van der Leun, JC, Tevini, M eds. United Nations Environment Programme , Nairobi, Kenya.

UNEP (1987) The ozone layer, United Nations Environment Programme, UNEP/GEMS Environmental Library No 2, UNEP, Nairobi.

UNEP - WMO (1989) Scientific assessment of stratospheric ozone: 1989 WMO Global ozone research and monitoring project, Report No 29. United

Nations Environment Programme, World Meteorological Organization, Geneva.

Urbach, F, Epstein, JH, & Forbes, PD (1974) Ultraviolet carcinogenesis: experimental, global and genetic aspects. In: Pathak, MA, Harber, LC, Seiji, M, & Kukita, A, eds, Sunlight and Man Normal and Abnormal Photobiologic Responses, Tokyo, University of Tokyo Press, 259-283.

Urbach, F, Davies, RE, & Forbes, PD (1966) Ultraviolet radiation and skin cancer in man. In: Montagna, W, & Dobson, RL, eds, Advances in Biology of Skin, Vol VII, Carcinogenesis, Oxford, Pergamon Press, 195-214.

Urbach, F (1989) Testing the efficacy of sunscreens: effect of choice of source 'and spectral distribution of ultraviolet radiation, and choice of endpoint. Photodermatology, **6**, 177-181.

Urbach F, (1987) Man and ultraviolet radiation in Human exposure to ultraviolet radiation - risks and regulations eds. Passchier WF and Bosnjakovic BFM (New York: Excerpta Medica).

Urbach, F (1987a) Cutaneous photocarcinogenesis. J Environ Sci Health-Environ Carcinogen Rev, **C5**, 211-34.

US Food and Drug Administration (1978) Sunscreen drug products for over-the-counter use. Fed Regis, **43**, 38206-28269.

US National Cancer Institute (1989) Sunscreens (Class Study Report; Contract No NO1-CP-71082 (7/89)), Rockville, MD, Tracor Technological Resources Inc.

Vågerö, D, Swerdlow, AJ, & Beral, V (1990) Occupation and malignant melanoma: a study based on cancer registration data in England and Wales and in Sweden. Br J Ind Med, **47**, 317-324.

Vågerö, D, Ringbäck, G, & Kiviranta, H (1986) Melanoma and other tumours of the skin among office, other indoor and outdoor workers in Sweden 1961-1979. Br J Cancer, **53**, 507-512.

Valerie, K, Delers, A, Bruck, C, Thiriatt, C, Rosenberg, H, Debouck, C and Rosenberg, M (1988) Activation of human immmunodefficiency virus type 1 by DNA damage in human cells. Nature **333,** 78-81.

Van der Leun, JC (1992) Interactions of UVA and UVB in photodermatology: what was photoaugmentation? In: Urbach, F, ed, The Biological Responses to Ultraviolet A Radiation, Overland Park, KS Valdenmar, 309-319.

Van der Leun, JC (1987) Principles of risk reduction and protection. In: Passchier, WF, & Bosnjakovic, BFM, eds, Human Exposure to Ultraviolet Radiation: Risks and Regulations, Amsterdam, Elsevier, 293-303.

Van der Leun, JC (1984) Yearly review: UV-carcinogenesis. Photochem Photobiol, **39**, 861-868.

Van der Leun, JC, & de Gruijl, FR (1993) Influences of ozone depletion on human and animal health. In: Tevini, M ed. UV-B radiation and ozone depletion. Effects on humans, animals, plants, microorganisms, and materials. Boc Raton, Lewis Publishers, 95-123.

Van der Schroeff, JG, Evers, LM, Boot, AJM, & Bos, JL (1990) *ras* oncogene mutations in basal cell carcinomas and squamous cell carcinomas of human skin. J Invest Dermatol, **94**, 423-425.

Van Weelden H and van der Leun J, (1987) UVA induced tumours in pigmented and albino hairless mice in Human exposure to ultraviolet radiation - risks and regulations eds. Passchier WF and Bosnjakovic BFM (New York: Excerpta Medica).

Van Weelden, H, de Gruijl, FR, & van der Leun, JC (1986) Carcinogenesis by UVA, with an attempt to assess the carcinogenic risks of tanning with UVA and UVB. In: Urbach, F, & Gange, RW, eds, The Biological Effects of UVA Radiation, New York, Praeger, 137-146.

Van Weelden, H, de Gruijl, FR, van der Putte, SCJ, Toonstra, J, & van der Leun, JC (1988) The carcinogenic risks of modern tanning equipment: is UVA safer than UVB? Arch Dermatol Res, **280**, 300-307.

Van't Veer, LJ, Burgering, BMT, Versteeg, R, Boot, AJM, Ruiter, DJ, Osanto, S, Schrier, PI, & Bos, JL (1989) N-*ras* Mutations in human cutaneous melanoma from sun-exposed body sites. Mol Cell Biol, **9**, 3114-3116.

Varghese, AJ and Wang, SY (1967) Ultraviolet irradiation of DNA in vitro and in vivo produces a third thymine-derived product. Science **156**, 955-957.

Verhoeff, FH, Bell, L, Walker, CB (1916) The pathological effects of radiant energy on the eye. Proc Am Acad Arts Sci, **510**, 1-810.

Vermeer M & Streilein JW (1990) Ultraviolet B light-induced alterations in epidermal Langerhans cells are mediated in part by tumor necrosis factor-alpha. Photodermatol Photoimmunol Photomed, **7**, 258-265.

Vermeer M, Schmieder GJ, Yoshikawa T, Van den Berg J-W, Metzman MS, Taylor JR, & Streilein JW (1991) Effects of ultraviolet B light on cutaneous immune responses of humans with deeply pigmented skin. J Invest Dermatol, **97**, 729-734.

Vile, GF, Basu-Modak, S, Waltner, C and Tyrrell, RM (1993) Haem oxygenase 1 mediates an adaptive response to oxidative stress in human skin fibroblasts. Proc Natl Acad Sci USA (in press).

Vincek V, Jurimoto I, Medema JP, Prieto E, & Streilein JW (1993) Tumor necrosis factor alpha polymorphism correlates with deleterious effects of ultraviolet B light on cutaneous immunity. Cancer Res, **53**, 728-732.

Vitale S, West S, Munoz B, Schein OD, Maguire M, Bressler, N & Taylor HR (1992) Watermen Study II: mortality and baseline prevalence of nuclear opacity. Invest Ophthalmol Vi Sci, **33**,1097.

Vitasa, BC, Taylor, HR, Strickland, PT, Rosenthal, FS, West, S, Abbey, H, Ng, SK, Munoz, B, & Emmett, EA (1990) Association of nonmelanoma skin cancer and actinic keratosis with cumulative solar ultraviolet exposure in Maryland watermen. Cancer, **65**, 2811-2817.

Volkenandt, M, Schlegel, U, Nanus, DM, & Albino, AP (1991) Mutational analysis of the human p53 gene in malignant melanoma. Pigment Cell Res, **4**, 35-40.

Vosjan, JH, Dohler, G, & Nieuwland G (1990) Effect of UVB irradiance on the ATP content of microorganisms of the Weddell Sea Antarctica, Neth J Sea Res **25**, 391-394.

Vuillaume, M, Daya-Grosjean, L, Vincens, P, Pennetier, JL, Tarroux, P, Baret, A, Calvayrac, R, Taieb, A and Satorin, A (1992) Striking differences in cellular catalase activity between two DNA repair-deficient diseases. Xeroderma pigmentosum and trichothiodystophy. Carcinogenesis **13**, 321-328.

Walker, GC (1987) The SOS response of Escherichia coli, in Escherichia coli and Salmonella typhimurium. Cellular and Molecular Biology (Niedhardt, FC, Ingraham, JL, Low, KB, Magasanik, B, Shaechter, M, Umbarger, HE, eds), pp 1346-1357. American Society of Microbiology, Washington DC.

Walter, SD, Marrett, LD, From, L, Hertzman, C, Shannon, HS, & Roy, P (1990) The association of cutaneous malignant melanoma with the use of sunbeds and sunlamps. Am J Epidemiol, **131**, 232-243.

Warfel AH, Moy JA, Meola T, Sanchez M, Soter NA, & Belsito DV (1993) Effett of ultraviolet B (UVB) on the expression of human immunodeficiency virus (HIV) in mice and humans, Photochem Photobiol, **57**, 755.

Waring GO, Roth AM, & Ekins MB (1984) Clinical and pathological description of 17 cases of corneal intraepithelial neoplasia. Am J Ophthalmol, **97,** 547-559.

Waterhouse, J, Muir, C, Correa, P, & Powell, J, eds (1976) Cancer Incidence in Five Continents, Vol III (IARC Scientific Publications No 15), Lyon, International Agency for Research on Cancer.

Waterhouse, J, Muir, C, Shanmugaratnam, K, & Powell, J, eds (1982) Çancer Incidence in Five Continents, Vol IV (IARC Scientific Publications No 42), Lyon, International Agency for Research on Cancer.

Webb, RB (1977) Lethal and mutagenic effects of near-ultraviolet radiation Photochem Photobiol Rev **2,** 169-261.

Wei, Q, Matanoski, GM, Farmer, ER, Hedayati, MA, & Grossman, L (1993) DNA repair and aging in basal cell carcinoma: A molecular epidemiology study. Proc Natl Acad Sci USA, **90**, 1614-1618.

Weinstock, MA, Colditz, GA, Willett, WC, Stampfer, MJ, Bronstein, BR, Mihm, MC, Jr & Speizer, FE (1989) Nonfamilial cutaneous melanoma incidence in women associated with sun exposure before 20 years of age. Pediatrics, **84**, 199-204.

Wellmann, E, (1991) Specific ultraviolet effects in plant development, J Exp Bot, (Suppl), **32, 42**.

Wellmann, E, (1971) Phytochrome mediated flavone glycoside synthesis in cell suspension cultures of Petroselinum hortense after preirradiation with ultraviolet light, Planta, **101**, 283-286.

Werner JS (1991) The damaging effects of light on the eye and implications for understnding changes in vision across the life span, in (P Bagnoli and W Hodos) The Changing Visual System, New York, Plenum Press.

West SK, Rosenthal FS, Bressler NM, Bressler SB, Munoz B, Fine SL, & Taylor HR (1989) Exposure to sunlight and other risk factors for age-related macular degeneration. Arch Ophthalmol, **107,** 875-879.

Wester A (1987) Ultraviolet transmission properties of sunscreens and sunglasses. In: eds Passchier W and Bosnjakovic B. Human exposure to ultraviolet radiation: risks and regulations, Elsevier, Amsterdam.

Westerveld, A, Hoeijmakers, JHJ, van Duin, M, de Wit, J, Odijk, H, Pavlink, A, Wood, RD and Bootsma, D (1984) Molecular cloning of a human DNA repair gene. Nature **310**, 425-529.

Whillock, MJ, McKinlay, AF, Kemmlert, J and Forsgren, PG (1990) Ultraviolet radiation emissions from miniature [compact] fluorescent lamps. Lighting Res Technol **22,** 125-128.

Whillock, MJ, Clark, IE, McKinlay, AF, Todd, CD & Mundy, SJ (1988) Ultraviolet radiation levels associated with the use of fluorescent general lighting, UVA and UVB lamps in the workplace and home. National radiological Protection Board, Research Report R221, London, HMSO.

Whitaker, CJ, Lee, WR, & Downes, JE (1979) Squamous cell skin cancer in the north-west of England, 1967-69, and its relation to occupation. Br J Ind Med, **36,** 43-51.

WHO (1989) Non-ionizing radiation protection. MJ Suess & DA Benwell-Morison eds., World Health Organization Regional Office for Europe, European series No 25, WHO, Copenhagen.

WHO/UNEP/IRPA (1979) Ultraviolet Radiation, Environmental Health Criteria 14, World Health Organization, United Nations Environment Programme, WHO, Geneva.

WHO (1977) Manual of the International Statistical Classification of Diseases, Injuries, and Causes of Death. International Classification of Diseases, 1975 rev, Vol 1, Geneva, p 102.

WHO (1948) International Statistical Classification of Diseases, Injuries and Causes of Death, Sixth Revision, Geneva.

Widmark J (1901) Ueber den Einfluss des Lichtes auf die Linse. Mitteil aus d Augenklin d Carol med chir Inst zu Stockholm **3,** 135-149.

Widmark (1889) Ueber den Einfluss des Lichtes auf die vorderen medien des auges. Skand Arch f physiol **1**, 264-330.

Wilesmith JW, Wells GA, Cranwell MP and Ryan JB (1988) Bovine spongiform encephalopathy : epidemiological studies. Vet Rec, **123,** 638-644.

Willis, I, Menter, JM, & Whyte, HJ (1981) The rapid induction of cancers in the hairless mouse utilizing the principle of photoaugmentation. J Invest Dermatol, **76**, 404-408.

Wittenberg S (1986) Solar radiation and the eye: a review of knowledge relevant to eye care. Am J Optom Physiol Optics, **63,** 676-689.

WMO (1993) World Meteorological Organization Report of the second meeting of the ozone research managers of the parties to the Vienna Convention for the protection of the ozone layer. Geneva 10-12 March.

Wolf, P, Donawho, CK, & Kripke, ML (1993a) Analysis of the protective effect of different sunscreens on ultraviolet radiation-induced local and systemic suppression of contact hypersensitivity and inflammatory responses in mice. J Invest Dermatol **100**, 254-259.

Wolfe P, Yarosh DB, & Kripke ML (1993b) Effects of sunscreens and a DNA excision repair enzyme on ultraviolet radiation - induced inflammation, immune suppression and cyclobutane pyrimidine dimer formation in mice. J invest Dermatol **101**, 523-527.

Wong L, Ho SC, Coggon D, Cruddas AM, Hwang CH, Ho CP, Robertshaw AM, & MacDonald DM (1993) Sunlight exposure, antioxidant status, and cataract in Hong Kong fishermen. J Epidemiol Comm Health, **47,** 46-49.

Wong CF, Fleming R & Carter SJ (1989) A new dosimeter for ultraviolet B radiation. Photochem Photobiol **50**, 611-615.

Wood, RD, Robbins, P and Lindahl, T (1988) Complementation of the Xeroderma pigmentosum DNA repair defect in cell-free extracts. Cell **53**, 91-106.

Wucherpfenning V (1931) Biologie und prackische verwenbarkeit der erythemschwelle des UV. Strahlentherapie **40**, 201-244.

Yannuzzi L, Fisher Y, Slakter J, Krueger A (1989) Solar retinipathy. A photobiologic and geophysical analysis, Retina, **9**, 28-43.

Yarosh, D, Alas, LG, Yee, V, Oberyszyn, A, Kibitel, JT, Mitchell, D, Rosenstein, R, Spinowitz, A, & Citron, M (1992) Pyrimidine dimer removal enhanced by DNA repair liposomes reduces incidence of UV skin cancer in mice. Cancer Res, **52**, 4227-4231.

Yasumoto S, Yoshinobu H, & Aurelian L (1987) Immunity to herpes simplex virus type 2: Suppression of virus-induced responses in ultraviolet B-irradiated mice. J Immunol, **139**, 2788-2793.

Yoshida A, Ishiguro S & Tamai M (1993) Expression of glial fibrillary acidic protein in muoller cells after lensectomy-vitrectomy. Invest. Ophthalmol. Vis. Sci. **34**, 3154-3160.

Yoshikawa T & Streilein JW (1990) On the genetic basis of the effects of ultraviolet B on cutaneous immunity. Evidence that polymorphisms at the Tnfα and Lps loci govern susceptibility. Immunogenetics, **32**, 398-405.

Yoshikawa T, Rae V, Bruins-Slot W, Van den Berg J-W, Taylor Jr, & Streilein JW (1990) Susceptibility to effects of UVB radiation on induction of contact hypersensitivity as a risk factor for skin cancer in humans. J Invest Dermatol, **95**, 530-536.

Young RW (1991) Age-related cataract. New York, Oxford University Press.

Young, AR, Potten, CS, Chadwick, CA, Murphy, GM, Hawk, JLM and Cohen, AJ (1991) Photo-protection and 5-MOP photochemoprotection from UVR-induced DNA damage in humans: the role of skin type. J Invest Dermatol, **97**, 942-948.

Young, AR, Walker, SL, Kinley, JS, Plastow, SR, Averbeck, D, Morlière, P, & Dubertret, L (1990) Phototumorigenesis studies of 5-methoxypsoralen in bergamot oil: evaluation and modification of risk of human use in an albino mouse skin model. J Photochem Photobiol B Biol, **7**, 231-250.

Young, AR, Magnus, IA, Davies, AC, & Smith, NP (1983) A comparison of the phototumorigenic potential of 8-MOP and 5-MOP in hairless albino mice exposed to solar simulated radiation. Br J Dermatol, **108,** 507-518.

Yu, CC, MacGregor, JM, Dublin, EA, Barnes, DM, MacDonald, DM, & Levison, DA (1992) Patterns of immunostaining for p53 in benign and malignant melanocytic lesions (meeting abstract). J Pathol, **167** (Suppl), 130A.

Zajdela, E, & Bisagni, E (1981) 5-Methoxypsoralen, the melanogenic additive in sun-tan preparations, is tumorigenic in mice exposed to 365 nm uv radiation. Carcinogenesis, **2**, 121-127.

Zamansky, G and Chou, I-N (1987) Environmental wavelength of ultraviolet light induce cytoskeletal damage. J Inv Dermatol **89**, 603-606.

Zanetti, R, Rosso, S, Faggiano, F, Roffino, R, Colonna, S, & Martina, G (1988) A case-control study on cutaneous malignant melanoma in the province of Torino, Italy (Fr). Rev Epidemiol Santé publ, **36**, 309-317.

Zanetti, R, Franceschi, S, Rosso, S, Colonna, S, Bidoli, E (1992) Cutaneous melanoma and sunburns in childhood in a southern European population. Eur J Cancer, **28A**, 1172-1176.

Zaridze, D, Mukeria, A, & Duffy, SW (1992) Risk factors for skin melanoma in Moscow. Int J Cancer, **52**, 159-161.

Zaunuddin D, Sasaki K (1991) Risk factor analysis in a cataract epidemiology survey in West Samatara, Indonesia. Dev Ophthalmol, **21,** 78-86.

Ziegler, A-M, Leffell, DJ, Kunala, S, Sharma, HW, Gailani, M, Simon, JA, Halperin, AJ, Baden, HP, Shapiro, PE, Bale, AE, & Brash, DE (1993) Mutation hotspots due to sunlight in the p53 gene of nonmelanoma skin cancers. Proc Natl Acad Sci USA, **90**, 4216-4220.

Zigman S (1993) Yearly review: ocular light damage. Photochem. Photobiol. **57**, 1060-1068.

Zigman S, Yulo T, & Schultz J (1974) Cataract induction in mice exposed to near UV light. Ophthalmol Res, **6**, 259-270.

Zigman S, Graff J, Yulo T & Vaughen T (1975) The response of mouse ocular tissue to continuous near-UV light exposure. Invest Ophthalmol, **14**, 710-713.

Zmudzka BZ & ... ency virus by ultravi...

Zuclich JA (19... ...cular tissues. Health ...

Zuclich, J, Ku... ...iolet induced cornea...

Zundorf, I, & H... ...sis of UV effects o... Arch Microbiol.

RA
565
A1
E58
VOL.
160

ULTRAVIOLET RADIATION

10057

This report contains the collective views of an international group of experts and does not necessarily represent the decisions or the stated policy of the United Nations Environment Programme, the International Labour Organisation, or the World Health Organization.

Environmental Health Criteria 147

PROPACHLOR

First draft prepared by Dr L. Ivanova-Chemishanska,
Institute of Hygiene and Occupational Health,
Sofia, Bulgaria

World Health Organization
Geneva, 1993

The **International Programme on Chemical Safety (IPCS)** is a joint venture of the United Nations Environment Programme, the International Labour Organisation, and the World Health Organization. The main objective of the IPCS is to carry out and disseminate evaluations of the effects of chemicals on human health and the quality of the environment. Supporting activities include the development of epidemiological, experimental laboratory, and risk-assessment methods that could produce internationally comparable results, and the development of manpower in the field of toxicology. Other activities carried out by the IPCS include the development of know-how for coping with chemical accidents, coordination of laboratory testing and epidemiological studies, and promotion of research on the mechanisms of the biological action of chemicals.

WHO Library Cataloguing in Publication Data

Propachlor.

(Environmental health criteria ; 147)

1.Acetanilides - adverse effects 2.Acetanilides - toxicity
3.Environmental exposure 4.Herbicides - adverse effects
5.Herbicides - toxicity I.Series

ISBN 92 4 157147 0 (NLM Classification: WA 249)
ISSN 0250-863X

Printed in Finland
93/9499 — Vammala — 5500

CONTENTS

WHO TASK GROUP ON ENVIRONMENTAL HEALTH CRITERIA FOR PROPACHLOR

Members

Dr L.A. Albert, Consultores Ambientales Asociados, Xalapa, Veracruz, Mexico

Dr S. Dobson, Institute of Terrestrial Ecology, Monks Wood Experimental Station, Abbots Ripton, Huntingdon, Cambridgeshire, United Kingdom

Dr L. Ivanova-Chemishanska, Institute of Hygiene and Occupational Health, Sofia, Bulgaria (*Joint Rapporteur*)

Dr J. Kangas, Kuopio Regional Institute of Occupational Health, Kuopio, Finland

Dr S.K. Kashyap, National Institute of Occupational Health, Meghaninagar, Ahmedabad, India

Professor A. Massoud, Department of Community, Environmental and Occupational Medicine, Faculty of Medicine, Ain Shams University, Cairo, Egypt (*Vice-Chairman*)

Professor Wai-on Phoon, Department of Occupational Health, University of Sydney, and Professional Education Program, National Institute of Occupational Health and Safety, Worksafe Australia, Sydney, Australia (*Chairman*)

Professor L. Rosival, Institute of Preventive and Clinical Medicine, Bratislava, Czechoslovakia

Dr K.C. Swentzel, Health Effects Division, US Environmental Protection Agency, Washington, D.C., USA (*Joint Rapporteur*)

Observers

Dr M. Carroll, Monsanto Services International, Brussels, Belgium

Dr B. Hammond, The Agricultural Group of Monsanto Company, St Louis, Missouri, USA

Secretariat

Dr K.W. Jager, International Programme on Chemical Safety, World Health Organization, Geneva, Switzerland (*Secretary*)

NOTE TO READERS OF THE CRITERIA MONOGRAPHS

Every effort has been made to present information in the criteria monographs as accurately as possible without unduly delaying their publication. In the interest of all users of the Environmental Health Criteria monographs, readers are kindly requested to communicate any errors that may have occurred to the Director of the International Programme on Chemical Safety, World Health Organization, Geneva, Switzerland, in order that they may be included in corrigenda.

* * *

A detailed data profile and a legal file can be obtained from the International Register of Potentially Toxic Chemicals, Palais des Nations, 1211 Geneva 10, Switzerland (Telephone No. 7988400 or 7985850).

* * *

The proprietary information contained in this monograph cannot replace documentation for registration purposes, because the latter has to be closely linked to the source, the manufacturing route, and the purity/impurities of the substance to be registered. The data should be used in accordance with paragraph 82-84 and recommendations paragraph 90 of the Second FAO Government Consultation (FAO, 1982).

ENVIRONMENTAL HEALTH CRITERIA FOR PROPACHLOR

A WHO Task Group on Environmental Health Criteria for Propachlor met at the World Health Organization, Geneva, from 4 to 8 November 1991. Dr K.W. Jager, IPCS, welcomed the participants on behalf of Dr M. Mercier, Director of the IPCS, and the three IPCS cooperating organizations (UNEP/ILO/WHO). The Group reviewed and revised the draft and made an evaluation of the risks for human health and the environment from exposure to propachlor.

The first draft was prepared by Dr L. Ivanova-Chemishanska of the Institute of Hygiene and Occupational Health, Sofia, Bulgaria, who also assisted in the preparation of the second draft, incorporating comments received following circulation of the first drafts to the IPCS Contact Points for Environmental Health Criteria monographs.

Dr K.W. Jager of the IPCS Central Unit was responsible for the scientific content of the monograph, and Dr P.G. Jenkins for the technical editing.

The fact that Monsanto Agrochemical Company, St Louis, USA, made available to the IPCS and the Task Group its proprietary toxicological information on their product is gratefully acknowledged. This allowed the Task Group to make its evaluation on a more complete data base.

The effort of all who helped in the preparation and finalization of the monograph is gratefully acknowledged.

ABBREVIATIONS

a.i.	active ingredient
AcP	acid phosphatase
ATPase	adenosine triphosphatase
CHO	Chinese hamster ovary
DMSO	dimethyl sulfoxide
GA	gibberillic acid
GGPT = GGT	gamma-glutamyltransferase
HGPRT	hypoxanthine-guanine phosphoribosyltransferase
LAP	leucine aminopeptidase
LDH	lactate dehydrogenase
MAC	maximum allowable concentration
MAP	mercapturic acid pathway
mCi	millicurie
MQL	minimum quantifiable limit
NOAEL	no-observed-adverse-effect level
NOEC	no-observed-effect concentration
NOEL	no-observed-effect level
OCT	ornithine carbamoyltransferase
ppb	parts per billion
ppm	parts per million
SAP = AP	alkaline phosphatase
SDH	succinate dehydroganase
SGOT = AST	aspartate aminotransferase
SGPT = ALT	alanine aminotransferase
UDS	unscheduled DNA synthesis
uv	ultraviolet
WP	wettable powder

1. SUMMARY AND EVALUATION

1.1 Identity, use pattern, physical and chemical properties, analytical methods

Propachlor is a pre-emergence and early post-emergence herbicide derived from acetanilide, and has been in use since 1965. The major formulations are as wettable powder, liquid flowable (suspension concentrate) and as granules. Its uses in agriculture include the control of annual grasses and some broad-leaved weeds in several crops including corn, sorghum, pumpkins, flax and flowers.

Propachlor is slightly soluble in water and readily soluble in most organic solvents. It has a low volatility, is non-flammable and is stable to ultraviolet radiation. The most practical method for analysis is gas chromatography with electron capture detection after suitable extraction and clean-up procedures.

1.2 Environmental transport, distribution and transformation

Propachlor is not known to photodegrade on soil surfaces. Volatilization of the compound occurs under windy conditions while the soil surface is still moist.

The adsorption of the compound to soil particles and organic matter is only moderate. This leads to the potential for leaching through the soil profile and into ground water. However, all studies show that this potential is unlikely to be realised in practice. Very high rainfall is required to move residues 30 cm down the soil profile. Most authors report that the great majority of residues remain within the upper 4 cm of soil. The characteristics of the soil greatly influence movement of the compound. Most leaching occurs in sandy soil with little organic matter.

Run-off of propachlor has been studied in both the laboratory and field. The organic matter in the soil reduced run-off from 7% to 1% of the applied herbicide in one study. Incorporation of propachlor into the soil also reduced loss through run-off (from 3% to 0.8% in one study).

By far the most significant factor in reducing propachlor levels in soil and water is degradation by microorganisms. Both bacteria and fungi have been shown to be involved in breakdown of the compound. Few bacteria appear to be able to use propachlor as the sole carbon source. Bacteria capable of utilizing soil metabolites of propachlor have also been isolated.

The predominant metabolites formed in soil are water-soluble oxanilic and sulfonic acids. A large number of other metabolites can be formed, but these represent a small proportion of the total.

Propachlor disappears rapidly from soil, half-lives of up to 3 weeks having been reported. Most studies report almost complete degradation within less than 6 months. Environmental conditions affect the rate of degradation, which is favoured by high temperature and soil moisture content. Those studies reporting longer persistence of propachlor in soil were conducted under conditions of low temperature or dry soil. Adequate nutrient levels in soil are also necessary for degradation.

The conjugated *N*-isopropylaniline metabolite is much more persistent than the parent compound. Residues of this metabolite have been found up to 2 years after the application of propachlor experimentally at higher rates than would normally be used in agriculture.

Under normal conditions of use, propachlor is not expected to leach through soil to ground water and will not persist in soil. Exceptional conditions of low temperature or dryness will lead to greater persistence of propachlor and its metabolites.

Under normal conditions, propachlor does not photodegrade significantly in water. In the presence of photosensitizers, photodegradation may take place. Propachlor is hydrolytically stable. Volatilization from water is unlikely because of the high water solubility and low vapour pressure of the compound.

As in soil, the major route of loss of propachlor from water is biotic degradation. The rate of loss of propachlor from water is, therefore, dependent on the microbial population. A study in water with few bacteria present yielded a half-life of about 5 months. Ring cleavage did not occur within six weeks in another study. Laboratory model ecosystem studies showed almost complete degradation of propachlor within 33 days.

In several studies on different plant species, propachlor was shown to be rapidly metabolized in both intact plants and excized plant tissues. The metabolic pathways were similar in all plants studied, at least for the first 6 to 24 h, producing water-soluble metabolites. No metabolic breakdown of the *N*-isopropylaniline moiety was observed. Only a very small proportion (< 1% in one study) of the metabolites was found in the fruit of the plants; the great majority was in the roots and foliage. The major metabolites produced in plants are identical with those produced in soil. Uptake of these metabolites from soil is known to take place and it is uncertain in some studies whether measured metabolites derive from the plant or the soil.

Although the octanol/water partition coefficient suggests a moderate potential for bioaccumulation, studies show that propachlor neither bioconcentrates nor biomagnifies in organisms.

1.3 Environmental levels and human exposure

Reported measurements of air concentrations of propachlor during application are few and inadequate.

Concentrations in surface and ground water in the USA were consistently low, the maxima being at 10 μg/litre in surface and 0.12 μg/litre in ground water. The highest water concentration recorded in a run-off study was 46 μg/litre.

Propachlor residues in food are usually below the detection limit of the analytical method (0.005 mg/kg). Experimental studies have identified residues in the order of 0.05 mg/kg in tomatoes, peppers, onions and cabbage.

Measurements of propachlor in the air of the working zone of tractor drivers applying the compound ranged between 0.1 and 3.7 mg/m^3.

1.4 Kinetics and metabolism

Propachlor can be absorbed into mammals through the respiratory and gastrointestinal tract as well as through the skin. It does not accumulate in the body. After 48 h it is not detectable in the organism.

Most animal species (rats, pigs, chickens) metabolize propachlor through the mercapturic acid pathway (MAP). Cysteine conjugates are formed by glutathione conjugation and this conjugate has been proposed as an intermediate in the metabolic formation of mercapturic acids. Bacterial C-S lyase participates in the further metabolism of the cysteine conjugate of propachlor and in the formation of the final methylsulfonyl-containing metabolites, which are mainly excreted in the urine (68% of the dose of propachlor), and insoluble residues, which are excreted in the faeces (19%). The propachlor C-S lyase is not active in germ-free rats.

Studies showed some differences in metabolism between the rat and pig. The bile is the major route of elimination of MAP metabolites in the rat, but it is has been proved that an extrabiliary route of metabolism exists in the pig.

Metabolic studies on calves showed that they may be unable to form mercapturic acids from glutathione conjugates, which may make them more susceptible to poisoning.

1.5 Effects on laboratory animals and *in vitro* test systems

Propachlor is slightly toxic in acute oral exposure (the LD_{50} in rats ranges from 950 to 2176 mg/kg body weight). Signs of acute intoxication are predominantly central nervous system effects (excitement and convulsion followed by depression). The acute inhalation toxicity in rodents is low (LC_{50} = 1.0 mg/litre). Propachlor caused severe irritation effects on eyes and skin.

Propachlor has been tested in short- and long-term exposure studies on rats, mice and dogs. The liver and kidneys are the target organs. In dogs, the no-observed-adverse-effect level (NOAEL) was 45 mg/kg body weight in a 3-month dietary exposure study. In a one-year study on dogs, the NOAEL was 9 mg/kg body weight (250 ppm in diet). The no-observed-effect level (NOEL) in a 24-month dietary exposure study on rats was 50 mg/kg diet (2.6 mg/kg body weight). In an 18-month dietary study in mice, the NOEL was 1.6 mg/kg body weight (10 ppm).

Propachlor was not found to be carcinogenic in mice and rats. It showed a negative mutagenic response in most of the mammalian test systems and positive results in a few assays. The experimental data available provide insufficient evidence of the mutagenic potential.

When tested as a single dose (675 mg/kg) in rats and mice, propachlor showed positive evidence of embryotoxicity. Embrytoxic effects were also observed in repeated dose regimens

(35.7-270 mg/kg). However, in another rat study using a dose range of 20-200 mg/kg, no embryotoxicity was observed.

At levels of 12 and 60 mg/kg body weight, propachlor (wettable powder) resulted in a decrease in protein content and an increase in ATPase and 5-nucleotidase activity in rat testis homogenate and degenerative changes in the testes. In a two-generation reproduction study there was no definite evidence of adverse effects.

1.6 Effects on humans

A few cases of contact and allergic dermatitis of farmers and production workers exposed to propachlor (Ramrod and Satecid) have been reported. Patch tests were carried out among some of them, revealing a positive patch test reaction, irritation reaction or mono- and bi-valent hypersensitivity.

There have been no reports of symptoms or diseases either among occupationally exposed humans or the general population other than the few reports of its effects on the skin of occupationally exposed workers.

1.7 Effects on organisms in the environment

In studies on soil microorganisms, nitrifying bacteria were the most sensitive group to the inhibitory effects of propachlor, their numbers being reduced by a factor of 3 to 4 after the application of 8 to 10 kg propachlor/ha. Cellulose-decomposing bacteria were the least sensitive. High adsorption to clay particles in soil and high temperature both reduce the inhibitory effects.

A 96-h EC_{50} of 0.02 mg/litre for growth and a no-observed-effect concentration (NOEC) of 0.01 mg/litre have been reported for the alga *Selenastrum capricornutum*. A second study using a formulation and conducted over 72 h suggested substantially less hazard for the same organism.

LC_{50} values of 7.8 and 6.9 mg/litre have been reported for the water flea *Daphnia magna* and a NOEC of < 5.6 mg/litre. The NOEC for reproduction was 0.097 mg/litre. LC_{50} values of 0.79 and 1.8 mg/litre have been reported for two species of midge larvae.

The 96-h LC_{50} for rainbow trout is 0.17 mg/litre and the NOEC in a 21-day study was 0.019 mg/litre.

Propachlor is considered to be moderately to highly toxic to aquatic organisms.

Propachlor is not toxic to earthworms at exposure concentrations in soil expected from normal use (the NOEC is 100 mg/kg soil). The contact LD_{50} for honey bees (311 μg/bee) shows that propachlor will not pose a hazard to these insects. Some beneficial parasitic insects have been reported to be adversely affected by propachlor in laboratory and field studies.

Propachlor is more toxic to birds when administered via the stomach than when fed in the diet. Acute LD_{50} values range between 137 and 735 mg/kg body weight for different bird species. The LC_{50} values from dietary exposure exceed 5620 mg/kg diet in birds.

Propachlor does not pose a hazard to birds in the field, even with the granular formulation.

2. IDENTITY, PHYSICAL AND CHEMICAL PROPERTIES, AND ANALYTICAL METHODS

2.1 Identity

Common name: Propachlor

Chemical structure

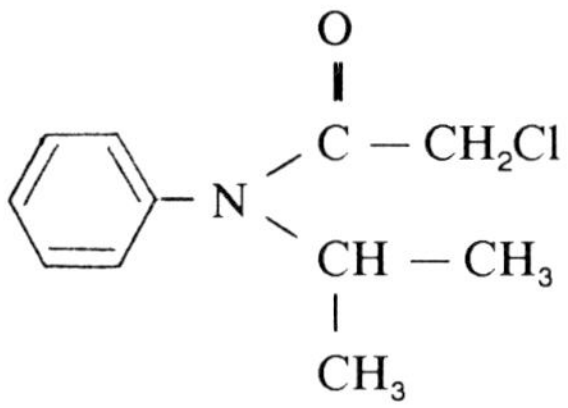

Chemical formula: $C_{11}H_{14}ClNO$

Common synonyms and trade names: Ramrod, Acylide, Bexton (discontinued by Dow Chemical Company), Niticid, Satecid

CAS chemical name: 2-chloro-*N*-(1-methylethyl)-*N*-phenyl acetamide

IUPAC name: 2-chloro-*N*-isopropylacetanilide (formerly alpha-chloro-*N*-isopropylacetanilide)

CAS registry number: 1918-16-7

RTECS registry number: AE1575000

Propachlor is available as a technical material containing 93% active ingredient for formulation of propachlor end-use products. It is available in the form of granules (200 g active ingredient/kg), wettable powder (WP, 650 g active ingredient/kg) and as a liquid flowable formulation (suspension concentrate), among others. Mixtures with other herbicides, e.g., atrazine and propazine are also used.

2.2 Physical and chemical properties

Some of the physical and chemical properties of propachlor are given in Table 1.

Table 1. Some physical and chemical properties of propachlor

Physical state		solid
Colour		tan
Relative molecular mass		211.7
Melting point (°C)		77
Boiling point (°C) at 0.03 mmHg		110
Decomposition (°C)		> 170
Vapour pressure (25 °C)		103 mPa
Solubility in water	(20 °C)	580 mg/litre
	(25 °C)	613 mg/litre
Solubility in organic solvents		readily soluble in most organic solvents except aliphatic hydrocarbons:
	acetone	448 g/kg
	benzene	737 g/kg
	chloroform	602 g/kg
	ethanol	408 g/kg
	xylene	239 g/kg
Log K_{ow}		1.62-2.30

It is non-flammable and stable to ultraviolet radiation.

2.3 Conversion factors

At 25 °C $\quad$ 1 mg/m^3 = 8.802 ppm

1 ppm = 0.1136 mg/m^3

2.4 Analytical methods

The analytical methods described in the literature, which are based on different types of determination of propachlor in different media, are given in Table 2.

Table 2. Analytical methods for the determination of propachlor and metabolites

Sample type	Method of detection	Extraction and clean-up	Detection limit	Reference
Soil and plants	thin-layer chromatography	2-h extraction with chloroform	0.02-0.04 mg/kg	Kofman & Nishko (1984)
Soil and plants	gas chromatography with electron-capture detection	extraction with benzene; clean-up by partition with hexane-acetonitrile followed by column chromatography (Florisil)	0.004-0.005 mg/kg	Balinova (1981)
Soil	gas chromatography with electron-capture detection	acetone extraction followed by alkane hydrolysis, steam distillation and concentration of anilines in toluene	0.01 mg/kg; recoveries at residual levels are generally better than 80%	Caverly & Denney (1978)
Soil	gas liquid chromatography with flame-ionization detection	extraction with isopropanol and benzene; column chromatography (Florisil)	< 0.05 mg/kg	Markus & Puma (1973)
Immature plants	gas-liquid chromatography with flame-ionization detection	extraction with isopropanol; column chromatography (Florisil)	< 0.05 mg/kg	Markus & Puma (1973)

Table 2 (contd).

Sample type	Method of detection	Extraction and clean-up	Detection limit	Reference
Mature grain	gas-liquid chromatography with flame-ionization detection	extraction with acetonitrile; column chromatography (Florisil)	< 0.05 mg/kg	Markus & Puma (1973)
Cabbage	gas chromatography with NP detection	extraction with acetone followed by alkaline hydrolysis to *N*-isopropyl-aniline; steam distillation and extraction with toluene	0.06 mg/kg (fresh weight)	Warholic et al. (1983)
Industrial and municipal waste water	gas chromatography with electron-capture detection	extraction with methylene chloride; clean-up on a Florisil column	1 ng/litre	Pressley & Longbottom (1982)
Urine metabolites of propachlor (glutathione conjugates)	gas or liquid chromatography and mass spectrometry	fractionation with lipophilic ion exchangers (Lipidex 1000, Lipidex DEAP SP-LH-20 and Sep pack C_{18})	not given	Sjovall et al. (1983)

High-pressure liquid chromatography with radioactive detection or liquid scintillation has been used to purify the metabolites from ^{14}C-labelled propachlor in several biological media, including egg yolk, egg white, edible tissues and excreta of laying hens, after extraction with organic solvents. The metabolites were characterized by gas chromatography with radioactive detection mass spectrometry (Bleeke et al., 1987). With liquid scintillation detection, the minimum quantifiable limit (MQL) was 0.01 to 0005 ppm.

3. SOURCES OF HUMAN AND ENVIRONMENTAL EXPOSURE

3.1 Production and uses

Propachlor was developed by the Monsanto Chemical Company and commercially introduced in 1965. Technical propachlor is produced in the USA by Monsanto and in Germany by BASF. There are other manufacturers of technical propachlor.

Propachlor is prepared by the reaction of chloracetyl chloride and *N*-isopropylaniline.

It is a pre-emergence, pre-planting (incorporated) or early post-emergence herbicide effective against annual grasses and some broad-leaved weeds (Worthing & Hance, 1991). It is used on field corn, hybrid seed corn, silage corn, grain sorghum (milo), green peas, soybeans, flax, pumpkins and flowers. In 1971, 10 000 tonnes were produced (US EPA, 1984a), but a more recent estimate of annual use in the USA is 1800 tonnes.

3.2 Methods and rates of application

Application rates range from 4 to 6 kg active ingredient in 150-300 litres of water per ha (6-9 kg wettable powder formulation/ha) in pre-emergence use. Some tests indicate that early post-emergence applications are equally effective for weed control. The best response occurred when broad-leaved weeds were between the cotyledonous stage and the 2½-leaf stage and when grassy weeds were up to the one-leaf stage.

Irrigation following application improves activity, particularly under dry soil conditions. The duration of weed control ranges from 4 to 6 weeks, depending on the soil structure and organic content (Humburg et al., 1989).

4. ENVIRONMENTAL TRANSPORT, DISTRIBUTION AND TRANSFORMATION

4.1 Transport and distribution between media

4.1.1 Soil

The fate and transport of propachlor in soil has been well studied. The principal aim has been to determine the rate and products of degradation, persistence, environmental factors and organisms participating in the biodegradation, and the conditions under which degradation takes place.

4.1.1.1 Abiotic factors

Beestman & Deming (1974) found that leaching did not contribute to dissipation since no residues were found below the upper 4-cm layer. The weak leaching ability was related to the high adsorption of propachlor by soil. The ultraviolet absorption spectrum of propachlor reveals no absorption at wavelengths longer than 280 nm. On the basis of these data it was suggested that photodecomposition of soil-applied propachlor would not be significant. Rapid herbicide volatilization occurred under windy conditions during the period that exposed soil surfaces remain moist.

In a study by Nesterova et al. (1980), propachlor was applied, under dry weather conditions, at a rate of 7 kg/ha for 4 consecutive years. The residues of propachlor in the soil were measured up to 4 weeks following the application. On the 5th day, residues were found in the upper layers (0-10 cm), and on the 15th day, after abundant rain (74 mm), they had reached 0-30 cm. There was rapid biodegradation, mainly in the first 5 days, followed by reduced degradation over the next 10 days. Between the 15th and 30th day, no residues were detected.

The mobility of ^{14}C-propachlor in the soil was investigated by Brightwell et al. (1981) by determining its leaching as well as its adsorption coefficient and desorption behaviour. Results were very variable and depended on soil type. With a sandy loam, 89.5% of the ^{14}C activity applied leached through laboratory soil columns, whereas only 5.4% leached through silty clay loam. A high organic matter content reduced the leachability of propachlor. Most of the radioactivity represented the parent compound. Propachlor was adsorbed only moderately, although the equivalent of 50 cm of rain was needed to desorb 40 to 70% of the activity previously bound to soil to a depth of 30 cm in the profile.

The mobility of propachlor in soil was the object of a study carried out by Ritter et al. (1973). The diffusion coefficient of propachlor in a silt loam soil was determined and was compared with the coefficients of two other pesticides, atrazine and diazinone. It was found that propachlor had the highest solubility and the largest diffusion coefficient, which allowed it to move rapidly in the soil. The movement increased with the temperature and moisture contents.

The run-off losses of propachlor have been studied by Baker & Laflen (1979), Baker (1980) and Baker et al. (1982). Rainfall simulation was used by Baker et al. (1982) to determine the effects of corn residue on herbicide run-off losses from the soil. Propachlor was applied to plots with 0, 375, 750 and 1500 kg corn residue per ha, and a 2-h rainfall of 127 mm was simulated. For plots with no corn residue, the average time to run-off was 11 min; run-off was 63 mm, soil loss 11 tonnes/ha, and herbicide loss 7% of the amount applied. Increased corn residue amounts increased time to run-off and decreased run-off, erosion and herbicide losses. Time to run-off for the largest corn residue amount was 30 min, run-off 18 mm, soil loss 1 tonne/ha, and herbicide loss 1%. At least 84% of the herbicide losses were in the dissolved phase. Herbicide placement had little or no effect on the concentrations of herbicide in run-off water and sediment. Herbicide concentrations in water and sediment were negatively correlated with time to run-off.

The effects of incorporation and surface application on run-off losses of propachlor were determined by measuring losses in water and sediment from small plots during 122 mm of simulated rainfall (Baker & Laflen, 1979). Losses of propachlor that was surface-applied to plots were 3%, whereas losses from plots where the herbicide was incorporated by disking were only 0.8%. Incorporation of herbicide has the potential to decrease run-off losses and may be considered the best application method.

In a laboratory study, propachlor was applied at rates of 0.4 and 1.8 kg/ha to corn (*Zea mays*) residue, which in turn was subjected to simulated rainfall (Martin et al., 1978). Initial concentrations in wash-off water were high (9 mg/litre for the high application rate), but this decreased rapidly with time. The mass balance showed that most of the applied dose was washed off and little was retained by the corn residue. Unexplained losses indicated the possibility of volatilization occurring between application of herbicide and application of wash-off water about 12 h later.

Gustafson (1989) described a method combining persistence and mobility parameters to assess the potential for leaching and contamination of ground water by propachlor. The author concluded that propachlor was unlikely to leach through the soil into subsoil water and ground water.

4.1.1.2 *Biotic factors*

Beestman & Deming (1974) carried out a large study to determine the dissipation rate under laboratory and field conditions from Ray silt and Wabash silty clay soils and to quantify the contributions of microbial decomposition, chemical breakdown, volatilization and leaching. Dissipation followed first-order kinetics with half-lives ranging from 2 to 14 days. In moist Ray silt the half-life of propachlor was 4.5 days. The important role of microbial degradation was clearly established. Dissipation from sterilized soil was 50 times slower ($T_{½}$ = 141-151 days) than from unsterilized soil under identical conditions.

Rankov & Velev (1977) conducted a model study over 120 days with 10 microscopic fungi from the genera *Penicillium*, *Aspergillus*, *Fusarium* and *Trichoderma* concerning the degradation and detoxication of propachlor in alluvial meadow soil at 28 °C and 65% soil humidity. The results confirmed the important role of microscopic fungi in increasing the rate of propachlor degradation and detoxication.

Villarreal et al. (1991) enriched microbial cultures from a pesticide disposal site to identify the range of metabolic capacity for propachlor and its metabolites and the species involved in breakdown of the compound. A single strain, corresponding most closely to the genus *Moraxella*, could grow on propachlor as its sole carbon source releasing a metabolite (2-chloro-*N*-isopropyl-acetamide) into the medium. A second strain, corresponding to the genus *Xanthobacter* grew on the metabolite. The *Moraxella* strain appears to use the aromatic carbon atoms of the propachlor for growth since there was induction of catechol 2,3-oxygenase activity in the cells and the growth rate was sustainable only from this source.

Novick et al. (1986) showed that suspensions of soil treated in the field with propachlor could mineralize 16-61% and 0.6-63% of ring-labelled propachlor in 30 days at propachlor concentrations of 0.025 and 10 mg/litre, respectively. A mixture of two bacteria mineralized 57.6% of propachlor within 52.5 h, producing *N*-isopropylaniline as a metabolite.

4.1.1.3 Metabolites

N-isopropylaniline, *N*-isopropylacetanilide, *N*-(1-hydroxyisopropyl)-acetanilide and *N*-isopropyl-2-acetoxyacetanilide are formed as metabolites of propachlor in soil (Lee et al., 1982). Frank et al. (1977) demonstrated the existence of a longer-lasting conjugated degradation product of propachlor in onions and in organic soils following soil application. This was conjugated *N*-isopropylaniline, which could be found in soil up to 2 years after application.

An extensive study on the environmental and metabolic fate of propachlor was conducted by Brightwell et al. (1981). A variety of soil metabolites was identified, the most significant resulting from the modification of the C-2 carbon to yield water-soluble oxanilic and sulfonic acids. The soil metabolism studies demonstrated the predominant proportion of the water-soluble metabolites, i.e. [(1-methylethyl) phenylamino] oxoacetic acid (IV), 2-[(1-methylethyl) phenylamino]-2-oxoethanesulfonic acid (V) and {{[(methylethyl) phenylamino] acetyl}sulfinyl}acetic acid (VI). These metabolites accounted for 25, 17, and 6% of the applied ^{14}C activity, respectively, at different sampling points during the studies. There was a decline in the level of these metabolites with time (Fig. 1).

In addition, several organic soluble metabolites were isolated and identified; these included *N*-(1-methylethyl)-2-(methylsulfinyl)-*N*-phenylacetamide (VII), *N*-(1-methylethyl)-2(methyl sulfonyl)-*N*-phenylacetamide and 2-hydroxy-*N*-(1-methylethyl)-*N*-phenylacetamide (II). These accounted for no more than 6% of the applied activity. The degradation products observed in the anaerobic soil metabolism study were comparable to those observed under aerobic conditions, but the rate of degradation in aerobic conditions was higher.

Lamoureux & Rusness (1989) studied the metabolism of propachlor and the cysteine conjugate of propachlor in sandy loam soil. Both compounds were metabolized at similar rates to three major products: *N*-isopropyloxanilic acid, 2-sulfo-*N*-isopropylacetanilide and 2-(sulfinylmethylenecarboxy)-*N*-isopropylacetanilide.

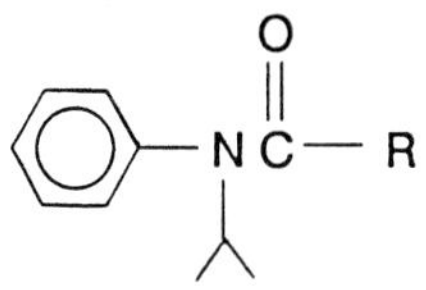

I. R = CH_2Cl
2-chloro-*N*-(1-methylethyl)-*N*-phenylacetamide = propachlor

II. R = CH_2OH
2-hydroxy-*N*-(1-methylethyl)-*N*-phenylacetamide

III. R = CH_3
N-(1-methylethyl)-*N*-phenylacetamide

IV. R = $\overset{O}{\overset{\|}{C}}OH$
[(1-methylethyl)phenylamino]oxoacetic acid

V. R = CH_2SO_3H
2-[(1-methylethyl)phenylamino]-2-oxoethanesulfonic acid

VI. R = $CH_2\overset{O}{\overset{\|}{S}}CH_2\overset{O}{\overset{\|}{C}}OH$
{{[(methylethyl)phenylamino]acetyl}sulfinyl}-acetic acid

VII. R = $CH_2\overset{O}{\overset{\|}{S}}CH_3$
N-(1-methylethyl)-2-(methylsulfinyl)-*N*-phenylacetamide

Fig. 1. Structures of propachlor degradation products.

4.1.1.4 Persistence

Fletcher & Kirkwood (1982) reported a half-life of 2-3 weeks for propachlor. Free propachlor disappeared rapidly in soil treated by Ritter et al. (1973); in 21-28 days residues of free propachlor declined 72-80%. In earlier laboratory studies and field bioassays carried out by Menges & Tamez (1973), the soil persistence (> 90% degradation) was found to be less than 6 months. According to Melnikov et al. (1985) and Zhukova & Shirko (1979), the period of propachlor degradation in soil to non-toxic products is about 2 months. The presence of an alkyl group attached to the nitrogen atom in its molecule prevents its decomposition to aniline or to azobenzolic residues, which could later be transferred into tetrachlorazobenzene (Panshina, 1985). Propachlor applied at 4-8 kg/ha was detoxified in peat soil within 59-63 days (Vasilev, 1982). When it was applied at 6.5, 9 and 11 kg/ha, it was still detectable after 113 days in two types of soil in the Voronezh and Krasnodar regions of the former USSR (Kolesnikov et al., 1980). The longer persistence determined in this study might be connected with the climatic conditions, particularly the low temperatures. Roberts et al. (1978) and Balinova (1981) confirmed that propachlor is rapidly decomposed in soil.

Field studies evaluating the degradation of propachlor in soil showed that 70 days after application, propachlor was detectable in insignificant quantities (0.04 mg/kg, i.e. 2% of the dose applied). Degradation was slower in dry than humid weather (Zhukova & Shirko, 1979) (Table 3). The conclusions of the authors were that degradation in soil is rapid and there is no possibility of propachlor accumulation in crops.

Table 3. Dynamics of dissipation of propachlor in soil (average data for 1974-1976)[a]

Dose application	After 10th day		On 30th day		On 50th day		On 70th day	
(kg propachlor/ha)	mg/kg	%[b]	mg/kg	%[b]	mg/kg	%[b]	mg/kg	%[b]
6	1.73	86.4	0.95	42.8	0.10	5.2	0.04	2
8	2.44	92.6	1.55	58.3	0.20	7.8	0.04	2
10	3.14	94.2	2.53	76.0	0.40	12.0	0.04	2

[a] From: Zhukova & Shirko (1979)
[b] Percentage of dose applied

In a study by Frank et al. (1977), soil with high organic matter content was treated with 19 kg propachlor/ha. The treatment times and rates are given in Table 4. Soil samples were collected to a depth of 20 cm and analysed. Residues of the conjugated metabolite *N*-isopropylaniline of up to 3.7 mg/kg soil were detected 2 years after the application. They were released from soil by hydrolysis, indicating the presence of active bonding sites for the metabolite in the soil. The authors concluded that using propachlor in successive years led to accumulation of long-lasting conjugated *N*-isopropylaniline. Applications made once every 3 years, however, did not lead to such accumulation and they recommended this type of application.

Table 4. Residues of conjugated *N*-isopropylaniline in organic soil treated with propachlor in 1971, 1972 and 1975[a].

Year	Time of application	Rate of application (kg/ha)[b]	*N*-isopropylaniline residues in oven-dried soil (mg/kg)
1971	May and June	9 + 10	not analysed
1972	untreated	none	3.67
	May, July, August	6.7 + 3.4 + 3.4	7.70
	May, July, August	6.7 + 6.7 + 6.7	9.47
1975	May and June	6.7 + 6.7	3.16

[a] From: Frank et al. (1977)

[b] Soil samples were collected in May 1973 and April 1976 and analysed in January and April 1976, respectively.

US EPA (1984b) re-evaluated the existing data concerning some environmental aspects of propachlor. It was concluded that microbes were the primary factor in its breakdown in soil and that its loss from photodecomposition and/or volatilization was low. Although this earlier assessment suggested a potential for propachlor to contaminate ground water, a later assessment (US EPA, 1988) concluded that "the rapid degradation of low levels of propachlor in soil is expected to result in a low potential for groundwater contamination by propachlor".

4.1.1.5 *Environmental conditions affecting distribution and breakdown*

Walker & Brown (1982, 1985) carried out laboratory studies and field trials in parallel. They found first-order kinetics dissipation of propachlor and confirmed the results of Beestman & Deming (1974). They also described a clear temperature dependence: an increase in temperature of 10 °C reduced the half-life by a factor of between 1.9 and 2.5. Soil moisture also influenced degradation: slower rates of loss were found in drier soil. The half-life in soil with a moisture content of 6% was about twice as long as at 15% (Table 5). In general, the time of persistence in the field was comparable to that measured in laboratory studies. The half-life of propachlor varied from 4 to 22 days (Table 5).

Table 5. Half-life for propachlor degradation (days)[a]

Temperature (°C)	25	25	25	25	15	5
Moisture (%)	6	9	12	15	12	12
Propachlor	7.7	4.6	4.2	3.7	9.2	21.7

[a] From: Walker & Brown (1985)

The persistence of propachlor in soil as a result of all microbial, chemical and physical processes has been studied by Zimdahl & Clark (1982). They measured the half-life of propachlor in clay loam and sandy loam soils in the laboratory, using different temperature and moisture conditions (Table 6). An increase in temperature (from 10 to 30 °C) and moisture content (from 20 to 80%) shortened the half-life.

Vasilev (1982) confirmed the importance of meterological conditions, type of soil, and rate and period of application on the degradation in soil. In dry weather, degradation took longer than in humid conditions. Based on field experiments where soil was treated with propachlor and carrots were then planted, the author reported the following residues (measured at the moment of harvest in the soil layer 0-20 cm) in soil: at an application rate of 4 kg/ha the propachlor residues were 0.05 mg/kg; at 6 kg/ha they were 0.15 mg/kg; and at 8 kg/ha they were 0.2 mg/kg.

Table 6. Half-lives of propachlor in clay loam and sandy loam as determined by bioassay[a]

Storage conditions		Half-life (days)	
Temperature (°C)	Soil moisture (%)	Sandy loam	Clay loam
10	50	16.7	14.3
20	50	3.3	5.3
30	50	1.9	1
20	20	23.1	21.5
20	50	3.3	5.3
20	80	3.3	4.1

[a] From: Zimdahl & Clark (1982)

Shirko & Belova (1982) found that residues of propachlor in soil and plants depended on the nitrogen and potassium content of the soil. At the moment of harvesting, no residues of propachlor were detected in soil after application at a rate of 4.5-6.5 kg/ha. According to the authors, a better supply of plants with nutrients (in this case, nitrogen and potassium fertilizers) leads to more intense detoxification and degradation of the herbicide and, conversely, an insufficiency delays the detoxification processes and leads to the accumulation of residues.

4.1.2 Water

Photodegradation of propachlor in aqueous media was studied by Tanaka et al. (1981) under laboratory conditions. They used a 10-ml sample with propachlor concentrations ranging up to 100 mg/litre, and the sample was irradiated for 135 min with a 300-nm sunlight lamp. Very weak photolysis was registered; by the end of the study only 1% of herbicide had been lost. Addition of a commercial surfactant (2% heterogeneous non-ionic Tergitol TMN, acting as photosensitizer) allowed 37% of propachlor to be photodegraded. It is difficult to make conclusions on this study because of certain deficiencies. The use of a commercial formulation in such studies should be avoided since some of the constituents may cause indirect photochemical reactions. No mention was made in the report of the purity of the compound studied. The test should preferably be carried out at constant temperature. The lack of data concerning the intensity of the irradiation source (US EPA, 1984a) does not allow any extrapolation of these data to the environment.

Rejtö et al. (1984) investigated the effects of ultraviolet irradiation of propachlor solutions and found that 5 h of irradiation led to 80% decomposition. The three photodecomposition products identified were: *N*-isopropyloxindole, *N*-isopropyl-3-hydroxyoxindole and a spiro compound. Irradiation of a solution of propachlor with visible light for 12 h led to almost complete decomposition in the presence of riboflavin as a photosensitizer. The photodecomposition products after visible light irradiation were found to be non-phytotoxic.

Monsanto (1987) demonstrated that propachlor is hydrolytically stable.

Volatilization of propachlor from aqueous media is of limited significance because of the high solubility in water and relatively low vapour pressure of the compound. In agreement with Henry's constant, the loss of propachlor by sorption and sedimentation in water bodies does not appear to be very significant (US EPA, 1984a).

The role of microbial biodegradation appears to be of major significance in water as well as in soil. Novick & Alexander (1985) studied the metabolism of low concentrations (10 μg/litre) of propachlor in sewage and lake water. They found that under aerobic conditions microbial populations from sewage and lake waters were not able to mineralize the carbon ring of propachlor in six weeks. However, propachlor was extensively metabolized, the products obtained were organic, and they were found to accumulate in the environment. In a parallel study, it was found that aniline was readily cleaved under similar conditions, indicating rapid mineralization of this compound. It was concluded that structural characteristics of propachlor, other than the ring, account for the mineralization of the compound. The presence of the three substituents on the nitrogen atom in propachlor may be the reason for its persistence. Steen & Collette (1989) determined microbial transformation rate constants for seven amides in natural pond water. A second order mathematical rate expression served to describe propachlor degradation, and a value of 1.1×10^{-9} litres/organism per h was calculated. Brightwell et al. (1981) presented data showing slow degradation of propachlor in lake water under aerobic conditions. After 30 days, 84.5% of the propachlor remained unchanged; under these conditions a half-life of about 5 months would be expected. The low rate of metabolism was due to a low level of microorganisms. Yu et al. (1975) studied the degradation of propachlor in water using a model ecosystem. An aquarium with 7-day-old sorghum plants was used with the addition of 50 μCi of ^{14}C ring-labelled propachlor. By the end of the 33-day experimental period, 7 degradation products in water were determined by thin-layer chromatography but were not identified. At that time only 0.4% of the radioactivity of the dose applied remained in the water.

4.1.3 Plants

The metabolism of propachlor in corn seedlings and in excized leaves of corn, sorghum, sugar cane and barley was studied by Lamoureux et al. (1971). Metabolism was rapid and similar in all mentioned plant species during the first 6-24 h following treatment. At least 3 water-soluble metabolites were produced in each species during this period. Two of these metabolites were isolated; the first one was identified as the glutathione conjugate of propachlor (compound I) and the second one appeared to be the gamma-glutamylcysteine conjugate (compound II). The primary mode of metabolism is a nucleophilic displacement of the alpha-chloro group of propachlor by the sulfhydryl group of a peptide. The metabolic reactions of propachlor proceed non-enzymatically *in vitro*, and the *in vivo* reaction may be enzymatic and/or non-enzymatic. The high percentage of propachlor converted to compounds I and II in corn seedlings during the first 18 h following treatment indicates that the reaction of propachlor with glutathione and/or gamma-glutamylcysteine is quite specific. This would be expected if the reaction is enzymatic. Some glutathione and gamma-glutamylcysteine conjugates in plants may be end-products, but, in the case of propachlor, these metabolites are transient intermediates. Further studies are needed to establish the final steps (Lamoureux et al., 1971).

Pantano & Anderson (1987) studied the metabolism of propachlor in sorghum (milo). Sorghum seeds were planted in soil treated with ^{14}C ring-labelled propachlor at a rate of 3.3 kg/ha and grown to maturity in a greenhouse. Following senescence, plants were separated into various anatomical parts, freeze-dried and analysed for activity. The uptake of ^{14}C in the foliage and grain was 9.5 and 0.5 mg/kg dry weight, respectively. Four metabolites were identified in the foliage extract; these represented 66.5% of the metabolites in foliage. The four metabolites were [(*N*-isopropyl) phenylamino]oxoacetic acid, {{[(*N*-isopropyl)-phenylamino]acetyl}sulfinyl}lactic acid, {{[(*N*-isopropyl)phenylamino] acetyl}sulfinyl}acetic acid and 2-[(*N*-isopropyl)phenylamino]-2-oxoethanesulfonic acid. In addition, other metabolites found at low levels in the foliage extract were characterized. Freeze-dried sorghum grain contained only 0.5 mg/kg of ^{14}C activity and only one metabolite was identified (the first compound mentioned above). This metabolite constituted at least 24.9% of the activity in grain. In all of the major metabolites identified in this study, no modification of the *N*-isopropylaniline moiety was observed. On the basis of metabolites identified in this study and known pathways for the metabolic transformations of related chloroacetamides, a scheme for the metabolic fate of propachlor in sorghum plants was postulated by the authors. The biotransformations include: 1) displacement of the chlorine by an oxygen-containing nucleophile followed by oxidation, and 2) conjugation with glutathione followed by further metabolic modification of this conjugate.

Lamoureux & Rusness (1989) studied the metabolism of propachlor in soybean and found that it was rapidly metabolized to homoglutathione conjugate in roots and foliage. This conjugate was rapidly metabolized to the cysteine conjugate and then slowly converted to a variety of other metabolites; four of these were present up to 72 days after application of propachlor. These four were malonylcysteine, malonylcysteine *S*-oxide, 3-sulfinyllactic acid and *O*-malonyl glucoside conjugates of propachlor. Less than 1% of metabolites was isolated from beans or pods, the great majority being in roots and foliage. The major metabolites found in plants were the same as those produced in soil. The authors suggested that it is difficult to differentiate between metabolites formed in the plant and those taken up from soil as to the relative importance of the two sites of metabolic degradation.

4.2 Bioaccumulation and biomagnification

The two published values for the log octanol/water partition coefficient (log K_{ow}) of propachlor, i.e. 1.62 and 2.3 (US EPA, 1984b, 1988), indicate a moderate potential for bioaccumulation.

Barrows & Macek (1974) used bluegill sunfish exposed to ^{14}C-labelled propachlor in a continuous-flow experiment in order to assess the potential for the compound to bioconcentrate in aquatic organisms. The fish were exposed for 35 days to a mean ^{14}C-propachlor concentration of either 0.54 mg/litre (high level) or 0.012 mg/litre (low level) in the water. Analysis of the fish tissues indicated bioconcentration factors (BCFs) in the edible tissue of 34 and 22 for the high and low levels, respectively, and in the non-edible tissue of 22 and 20. When the fish were placed in clean water the activity was rapidly eliminated from the non-edible portion of the fish and at a somewhat slower rate from the edible tissue. Because of the polar, water-soluble nature of the soil metabolites (section 4.1.1), they would be less likely to bioconcentrate in aquatic organisms. The results of a static study on catfish by Malik (1982) showed that BCFs for both edible and non-edible tissues were 0.23 and that the low level of accumulated activity was eliminated rapidly when the fish were placed in clean water.

Yu et al. (1975) studied ^{14}C-propachlor in a model ecosystem containing seven species. There was no indication of either bioconcentration or biomagnification; total radioactivity declined from 0.21 to 0.015 mg propachlor/kg through the seven stages of the food chain.

5. ENVIRONMENTAL LEVELS AND HUMAN EXPOSURE

5.1 Environmental levels

The application of propachlor as a herbicide in plant protection results in its presence in air, soil and water. It is taken up from the soil into plants through the root system.

5.1.1 Air

Propachlor application resulted in its presence in the ambient air 300 m away from the treated field at concentrations ranging from 0.02-0.6 mg/m^3 (Panshina, 1976). No details on the analytical method or quantity of propachlor sprayed were given in this report.

5.1.2 Water

Propachlor was found in 34 of 1690 surface water samples analysed in the USA (US EPA, 1988). Samples of surface water were collected at 475 locations and groundwater samples at 94 locations. The compound was detected in eight different states. The maximum concentration found was 10 μg/litre in surface water and 0.12 μg/litre in groundwater (the 85th percentile for all non-zero samples was 2 μg/litre in surface water and 0.12 μg/litre in ground water). Spalding & Snow (1989) detected propachlor at a maximum concentration of 46 μg/litre in stream water receiving its flow from agricultural land planted principally with corn. The monitoring was carried out during a spring period of high water flow and run-off.

5.1.3 Food

The residues of propachlor in potato tubers and tomatoes were lower than 0.005 mg/kg (the limit of detection) approximately 60-70 days after application of the recommended dose of 4-6 kg/ha (Balinova, 1981). Warholic et al. (1983) could not detect propachlor (detection limit, 0.06 mg/kg fresh weight) in cabbages grown on soil treated with propachlor at 0.6 kg a.i./ha (wettable powder).

Frank et al. (1977) reported the results of a study on the fate of propachlor applied to onions. Planted in May, the onions were harvested in September and analysed in January the following year. Conjugated *N*-isopropylaniline was present in onion tissue after harvest and after a normal storage period for the crop before sale. Bearing in mind the reports of other authors (Lamoureux et al., 1971), Frank et al. (1977) suggested that 2-chloro-*N*-isopropylacetanilide could be hydrolysed to 2-hydroxy-*N*-isopropylacetanilide and bonded to glutathione. It is probable that alkaline hydrolysis cleaved the weaker N-carbonyl C linkage to given *N*-isopropylaniline rather than the stronger C-S bond which would have resulted in 2-hydroxy-*N*-isopropylaniline. Tissue residues of *N*-isopropylaniline increased as the rate of application of propachlor was increased, and the later the application was made the higher the tissue residues (see Table 7).

Table 7. Residues of conjugated *N*-isopropylaniline[a]

Year	Time of application	Rate of propachlor application (kg/ha)	*N*-isopropylaniline residues (mg/kg)
1974	untreated	0	0.03
	pre-emergence	7.2	0.05
		12.0	0.09
	pre-emergence and early post-emergence (21 May and 13 June, respectively)	7.2 + 7.2	0.17
		12.0 + 12.0	0.15
	pre-emergence and late post-emergence (21 May and 9 July, respectively)	7.2 + 7.2	0.28
		12.0 + 12	0.40

[a] From: Frank et al. (1977). Onions were planted 6 May 1974 and harvested 4 September 1974. Analyses were performed in January 1975.

Propachlor has been used for soil treatment (6 kg/ha) before planting tomatoes and peppers. Sampling was performed at 15-day intervals and the samples were analysed by gas chromatography (detection limits, 0.005 mg/kg). Small quantities of propachlor (of the order of 0.04 mg/kg) were found in tomatoes on the 70th and 85th days after soil treatment. On the 73rd day, 0.07 mg/kg was found in peppers, and on the 88th and 108th days the residues had decreased to 0.05 and 0.04 mg/kg, respectively. No herbicide residues were found in the following years (Balinova & Konstantinov, 1975).

In a study where soil was treated (8 kg/ha) before the seedlings were planted, samples of cabbages contained propachlor residues 0.6-0.8, 0.3-0.4 and 0.1-0.16 mg/kg after one, two and three months, respectively (Medved, 1977). No residues were detected in cabbages 96 days after the application of propachlor, at harvesting (Kolesnikov et al., 1979). A decrease in dose and application by conveyor belt perceptibly reduced the residues (Table 8).

Table 8. Residues (mg/kg) of propachlor in cabbages (type Amager 611)

Propachlor application rate	Date of application	Sampling time (no. of days after application)			
		13	33	64	96
8 kg/ha (before setting out)	31 May	0.6	0.3	0.1	No
8 kg/ha (after prior application of 5 kg/ha)	31 May	0.8	0.4	0.16	No
4 kg/ha (conveyor-belt application after setting out)	7 June	0.4	0.2	0.03	No

In a study by Nesterova et al. (1980), a dry soil area planted with cabbages was treated with propachlor (7 kg/ha) each year. In the second year no residues were detectable two months after application. In the third year, when the moisture content of the soil had increased, propachlor degradation was more rapid and no residues were detectable 15 days after the application. The soil was dry in the fourth year, and residues were detectable in cabbages up to two months after application.

Lottman & Cowell (1986) reported propachlor residues in sorghum grains of between < 0.02 and 0.24 mg/kg after treatment of soil at 4.4 kg/ha. Lottman & Cowell (1987) found residues in corn grain of < 0.02 to 0.04 mg/kg after soil treatment with propachlor at 4.4 kg/ha and of < 0.02 to 0.19 mg/kg after treatment at 6.6 kg/ha.

5.2 Occupational exposure

Only limited data are available on occupational exposure to propachlor. Its application by a tractor-mounted sprayer to cabbages resulted in its presence in the breathing zone of the tractor drivers at levels of 0.8 to 2.1 mg/m^3 (Panshina, 1977) and 0.1 to 3.7 mg/m^3 (Panshina, 1976).

6. KINETICS AND METABOLISM

6.1 Absorption

Propachlor may be absorbed through the respiratory and gastrointestinal tracts as well as through the skin. Following a single oral administration in mammals, it is rapidly taken up into the blood and internal organs, reaching its maximum blood concentration in 1 h. After 48 h it is no longer detectable in the organs (Panshina, 1985). An estimated 68% of a single 10 mg dose of ring-labelled ^{14}C-propachlor administered to 12 rats was recovered in urine 56 h later (Malik, 1986). These results are supported by those of other studies in which 54-64% (Lamoureux & Davison, 1975) and 68.8% (Bakke et al., 1980) of the administered dose was recovered in urine 24 h and 48 h after dose administration, respectively.

6.2 Metabolic transformation

Propachlor is rapidly metabolized. Its metabolism in animal species has been studied by Bakke & Price (1979), Pekas et al. (1979), Bakke et al. (1981a,b,c), Rafter et al. (1983a,b), Aschbacher & Struble (1987) and Davison et al. (1988, 1990). Most of the animal species studied metabolize propachlor through the mercapturic acid pathway (MAP). The intestinal microflora is involved in the metabolism of MAP intermediates (Bakke et al., 1981c). Metabolites of propachlor, in which chlorine from the parent compound (2-chloro-isopropylacetanilide) is removed by a nucleophilic displacement (Rafter et al., 1983a) by a cysteine group or methylsulfonyl group (CH_3SO_2), are present in the urine of rats dosed orally with propachlor (Larsen & Bakke, 1979). It has been shown that a cysteine conjugate of propachlor is the source of sulfur in methylsulfonyl-containing metabolites, but that the carbon in the methylsulfonyl group does not come from the cysteine moiety. Propachlor is conjugated firstly with glutathione and the reaction is mediated by glutathione transferases. The glutathione conjugation provides a means for inactivation of reactive electrophiles. Glutathione conjugates have the required physico-chemical properties for biliary excretion and will generally be present, together with their catabolites cysteinyl-glycine, cysteine and *N*-acetylcysteine-mercapturic acid, in relatively high concentrations in the bile (Rafter et al., 1983a). After excretion with the bile, they are metabolized in the intestine where the C-S lyase present cleaves the cysteine conjugate, allowing further metabolism of sulfur to a methylsulfonyl-containing moiety (Larsen & Bakke, 1979).

The C-S lyase enzyme systems have been isolated in rat liver and bacteria demonstrating that they are of bacterial origin. As a good example, C-S lyase from *Fusobacterium necrophorum*, one of the pure intestinal bacteria, has been isolated and characterized as a key enzyme in mammalian metabolism (Larsen et al., 1983). This is confirmed by the fact that in germ-free rats (Bakke et al., 1980) (Fig. 2) and rats treated by antibiotics (Larsen & Bakke, 1981) ^{14}C was excreted from ^{14}C-propachlor as MAP metabolites, but there were no methylsulfonyl-containing metabolites in urine. Inextractable residues were eliminated in the faeces. This shows that MAP metabolites are available as substrates for the intestinal microflora. Of the MAP metabolites studied, the glutathione and cysteine conjugates are the best substrates both for production of 2-mercapto-*N*-isopropyl-acetanilide and for parallel formation of insoluble ^{14}C residues (Larsen & Bakke, 1983) which are excreted in the faeces.

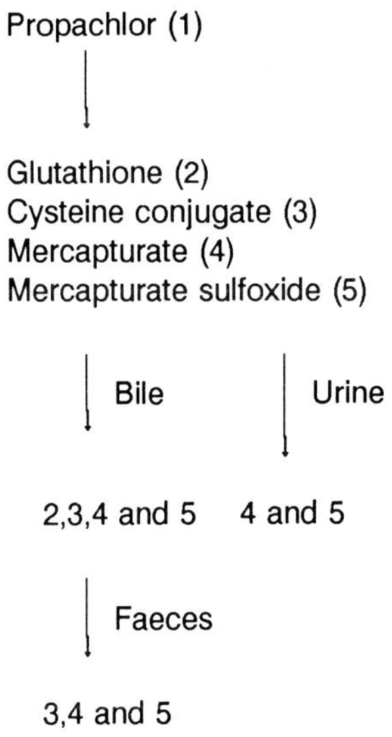

Fig. 2. Summary of the metabolism of propachlor in germ-free rats.
From: Bakke et al. (1980).

In normal rats dosed with propachlor, the above-mentioned final metabolites were formed when MAP metabolites underwent a number of reactions: carbon-sulfur bond cleavage by microflora, S-methylation, S-oxidation, ring and alkyl-hydroxylation, glucuronide conjugation, N-dealkylation and amide cleavage (Rafter et al., 1983b).

Fig. 3 shows the proposed metabolic pathway for the formation of methylsulfonyl metabolites in rats and pigs (Aschbacher & Struble, 1987) and Fig. 4 the metabolism in normal rats treated with propachlor proposed by Bakke et al. (1980).

The tissue in which propachlor enters the mercapturic acid pathway has not been determined. The liver is an obvious site for glutathione conjugation, but the intestine cannot be excluded (Bakke et al., 1980). Organ perfusion studies have demonstrated that all enzymes necessary for the formation of mercapturic acid conjugates are present in the kidneys of both chickens and rats (Davison et al., 1988, 1990) and in the livers of rats (Davison et al., 1990). Rat caecal contents are similar to those of the pig with respect to C-S lyase activity, which explains the general similarity of their metabolic transformations (Larsen & Bakke, 1983).

When pig caecal contents were incubated with the glutathione conjugate of propachlor, the formation of both insoluble residues and the thiol increased with increase in incubation period (Table 9). Digestive peptidases extracted during isolation of the metabolites were thought to be the explanation for the presence of the cysteine conjugate in the zero time samples, because no cysteine conjugate was isolated from heat-treated caecal contents. A decrease in glutathione concentration with increased incubation time was also evident and was confirmation of a product-precursor relationship. This decrease in glutathione conjugate concentration was assumed to be caused by formation of cysteine conjugate (82%), due to cleavage by peptidase activity, in the caecum (Larsen & Bakke, 1983).

In summary, three or more enterohepatic cycles for propachlor metabolism in normal rats have been described. In the first, propachlor is metabolized via the mercapturic acid pathway and the conjugates are excreted in the bile. The second cycle is initiated when the biliary mercapturic acid pathway metabolites are metabolized by microbial/intestinal C-S lyase into reabsorbable metabolites (possibly 2-mercapto-*N*-isopropylacetanilide). The reabsorbable metabolites are further metabolized to

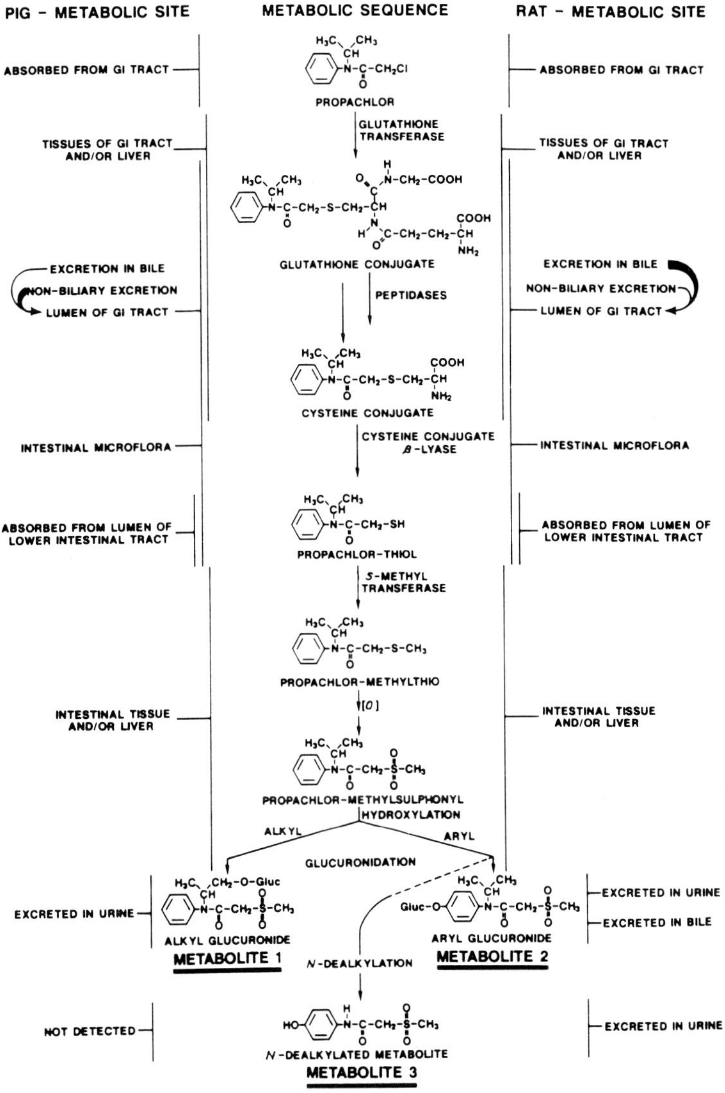

Fig. 3. Proposed metabolic sequence in the formation of methylsulfonyl metabolites by rats and swine.
From: Aschbacher & Struble (1987)

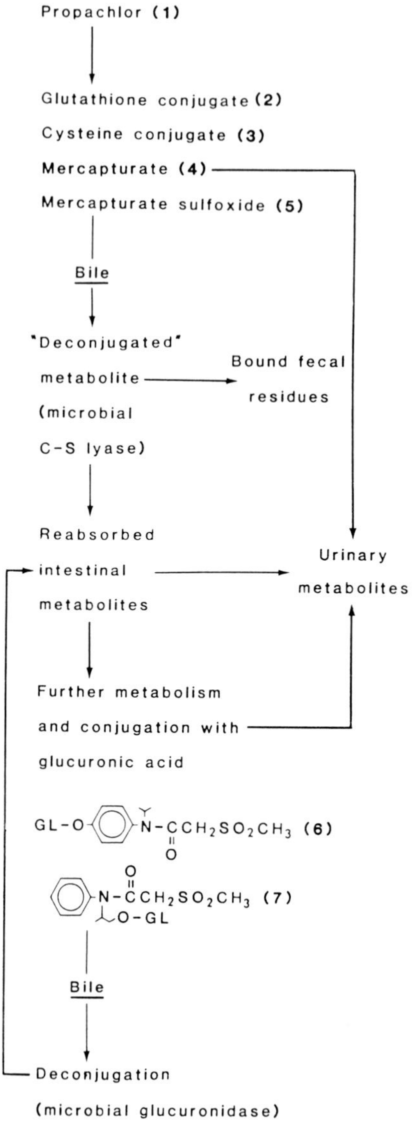

Fig. 4. A diagrammatic representation of the metabolism of propachlor in normal rats treated with propachlor.
Metabolites 6 and 7 are glucuronides.
From: Bakke et al. (1980)

Table 9. Incubation of the glutathione conjugate of propachlor with pig caecal contents for various durations[a]

Metabolites recovered	Incubation time					
	0	20 min	40 min	1 h	2 h	4 h
2-Mercapto-*N*-isopropyl-acetanilide	7.7[b] (5.1-10.6)	14.5[b] (5.5-22.8)	23.0[b] (15.8-36.0)	28.3[b] (22.9-38.7)	34.7[b] (21.8-44.0)	43.4[c] (38.7-49.2)
Glutathione conjugate of propachlor	26.8 (15.8-38.1)	36.0 (18.1-51.6)	20.8 (13.3-25.3)	28.8 (16.6-42.3)	21.5 (14.0-32.2)	16.5 (14.8-19.2)
Cysteine conjugate of propachlor	47.5 (36.0-51.5)	32.5 (21.3-43.7)	35.1 (30.5-41.9)	20.9 (12.0-27.9)	11.9 (10.9-12.5)	3.8 (2.2-5.6)
Non-extractable ^{14}C residues	13.1 (13.0-13.4)	12.9 (9.9-17.8)	16.0 (13.5-20.5)	16.6 (15.0-18.9)	25.4 (22.8-28.2)	33.9 (31.5-35.8)

[a] From: Larsen & Bakke (1983).
[b] Isolated as 2-carboxymethylthio-*N*-isopropylacetanilide
[c] Isolated as 2-(^{13}C)-carboxymethylthio-*N*-isopropylacetanilide
Pigs were gilts. Results are shown as a percentage of the substrate. Values given in parentheses represent the range of values obtained from ^{14}C-recovery measurements.

glucuronides by glucuronidase enzymes, and these are secreted with the bile. These biliary glucuronides subsequently initiate the third cycle in the enterohepatic circulation of propachlor metabolites.

No doubt the intestinal microorganisms complicate the metabolism of propachlor (in comparison with the situation in germ-free and antibiotic-treated rats) and create new non-polar compounds from the products of the mercapturic acid pathway, which are reabsorbed into the blood. These new compounds have to be converted again into polar products in order to be excreted (Bakke et al., 1980).

More recent studies carried out by Aschbacher & Struble (1987) on the metabolism of propachlor in pigs have proved the similarity, i.e. the formation of methylsulfonyl-containing metabolites, with the metabolism of rats, but have also revealed some differences.

A pig with a cannulated bile duct, which was dosed orally with ^{14}C-propachlor, excreted 7.6% of the dose in the bile compared with approximately 75% in the case of the rats. When enterohepatic circulation was prevented in the bile of cannulated pigs, CH_3SO_2-containing metabolites of propachlor were excreted in the urine. As mentioned above, enterohepatic circulation is necessary for the production of methylsulfonyl-containing metabolites in rats. In experiments with germ-free pigs dosed orally with ^{14}C-propachlor, it was shown that they did not excrete urinary CH_3SO_2 metabolites, which indicated involvement of the intestinal flora in the production of these metabolites, as occurs in rats. Non-biliary excretion of metabolites of propachlor into the lumen of the intestine probably occurred. It is presumed that propachlor is absorbed by the mucosal cells and conjugated with glutathione and that some of this conjugate moves directly into the lumen of the intestinal tract by simple diffusion, where it becomes the substrate of bacterial beta-lyase. The presence of glutathione transferase has been demonstrated previously in subcellular fractions of mucosal tissue homogenates.

In situ intestinal absorption of propachlor and non-biliary excretion of metabolites into the intestinal tract of rats, pigs and chickens was studied by Struble (1991). Propachlor was absorbed from *in situ* intestinal loops of rats and pigs, the absorption half-times being 7.5 and 16.5 min, respectively. Water-soluble ^{14}C-labelled metabolites that accumulated in the intestinal loops accounted for 31%, 53% and 25% of the initial ^{14}C in rats, pigs and chickens, respectively. Propachlor-S-cysteine was identified as the major metabolite in the pig intestinal lumen (43% of the water-soluble ^{14}C). It was concluded that the intestinal metabolism and intestinal excretion of water-soluble metabolites of propachlor are important physiological processes that occur in a variety of animal species. These processes provide a route by which metabolites of xenobiotics may reach the intestinal lumen in animals that are poor biliary excretors. These studies demonstrated that although bile may be the major route by which MAP metabolites are made available to the intestinal microflora in the rat, an extrahepatic route exists in the pig.

Davison (1991) conducted a study using six anaesthetized 2- to 21-day-old male Guernsey calves weighing 28 to 61 kg in which either the left kidney was perfused (via the left renal artery) or the left ureter was perfused with metabolites of propachlor. The glutathione conjugate of propachlor (2-*S*-glutathionyl-*N*-acetyl-acetanilide) was metabolized in both kidney and ureter to the cysteine conjugate. When the mercapturic acid conjugate of propachlor was presented to the kidney, it was eliminated in urine. First-pass metabolism and elimination of the glutathione conjugate by the kidney was 16% of the dose, whereas first-pass elimination of the mercapturic acid was 33%. Absorption of the glutathione conjugate of propachlor or its metabolites, or of glycine by the ureter was nil. The cattle may be unable to form mercapturic acids from glutathione conjugates of some xenobiotics, which may result in their being more easily poisoned by these xenobiotics than chickens, pigs and rats.

The glutathione conjugate of 2-chloro-*N*-isopropyl[1-^{14}C]acet-anilide (^{14}C-propachlor) was perfused through a calf kidney *in situ* by Bakke et al. (1990). Twenty-three per cent of the dose was excreted in the perfused kidney urine as the cysteine conjugate; no mercapturic acid was detected. A 5-day-old calf dosed orally with ^{14}C-propachlor excreted 70% of the dose in the urine as the cysteine conjugate; again no mercapturic acid was detected. Rumen microflora were established in the calf when it was 5 weeks older and the experiment was repeated. The same results were obtained.

6.3 Elimination and excretion

When ^{14}C-propachlor was given to rats, 56-64% of the dose was excreted in urine in the first 24 h and 5.7-7.0% in 24-48 h. In the faeces, 8-13% and 2.2-7.7% were eliminated in 0-24 h and 24-48 h, respectively; 0.4% of the ^{14}C was eliminated as CO_2 and 5-11% was in the carcass. In total 80-97% was eliminated in 48 h (Lamoureux & Davison, 1975).

According to Bakke et al. (1980), the metabolites of propachlor formed in normal rats treated with propachlor are excreted mainly through urine (68%) and faeces (19%). Eleven urinary metabolites were isolated from rats given ^{14}C-labelled propachlor orally. The major metabolite was the mercapturate (17%), and six of the metabolites were 2-methylsulfonylacetanilides. Faecal residues (19%) of the administered dose, insoluble in common solvents or by treatment with diluted acid or base, were also determined.

Rats with cannulated bile ducts secreted 66% of an oral dose of propachlor in the bile as the glutathione conjugate (2), cysteine conjugate (3), mercapturate (4) and the mercapturate sulfoxide (5) (see Table 10). Germ-free rats given orally ^{14}C-labelled propachlor excreted 98% of the dose in the urine and faeces within 48 h. Three metabolites were isolated from the excreta and the faecal radioactive metabolites were water soluble. The major metabolite was mercapturate (4) and the other metabolites were the cysteine conjugate (3) (present only in the faeces) and mercapturate sulfoxide (5) (Bakke et al., 1980). Mercapturate sulfoxide was isolated from the excreta of germ-free rats by Feil et al. (1981), who also demonstrated its presence in the bile of rats and urine of chickens and pigs dosed with propachlor. The metabolite was characterized by mass and nuclear magnetic resonance spectrometry on samples isolated from rats.

As in the case of the glutathione and cysteine conjugates, the sulfoxide is not excreted at detectable levels by normal rats and was detected only in the bile (Bakke et al., 1981a). It may become a substrate for the intestinal flora, but the ultimate *in vivo* fate of this metabolite is unknown.

Bakke et al. (1981c) reported differences between some species concerning the metabolism of propachlor in the MAP. Clear but unexplained differences are that rats excrete no cysteine conjugate and chickens form no methylsulfonyl-containing metabolites, whereas sheep excrete large amounts of cysteine conjugate in urine.

Nadeau & Pantano (1986) carried out a study to determine the rates and routes of excretion of orally administered synthetic

Table 10. Comparison of the excretion of single oral doses of ^{14}C-propachlor by control rats with fistulated bile ducts, and germ-free rats[a]

Metabolite	Recovery of ^{14}C (% dose)[b]				
	Control rats		Bile-fistulated rats	Germ-free rats	
	Urine	Faeces	Bile	Urine	Faeces
Glutathione conjugate (2)[b]			37		
Cysteine conjugate (3)			13		19
Mercapturate (4)	17		12	63.1	3.7
Mercapturate sulfoxide (5)			4	5.7	5.4
Non-extractable residues		19			
Other metabolites	51				
Total	68	19	66	68.8	32.1

[a] From: Bakke et al. (1980)

[b] Metabolite designations are those used in Figs. 1 and 3.

^{14}C-labelled propachlor plant metabolites in lactating goats and to quantify and identify the radioactive metabolites in the goat milk, tissues, urine and faeces. The daily dose level for the three treated goats was 15 mg/kg administered on 5 consecutive days (the actual dose levels for the treated goats were 13, 14.5 and 13 mg/kg, respectively). Each treated goat received a total of 130.5 mg of the $^{13}C/^{14}C$-labelled propachlor plant metabolites mixture during the dosing period. A control animal received placebo capsules. The radioactivity eliminated in faeces accounted for 72.1, 64.5 and 57.9% of the administered dose, respectively (average 64.8%), and that excreted in urine accounted for 35.8, 28.1 and 32.3% (average 32.1%). The percentage of the dose eliminated through faeces and urine averaged 96.9%.

The radioactivity found in the milk accounted for only 0.084, 0.10 and 0.13% (average 0.10%) of the administered dose. These values corresponded to metabolite concentrations in the milk of 11.9, 14.8 and 18.0 μg/litre (average 14.9 μg/litre). The metabolic concentrations (μg/kg) in the tissues were: kidney 51.9, liver 30.4, muscle 8.5, fat 19.5 and blood 50.1. The loss of radioactivity from tissues, milk and excrement occurred rapidly, and after 5 days of depuration the milk and tissue radioactivity levels were below the limit of detection, except in the case of the liver (5.7 μg/kg).

6.4 Metabolism in laying hens

Since crops treated with propachlor are used in animal feed, it is important to know the fate of propachlor in animal feed.

The purpose of the study by Bleeke et al. (1987) was to examine the metabolic fate of propachlor plant metabolites in laying hens and to determine whether they accumulate or persist in the eggs or edible tissues. The compounds used for feeding were the three major metabolites of propachlor found in sorghum, i.e. [(*N*-isopropyl)-phenylamino] oxacetic acid, sodium salt (I), {{[(*N*-isopropyl)-phenylamino]acetyl}sulfinyl} lactic acid, sodium salt (II) and 2-[(*N*-isopropyl)-phenylamino] 2-oxoethane sulfonic acid, sodium salt (III).

The first study involved dosing chickens at a level of 5 mg/kg diet for 6 consecutive days. Data for bioaccumulation and excretion of plant metabolites were obtained from this study. A second group of chickens, dosed at a level of 25 mg/kg diet (nominal dose) on 6 consecutive days, provided eggs and tissues with higher residues for metabolic characterization. Each group consists of five hens. Control groups received a single gelatine capsule per day. The total recovery of ^{14}C radioactivity was good in both studies.

An average of 87.4% of the total administered dose was recovered from the chickens fed 5 mg/kg approximately 1 day after the last dose, and 97.9% was recovered from the chickens fed 25 mg/kg, primarily in the excreta. The eggs contained low residue levels; those from chickens fed 5 mg/kg contained residues below the minimum quantifiable limit (MQL) of 1.7 μg/kg. The level in the egg yolks reached an average of 5.5 μg/kg by day 6 but by day 12 the residues in the yolk had fallen below 1.6 μg/kg.

In the high-dose group, the residues in the egg white levelled off at about 4 μg/kg on day 2, while those in the egg yolk increased to a level of 27.3 μg/kg on day 6.

Tissues also contained low levels of residues. In the low-dose group, the highest levels were found in the kidney and they averaged only 6 μg/kg. The residue levels in the liver measured an average of 1.9 μg/kg and those in the fat 3.5 μg/kg. The residues in other fat samples and organs were below the MQL (1.4-1.6 μg/kg). Residues in the breast muscle were below the minimum detectable limit (7 μg/kg) and those in the blood were 6-7 μg/kg.

7. EFFECTS ON LABORATORY MAMMALS AND *IN VITRO* TEST SYSTEMS

7.1 Single exposure

7.1.1 Oral

The acute oral toxicity of propachlor for the rat, mouse and the rabbit has been examined. According to the WHO hazard classification of pesticides and as far as its acute oral toxicity to rats is concerned, propachlor is slightly hazardous (Group III) (WHO, 1990). LD_{50} values in various animal species reveal a higher susceptibility for the mouse and the rabbit than for the rat (Table 11). The LD_{50} for rats ranges from 950 to 2176 mg/kg.

The clinical picture of acute oral intoxication by propachlor has been described in three species of experimental animals: mice, rabbits and rats (Panshina, 1973). When propachlor is given at lethal or toxic doses, the main symptoms concern the central nervous system. In mice and rabbits, a state of excitement, trembling and light convulsions is observed 15 min after a toxic or lethal dose of propachlor. This gradually increases, breathing becomes difficult and death follows in several hours. Intoxication in rats takes a different course: a state of immobility and head and body tremors are accompanied by the sudden onset of convulsions and death occurs within 24 h. This clinical picture was confirmed by Strateva (1974,a,b).

Kronenberg (1988) reported clear signs of irritation to the gastrointestinal tract and lungs that were evident at necropsy in animals that died during the study. Histoenzymological changes expressed as decreased enzyme activity were in full agreement with the morphological picture (Strateva et al., 1974a,b).

7.1.2 Dermal

Results of studies in rabbits on the acute dermal toxicity of propachlor and its formulations indicate that the dermal LD_{50} ranges from 4000 mg/kg for a 65% WP formulation (Auletta & Rinehart, 1979) to 20 000 mg/kg for technical propachlor (94.5%) (Braun & Rinehart, 1978). Test animals exhibited moderate to severe erythema, severe oedema and necrotic skin at the dermal application sites at a dose level of 2800 mg/kg. Motor activity decrease and ataxia were noted at dose levels of 2000 to 5600 mg/kg.

Table 11. Oral LD_{50} values for laboratory mammals

Species	LD_{50} (mg/kg)[a]	Reference
Rat	1056 (834-1278)	Panshina (1973, 1977)
	950 (860-1050)	Strateva (1974b)
	1340	Mirkova (1975)
	2176 ± 220	Lehotzky et al. (1979)
Rat (Sprague-Dawley)	840 (419-1261) (in corn oil)	Blaszcak (1988)
	1700 (1265-2135) (in 1% methylcellulose)	Blaszcak (1988)
Rat (Fischer-344)	550 (252-848) in corn oil	Blaszcak (1988)
	1359 (1009-1691) (in 1% methylcellulose)	Blaszcak (1988)
Rat (both sexes)	4000	Heenehan et al. (1979)
Rat (both sexes)	3269	Branch et al. (1982a)
Mouse	306 (275-337)	Panshina (1973, 1977)
	290 (240-350)	Strateva (1974b)

[a] The concentration is based on the percentage active ingredient. Figures in parentheses indicate the range of values.

Using groups of 16 Wistar rats, Baynova et al. (1977) studied the acute dermal toxicity of a single application of propachlor 65 WP (10-20% in aqueous suspension) with doses of 1500-4000 mg/kg body weight (active ingredient). There was no mortality, and no signs of intoxication were observed. No haematological or biochemical tests were performed.

Propachlor and Satecid 65 WP caused severe dermatitis, ulceration and necrosis in the skin of rabbit and ears of mice. None of the compounds exhibited contact sensitization effects on guinea-pigs (Lehotzky et al., 1979).

7.1.3 Inhalation

In a study by Bechtel (1991), technical propachlor (96.8%) was dissolved in dimethylsulfoxide (DMSO) to generate an aerosol and administered to five male and five female Sprague-Dawley rats in a nose-only chamber at an analytically determined concentration of 1.2 mg/litre for 4 h. Control rats (five of each sex) were exposed to an atmosphere of aerosolized DMSO for the same duration. Particle size measurements on the propachlor/DMSO aerosol indicated a mass median aerodynamic diameter of 3.5 μm, with 96% of the particles being less than 10 μm and 1.8% less than 1 μm in diameter (Bechtel, 1991). No treatment-related deaths occurred. Clinical signs included laboured respiration and nasal discharge; all animals appeared normal by post-exposure day 2. A transient weight loss was noted in both treated and control animals during the first two days of the study, but normal body weight was observed thereafter. No abnormalities were apparent during postmortem examination of the animals.

In another acute inhalation study, three groups of Charles River CD rats (five rats of each sex per group) were exposed to test atmospheres of a propachlor formulation (44% active ingredient) for 4 h (Kaempfe, 1991). During the exposure period, animals were housed in a 250-litre New York University style stainless steel chamber, and were exposed to analytically confirmed concentrations of 0.18, 0.67 and 1.0 mg propachlor/litre in the breathing zone of the chamber. At least 82% of the particles were less than 10 μm in diameter. No animals died at the two lower exposure levels, whereas four out of ten rats died at 1.0 mg/litre. Clinical observations during the post-exposure period included ocular opacities, perinasal encrustation, rapid or shallow respiration, perioral wetness and focal loss of hair from animals in the highest exposure group. Fourteen days after exposure, all surviving animals had body weights higher than the pre-exposure (day 0) values with the exception of females in the 1.0-mg/litre group, which exhibited body weight depression. There were no abnormal findings in rats that died during the test or were sacrificed at 14 days. Based on the mortality observed, the LC_{50} was slightly greater than 1.0 mg/litre.

7.2 Short-term exposure

7.2.1 Oral

7.2.1.1 Dogs

To assess potential subchronic toxicity, propachlor (96.1% pure) was administered via the diet to five groups of two male and two female beagle dogs for 4 weeks (Daly & Knezevich, 1984). Dietary concentrations of propachlor were 0, 100, 500, 1000 and 1500 mg/kg (equivalent to 0, 2.5, 12.5, 25, and 37.5 mg/kg body weight per day). No mortality or clinical signs of toxicity related to treatment occurred during this study. Food consumption was initially decreased, but only in the females treated with 1000 and 1500 mg/kg (equal to 25 and 37.5 mg/kg body weight) and the males treated with 1000 mg/kg. The consumption had returned to normal by the end of the study. Body weight varied markedly. The decreased body weight and/or weight gain noted in males fed 12.5 or 25 mg/kg body weight per day, and females fed 37.5 mg/kg per day could have been treatment related. Haematological examination showed slightly increased platelet counts in high-dose males. No treatment-related gross pathological effects were noted at sacrifice.

Following the 4-week pilot feeding study in beagle dogs, a 90-day feeding study was undertaken (Naylor & Ruecker, 1986). Propachlor (96.1% purity) was administered in the diet to groups of six dogs of each sex per group for 90 days. Nominal dietary concentrations were 0, 100, 500 and 1500 mg/kg. There was no mortality or clinicopathological or histopathological changes related to the treatment. The dose level of 1500 mg/kg (45 mg/kg body weight) was a no-observed-adverse-effect level (NOAEL).

7.2.1.2 Rodents

Propachlor (65% WP) was given orally by gavage to white rats at daily doses of 21, 53 and 106 mg/kg body weight for 4 months, and its cumulative effect was studied by Panshina (1973). Later, Strateva (1974a, 1976) carried out a short-term study (45 days) at dose levels of 50, 100 and 200 mg/kg body weight given orally by gavage to 104 Wistar rats (divided into four groups (three experimental and one control) with equal numbers of both sexes), and a long-term oral study (6 months) at dose levels of 0.05, 0.5, 5 and 20 mg/kg body weight given to 220 Wistar rats divided into five groups (four experimental and one control).

Strateva (1976) found a decrease in haemoglobin content and number of erythrocytes, slight leucocytosis and an increased number of neutrophils. The threshold dose for rats in long-term studies was 5 mg/kg body weight.

Panshina (1976) carried out a 10-month study on white rats given propachlor by gavage at doses of 1, 3.5 and 10.6 mg/kg body weight. Slight leucocytosis was found within 4-7 months. The first two doses provoked a decreased activity of catalase and peroxidase as well as an increase in nicotinamide adenine dinucleotide in brain and heart tissue homogenates. No changes in haemoglobin content or number of erythrocytes were noted. There were no alterations to the pathomorphological picture.

Baynova et al. (1978a) compared the effects of continuous and intermittent oral dosing of propachlor (65% WP) on white rats (equal numbers of both sexes). The number of animals per group was not given. The scheme of the experimental design is given in Table 12.

Table 12. Experimental design of the study by Baynova et al. (1978a)

Group	Duration of study	Daily dose (mg/kg)	Dose (fraction of the LD_{50})
Control	4 months	-	-
I (dosing every week)	4 months	70	1/20
II (dosing every second week)	4 months	140	1/10
III (dosing every second week)	8 months	70	1/20
Control	8 months	-	-

Continuous administration of propachlor led to more marked changes in the main parenchymous organs than intermittent administration. These changes were characterized by decreased activity of oxido-reductive tissue enzymes. The hexabarbital sleeping time, which characterized the detoxification function of the liver, showed a statistically significant reduction. Propachlor administration at 120 mg/kg body weight for 6 consecutive days to male and female rats increased the levels of both cytochrome and microsomal protein content (Nenov & Baynova, 1978) as a result of the induction of mixed-function oxidase in the liver (Baynova et al., 1978a).

A special study on the morphological changes in kidneys was carried out. Propachlor (65% WP) was administered by gavage to male white rats (10 animals per group and 1 control) at doses equivalent to 6, 12 and 60 mg/kg body weight for 3 months (Maleva & Zlateva, 1982). Dose-dependent morphological changes were found in the proximal convoluted renal tubules. The tubules were deformed and the epithelial cells were vacuolized and dystrophic. A decreased cellular content of ribonucleoproteins was also observed and pycnosis and caryolysis of nuclei were seen. In the lumen, desquamated epithelia and hyalin cylinders were found. The intestine was slightly swollen in certain areas.

The subchronic toxicity of propachlor (96.1% purity) has also been evaluated in Sprague-Dawley CD rats (30 of each sex per group) fed diets containing 0, 300, 1500 or 7500 mg/kg for 90 days (Reyna & Ribelin, 1984a). No animals died. A statistically significant reduction in body weight was observed in animals fed 1500 mg/kg (8% for males and females) and 7500 mg/kg (59% for males and 36% for females). Food consumption was significantly depressed for animals at the highest dose level for the first month of the study, but recovered during the remainder of the study. After 6 weeks, reduced haemoglobin, haematocrit, mean corpuscular haemoglobin and haematocrit, and an increase in reticulocytes were observed in females at all dose levels and in high-dose males. The anaemia was less evident in high-dose males and was only present in high-dose females at study termination. Significantly reduced lymphocyte counts were observed at week 6 for high-dose males and mid- and high-dose females, and at study termination for all groups. Levels of serum enzymes (SGPT, SAP, GGT), cholesterol and total bilirubin were significantly increased for high-dose animals at weeks 6 and 13 and there were significant reductions in total protein, glucose, creatinine and albumin. No histological changes were observed in the liver. Organ weights (with the exception of female livers) were reduced, relative to controls, for high-dose animals, and spleens were extremely small and treatment-related in size in about 65% of the animals. No histological changes were observed in the tissues examined, which included the spleen.

7.2.1.3 Mice

The subchronic toxicity of propachlor (96.1% pure) was evaluated in four groups of Charles River CD-1® mice (30 mice of each sex per group) (Reyna & Ribelin, 1984b). Dietary levels were 0, 500, 1500 and 5000 mg/kg. No mortality or adverse clinical signs were observed during the study. A statistically significant reduction (10%) in body weight was observed in the mid- and high-dose males and females during the study. Food consumption was also reduced during the first month for mid- and high-dose animals. A dose-related statistically significant reduction in the number of white blood cells was observed in both sexes at all dose levels, except low-dose females, at the 7-week sampling period. At study termination, this reduction was evident in mid- and high-dose animals but was statistically significant only for high-dose males. Liver weights were increased for males at all dietary levels and for mid- and high-dose females. There was an accompanying statistically significant increase in the incidence of centrilobular hepatocellular hypertrophy for mid- and high-dose males, based on histological examination. No other microscopic changes that could be considered treatment related were evident in tissues. For males, the kidney to body weight ratio was decreased at the high-dose level.

7.2.2 Dermal

A 21- and 90-day short- and longer-term dermal toxicity study on Wistar rats (12 animals in each tested group plus 1 control) using propachlor (65% wettable powder) administered 5 days per week was carried out by Baynova et al. (1977). The doses applied were 50, 200 and 500 mg/kg in aqueous suspensions in the 21-day experiment, and 10, 25 and 50 mg/kg in the 90-day study. The dermal application was performed uncovered (Draize, modification of Noakes). By the end of day 21, anaemia was found at dose levels of 200 and 500 mg/kg, but there was no methaemoglobinaemia. The same doses induced a statistically significant decrease in the activity of certain enzymes (SGOT, SGPT, OCT and AP). Dermal application of propachlor at dose levels of 25 and 50 mg/kg to the skin of white rats (two groups of 12 animals) for 90 days did not provoke any changes in concentrations of red blood cells and haemoglobin, but there were decreases in SGOT, SGPT, LAP, AP and catalase. Decreased sulfur-containing enzymes were found in tissue homogenates (liver and kidney). Decreases in the levels of LDH, SDH, AcP and glucose-6-phosphate dehydrogenase were determined histochemically. There was no evidence of clinical signs of intoxication after repeated dermal application of the herbicide, but the occurrence of the above-mentioned enzymatic changes demonstrated the penetration of this herbicide through the dermal barrier. The hexabarbital sleeping time was statistically significantly shortened at the mid- and high-dose levels, thereby confirming the induction of mixed-function oxidases reported by Nenov & Baynova (1978).

A threshold dermal dose of 25 mg/kg (1% aqueous suspension of propachlor 65 WP) and a no-observed-effect level (dermal) of 10 mg/kg (0.5% aqueous suspension) were determined in 90-day experiments by Baynova et al. (1977).

7.3 Skin and eye irritation; sensitization

7.3.1 Skin irritation

Single application to Wistar rats (three rats of each sex per group) of propachlor 65 WP at doses of 1500, 2000, 3000 and 4000 mg/kg in 10 or 20% aqueous suspension, under the open modified method of Noakes, did not cause any local irritative effects (Baynova et al., 1977).

Panshina (1973) reported a strong irritative effect of propachlor after single and repeated application. Single applications to rabbits of 16% propachlor 65 WP in aqueous suspension at doses of 500, 700, and 1000 mg/kg led to hyperaemia and even ulceration in the skin of some animals. Ten applications of a 32% aqueous suspension of propachlor at a level of 200 mg/kg had the same effect on the skin. Seventeen applications of a 6.5% aqueous suspension at 100 mg/kg did not result in mortality, and only slight hyperaemia was seen in the treated skin area of the rabbits.

Primary irritation and contact sensitization effects of Satecid 65 WP containing 65% propachlor were investigated in rabbits, mice and rats, and these were compared with the effects of technical grade propachlor, propachlor with analytical purity, and the vehicle alone (Lehotzky et al., 1979). Propachlor had strong to very strong irritating effects on intact and scarified skin as well as on the eye mucosa of rabbits and mice. The symptoms included erythema, oedema and penetrating ulcer. Technical grade propachlor had the most potent irritating effect.

Heise et al. (1983) conducted parallel experiments with two propachlor preparations, one produced in the USA and the other in Hungary, using an aqueous suspension applied under occlusion to the skin of rabbits for 24 h. The irritant dose (ID_{50}) for the USA preparation was 2% and for the Hungarian preparation 0.6%.

Several dermal irritation studies have been carried out with technical propachlor and its formulations, each of which involved the use of six New Zealand white rabbits (2.5 to 3.5 kg). All application sites were scored for erythema, eschar and oedema formation. For technical propachlor (94.5% pure) a slight degree of dermal irritation was observed (2.5/8.0 score) (Braun et al., 1979a); for a 20% formulation of propachlor (again 94.5% pure) there was a slight degree of dermal irritation (1.8/8.0 score) (Braun et al., 1979b); for a 65% formulation a moderate degree of dermal irritation (3.4/8.0 score) (Braun et al., 1979c); and for a 42% formulation corrosive effects were observed (Branch et al., 1982b).

7.3.2 Skin sensitization

A modification of the maximalization test of Magnusson & Kligman (1969) for identification of allergens was used by Heise et al. (1983). Guinea-pigs (12 female and 12 male) were treated by intramuscular injection of 0.2% propachlor aqueous suspension (using preparations from both the USA and Hungary together with Freund adjuvant), by subcutaneous injection of 0.05% aqueous suspension and by epicutaneous application of a 1% water suspension of both preparations for 6 weeks, both on healthy and scarified skin. A challenge single application was given two weeks after the last application using 0.2 ml of an 1% aqueous suspension of each formulation. There was no significant difference between the reactions to the two preparations. A challenge dose did not induce a reaction.

The dermal sensitization potential of propachlor was evaluated in guinea-pigs using the Buehler procedure (Auletta, 1983). For the induction phase, 0.2 ml of undiluted propachlor (95.7% purity) was applied dermally using the closed patch technique to the shaved backs of five male and five female Hartley albino guinea-pigs. The applications were made for 6 h/day, 3 days/week, for 3 weeks. Two weeks after the final dose, additional 0.2 ml doses of 25% propachlor in ethanol (challenge dose) were applied to previously untreated areas on those guinea-pigs that had received the induction doses and to six others (three males and three females) which served as irritation controls. Two positive control groups, treated with 1-chloro-2,4-dinitrobenzene (DNCB) as positive control, were used. The negative control group (five males and five females) was treated with saline for the induction doses and challenged with acetone. All animals had slight to moderate dermal irritation following the third induction dose of propachlor, and some of them exhibited severe irritation, including oedema, necrosis and exfoliation. Following application of the challenge dose, one out of ten animals had an irritation score of 1 (slight), eight animals had a score of 2 (moderate) and one animal had a score of 3 (severe) at 24 h. Nine of these animals exhibited oedema. At 78 h, two animals had very low scores, six animals had scores of 1, and two scores of 2. Six of these animals exhibited oedema. Similar results were obtained when 20 and 40% propachlor formulations were tested for sensitization in guinea-pigs (Auletta et al., 1984a,b).

7.3.3 Eye irritation

Molnar & Paksy (1978) studied the effect of Satecid 65 WP on the eye mucosa of CFY male albino rats using the Evans blue diffusion technique. The aqueous suspension caused strong conjunctivitis at the minimum concentration of 0.01%.

In a study by Auletta (1984), technical propachlor (96.1% pure) was ground to a fine powder and introduced in the conjunctival sac of the right eye of six (two males and four females) albino New Zealand White rabbits. The left eye served as the control. The treated eyes were rinsed 24 h later. Five of the animals exhibited severe conjunctival irritation (redness, necrosis, chemosis and discharge), five exhibited opacity and/or ulceration, and five had iridial damage. Two animals exhibited neovascularization of the cornea and one bulging of the cornea, indicative of increased intraocular pressure. After 21 days of observation one animal continued to exhibit conjunctival redness and one corneal opacity and bulging of the cornea. The eyes of the remaining animals had minimal conjunctival irritation.

In an eye irritation test on six New Zealand white rabbits using technical propachlor (94.5%), 0.1 cm^3 was instilled into one eye of each rabbit and ocular reactions were observed on days 1, 2, 3, 4, 7, 10 and 14. According to Draize scores, all treated eyes were assigned positive scores for corneal opacity and ulceration, conjunctival redness, chemosis and necrosis. Two eyes were assigned positive scores for iritis. Three eyes exhibited pannus, and corneal bulge was observed in two eyes. Four eyes were clear of signs of irritation by day 14 and two eyes showed signs of irritation at the termination of the study (Braun, 1979).

US EPA (1984b) reviewed the existing data and concluded that propachlor is corrosive to the rabbit eye, corneal opacity being irreversible after 7 days.

7.4 Reproduction, embryotoxicity and teratogenicity

7.4.1 Reproduction

7.4.1.1 Biochemical and histopathological studies on gonads

The effect of propachlor 65 WP on protein content, activity of 5-nucleotidase and ATP in testis homogenate was evaluated by Maleva & Stereva (1977), Stereva & Maleva (1977) and Zlateva & Maleva (1978, 1979). Each test group consisted of 20 male Wistar rats, administered orally (by gavage) 12 or 60 mg propachlor/kg body weight per day for 6 months. A control group consisted of the same number of animals. At the end of the experiment, there were dose-dependent statistically significant changes in the biochemical indices studied (a decrease in protein content and an increase in 5-nucleotidase and ATPase activity) and these were accompanied by histomorphological changes, i.e. disorganization of the seminiferous epithelium. After prolonged dosing some dystrophic and degenerative changes in the gonad tissue and the appearance of multinuclear giant cells with central chromatolysis were observed. Adverse effects on the mitotic division of spermatogonia and blockage of meiosis in the earlier phases were found (Zlateva & Maleva, 1978, 1979).

In subchronic toxicity studies, there was no microscopic evidence of testicular pathology in dogs administered the equivalent of 45 mg propachlor/kg diet per day (Naylor & Ruecker, 1986), in rats fed the equivalent dose of 250-310 mg/kg diet per day in the food (Reyna & Ribelin, 1984a), or in mice fed the equivalent of 400 to 600 mg/kg diet per day (Reyna & Ribelin, 1984b).

7.4.1.2 Reproduction studies

A two-generation rat reproduction study was undertaken to evaluate the effects of propachlor (96.3% pure) (Rao, 1981). Four groups of 30 male and 30 female 6-week-old Fischer-344 rats (F_0 generation) were exposed to diets adjusted weekly to provide dose levels of 0, 0.3, 3 and 30 mg propachlor/kg body weight per day for 100 days and were then allowed to mate to produce the F_1 generation. The F_1 weanlings were similarly dosed for 120 days prior to breeding. The F_1 adults were mated twice to produce F_{2a} and F_{2b} litters. At weaning of F_1, F_{2a} and F_{2b} litters, 10 pups of each sex at each dose level were sacrificed and selected organs were examined histologically. No signs of toxicity in any animals were found during the study. A significant decrease in food consumption and body weight of adult F_1 males dosed with 30 mg/kg per day was found. No adverse effects in any of the treated groups over two generations were noted with respect to gestation length, number of live pups delivered, neonatal survival, litter weight and sex ratio. Decreased pregnancy rates (fertility index) were observed in mid-dose (60%) and high-dose (63%) F_1 females following the first mating (F_{2a} litter), in comparison with 83% in the control rats. Test animals continued to be treated with propachlor and were remated to produce a second (F_{2b}) litter. Pregnancy rates for the F_{2b} litter were 83% for controls and 83, 83 and 80% for low-, mid- and high-dose groups, respectively.

No treatment-related gross necropsy findings were noted. Slight increases in absolute and/or relative liver weights were noted in high-dose F_0 adults, mid- and high-dose F_1 adults and high-dose F_{2a} weanlings. Hypertrophy of the centrolobular hepatocytes was noted during microscopic examination of livers from the high-dose F_0 and F_1 adult females. There was no evidence of compound-related microscopic changes in the testes and ovaries of test animals for either generation.

7.4.2 *Embryotoxicity and teratogenicity*

7.4.2.1 *Rats*

a) *Single dose treatment*

Mirkova (1975) reported embryotoxic and teratogenic effects of propachlor 65 WP in Wistar rats following single-dose treatment (675 mg/kg body weight) on each of the first 16 days of gestation. Significantly increased lethality and frequency of haematomas, predominantly in the head of the fetuses, and reduced cranio-caudal size were observed when the treatment was performed from days 1 to 4 and on days 8, 10 and 12 of gestation (8 to 12 animals per test group and 57 controls). The effect was more marked following treatment on the first day of pregnancy. A weak teratogenic effect was observed with a single dose, which included the induction of external malformations (day 11, brachygnatia), abnormality of internal organs, i.e. hydrocephalus (days 9, 11, 12 and 13 of gestation), defects in skeletal ossification, i.e. non-ossification of sternum (day 9), and delayed ossification of parietal bones (days 11, 12 and 13 of gestation).

b) Repeated dose treatment

Wistar rats were treated daily with 67.5, 135 or 270 mg propachlor/kg body weight on days 1-7 or 8-16 of gestation (six test groups of 10 animals each). In a second set of experiments, a daily treatment of 33.7, 67.5, 135 and 270 mg/kg body weight was given throughout the gestation period (1-21 days) (Mirkova, 1975). Propachlor induced embryotoxicity at all dose levels of repeated treatment during the pre-implantation stages of embryogenesis (days 1-7 of gestation). This was expressed as raised lethality and haemorrhages, predominantly in the head of the fetus, and reduced weight and cranio-caudal size. The effects were significantly reduced when administration was performed during the period of organogenesis (8-16 days). Propachlor showed low teratogenic activity, producing external malformations of the tail (short, curved tail), skeletal abnormalities (non-ossified parietal and occipital bones) and hydrocephalus, at all three dose levels during the pre-implantation stage (days 1-7 of gestation). A slight degree of internal hydrocephalus was observed with doses of 135 and 270 mg/kg on days 8-16 of gestation.

Using a similar treatment regimen, Ivanova-Chemishanska et al. (1975) reported similar changes. No embryotoxic or teratogenic effect was seen at a dose level of 10 mg/kg body weight given daily to rats throughout the pregnancy (Medved, 1977; Panshina, 1985).

Teratogenic effects of technical propachlor were assessed in pregnant Charles River COBS CD rats using a control and three treatment groups consisting each of 25 females (Schardein & Wahlberg, 1982). Propachlor (96.5% pure) levels of 20, 60 and 200 mg/kg body weight were administered orally by gavage as a single daily dose on days 6-19 of gestation in a constant volume of 10 ml/kg corn oil. The control group received the same dose of corn oil. Survival in the control, low-dose and mid-dose groups was 100%. One female in the high-dose group died on gestation day 18 due to an intubation error. There were no differences in mean maternal body weight gain. No changes were evident at gross necropsy that could be considered treatment related. There were no differences between treated and control groups with respect to the mean number of viable fetuses, post-implantations loss, total implantations, corpora lutea, fetal body weights, sex ratio distribution, and in the number of litters or fetuses with external, visceral or skeletal malformations and/or developmental and genetic variations.

7.4.2.2 *Mice*

When Balb/c mice (8-12 in each test group and 18 control pregnant females) were treated with a single dose of 675 mg propachlor/kg body weight on each of days 8-13 of gestation, and at dose levels of 33.7, 67.5, 135 and 270 mg/kg body weight per day from days 1 to 21, a significant increase in post-implantational lethality and reduced fetal weight and cranio-caudal size were observed at all dose regimens. With both single and repeated doses, there was a statistically significant increase in the frequency of internal hydrocephalus, but only at a dose level of 675 mg/kg in a single application on days 9 and 11 of gestation and on daily application at 270 mg/kg from days 1 to 18 of pregnancy (Mirkova, 1975).

7.4.2.3 *Rabbits*

Pregnant New Zealand White rabbits randomly assigned to a control and three treatment groups (each consisting of 16 rabbits) were used to determine the teratogenic potential of propachlor (95.6% pure) (Schardein, 1982). Dose levels of 5, 15 and 50 mg/kg were administered orally by gavage as a single daily dose on days 7-19 of gestation at a constant volume (0.5 ml/kg dissolved in corn oil). The control group received only 0.5 ml/kg corn oil. On gestation day 29, the number and location of viable and non-viable fetuses, early and late resorptions, number of total implantations and the number of corpora lutea were recorded. All fetuses were examined for external, soft tissue and skeletal malformations and for genetic or developmental variations.

Mortality (between 3 and 26 days of gestation) was recorded in the control as well as the treated groups, i.e. two in the control group, three at 5 mg/kg, three at 15 mg/kg and two at 50 mg/kg. Two rabbits from the low-dose group and one from the mid-dose group aborted on gestation days 22 to 25. Ante-mortem observations gave no indication of a treatment-related effect at any dosage level.

Results of the reproductive parameters revealed slight to moderate increases in the number of post-implantation losses and the number of early resorptions in the mid- and high-dose groups when compared with controls (Table 13). Single animals with resorptions only were also found at the two highest dose levels. This resulted in a subsequent decrease in the average number of viable fetuses in the mid- and high-dose groups when compared with controls. Although the number of post-implantation losses fell within the range of historical control frequencies, all the above parameters were considered to imply a mild embryotoxic response. No effects were observed in the number of late resorptions, total implantations, number of corpora lutea, fetal sex distribution or the mean fetal body weights. Examination of the fetuses revealed no external, skeletal or soft tissue malformations, or genetic and developmental variations that could be considered to be related to treatment. These abnormalities observed were low in frequency and within the range of historical control values. A statistically significant increase in the total number of litters with malformations was observed in the mid-dose group when compared to the control group. This trend, however, was not found in the high-dose group and the malformations in the group given 15 mg/kg per day were considered to be incidental to treatment.

Table 13. Mean number of resorptions (late and early), post-implantation losses and total implantations in New Zealand rabbits (Schardein, 1982)

Dose (mg/kg)	Fetuses viable	Fetuses non-viable	Resorptions late	Resorptions early	Post-implantation losses	Total implantations
0	8.0	0.0	0.3	0.3	0.6	8.6
5	7.9	0.0	0.0	0.4	0.4	8.3
15	5.2[a]	0.1	0.0	1.4	1.4	6.6
50	5.9	0.0	0.2	0.9	1.1	7.0

[a] $P < 0.05$

7.5 Mutagenicity and related end-points

Appraisal

Many in vitro *and* in vivo *studies on the genotoxicity of propachlor have been reported. It has been found to be clastogenic in* in vivo *lower test systems and plant assays. It is cytotoxic and also shows a weakly positive clastogenic response in* in vitro *mammalian tests, inducing chromosomal aberrations in Chinese hamster ovary cells. Variable results do not allow any definite conclusions to be drawn. However, on the basis of negative results in many* in vivo *assays in mammalian test systems, the available experimental data provide insufficient evidence of a mutagenic potential. Data on mutagenicity testing are summarized in Table 14.*

7.5.1 Bacterial test systems

Salmonella mutation assays using standard tester strains (TA1535; TA1538; TA98 and TA100), both with and without metabolic activation with rat liver S9, were negative for formulations and technical grades of propachlor (Plewa et al., 1984; Flowers, 1984). No mutagenicity was observed with extracts of plants treated with propachlor.

Negatives results for propachlor in spot tests using *Salmonella typhimurium* test strains were also reported by Njagi & Gopalan (1980) and Eisenbeis et al. (1981).

7.5.2 Yeast assays

Propachlor was not recombinogenic when tested at 1000 mg/litre in *Saccharomyces cerevisae* strain D4 (ade 2-1, ade 2-2; trp 5-12, trp 5-27) either with or without a liver microsomal activation system (Gentille et al., 1977).

Extracts of plants treated with propachlor cause a weak recombinogenic activity (Gentille et al., 1977). Maize extracts treated with 25 ppm propachlor increased the rate of mitotic gene conversion at the ade locus in *S. cerevisae* strain D4 approximately 4-fold over the control levels. Extracts of plants treated with a technical grade of propachlor (1.306×10^{-4} mol/litre) and formulated grade (1.306×10^{-3} mol/litre) induced a significant increase in gene conversion at the ade locus and a lower increase at the trp locus in *S. cerevisae* D4. Results for both formulated and technical grades of propachlor were negative after mammalian S9 activation (Plewa et al., 1984).

7.5.3 Plant assays

Njagi & Gopalan (1981) studied the cytogenic and cytological effects of propachlor at a wide range of concentrations (10, 50,

Table 14. Summary of mutagenicity testing

Test material[a]	Test system	Result[c]			Reference
		-S9	+S9	1S	
Gene mutation in Prokaryotes					
Propachlor U	Ames spot test	-			Njagi & Gopalan (1980)
Propachlor U	Ames spot test	-	-		Eisenbeis et al. (1981)
Propachlor T	Ames plate test	-	-		Flowers (1984)
Propachlor T	Ames plate test	-	-	-	
Propachlor + Cyanazine[b]	Ames plate test			+	Plewa et al. (1984)
Gene mutation in plants					
Propachlor C	maize Wx locus	-			Plewa et al. (1984)
Gene mutation in mammals (*in vitro*)					
Propachlor T	CHO/HGPRT	-	-		Flowers (1985)
Chromosome effects in plants					
Propachlor U	*Vicia faba* cytogenetics	+			Njagi & Gopalan (1981)
Propachlor U	maize cytogenetics	+			Lapina et al. (1984)
Propachlor U	maize chlorophyll mutations	+			Lapina et al. (1984)

Table 14 (contd).

Test material[a]	Test system	Result[c]			Reference
		-S9	+S9	1S	
Chromosome effects in mammals (*in vitro*)					
Propachlor T	CHO cytogenetics	-	+		Li & Meyers (1987)
Chromosome effects in mammals (*in vivo*)					
Propachlor U	*in vivo* mouse bone marrow cyt.	+			Pilinskaya et al. (1980)
Propachlor T	*in vivo* rat bone marrow cyt.	-			Ernst & Blazak (1985)
DNA damage/recombination in yeast					
Propachlor T	gene conversion	-		+	Gentile et al. (1977)
Propachlor T	gene conversion	-	-	+	Plewa et al. (1984)
Propachlor C	gene conversion	-	-	+	Plewa et al. (1984)
Propachlor + Cyanazine	gene conversion			-	Plewa et al. (1984)
DNA damage in mammals (*in vitro*)					
Propachlor T	*in vitro* hepatocyte UDS	-			Steinmetz & Mirsalis (1984)
Propachlor T	*in vivo/in vitro* hepatocyte UDS	-			Steinmetz & Mirsalis (1986)

[a] T = technical grade; C = commercial grade; U = unspecified grade
[b] Propachlor and cyanazine were both of commercial grade.
[c] +S9 and -S9 = with or without rat liver S9 activation mixture;
1S = with maize 1S fraction

100, 500, 1000, 5000 and 10 000 ppm) in root-tip meristematic cells of *Vicia faba*. At a concentration of 100 ppm, propachlor induced, within 2 h, chromosomal aberrations, such as anaphase bridge formation, micronuclei as well as inhibition of mitosis, formation of highly pycnotic nuclei and premature chromosome condensation. The mutagenic properties of propachlor were not detectable in the field experiments using reverse mutations at the wx-C locus in maize as the genetic end-point. Lapina et al. (1984) also reported that propachlor induced mitotic chromosomal aberrations in the root-tip meristematic cells of an inbred F_2 strain of maize. At a concentration of 10^{-3} mol/litre and within 2 h of treatment of maize grains, propachlor increased the rate of mitotic chromosomal aberrations more than 4-fold over the control levels. The main types of cytogenetic damage included single bridges (72%) and fragments (28%). Propachlor did not show evidence of being significantly cytotoxic.

7.5.4 *Cultured mammalian cell CHO/HGPRT assay*

Propachlor (96.1%) was tested in a gene mutation assay in cultured mammalian cells (CHO/HGPRT assay), both in the presence and absence of mammalian metabolic activation, at doses ranging from 10-60 mg/litre. It was found to be cytotoxic at some of the higher concentrations tested, but no mutagenicity was observed (Flowers, 1985).

7.5.5 In vitro *unscheduled DNA synthesis in primary rat hepatocyte cultures*

Steinmetz & Mirsalis (1986) studied the potential of propachlor to induce unscheduled DNA synthesis (UDS) in primary rat hepatocyte cultures. They used ten concentrations of propachlor (95.8% pure) ranging from 0.1 to 5000 mg/litre and, in another assay, five concentrations ranging from 0.1 to 50 mg/litre. Results of this study showed a cytotoxic effect of propachlor at concentrations of 50 mg/litre or more, but there was no evidence of UDS induction.

7.5.6 In vitro *test for induction of chromosomal aberrations using Chinese hamster ovary cells*

Propachlor was tested for its potential to induce chromosomal aberrations in cultured Chinese hamster ovary (CHO) cells treated with propachlor (97.4% pure) at concentrations of 5, 10 or 15 mg/litre for 5 h both in the presence and absence of exogenous activation (Li & Meyers, 1987). As indicated both by decrease in mitotic index and lengthening of average cell generation times, the highest treatment level was cytotoxic both in the presence and absence of activation. In the non-activated study, no statistically significant increases in the percentage of cells with structural aberrations or in average structural aberrations per cell were observed at any treatment level. In the study with S9 activation (15 mg propachlor/litre), the average number of aberrations per cell was statistically elevated at 12 h and 24 h ($P < 0.05$ test). Chromatid and chromosome gaps were not included. The percentage of cells with structural aberrations following treatment at 15 mg/litre was statistically elevated at 12 h but not at 24 h. No apparent dose-response relationship was observed at either harvest time. Under these conditions, propachlor was considered to be negative in the assay without exogenous metabolic activation and a weak clastogen with activation.

7.5.7 In vivo *rat bone marrow cytogenetic assay*

Ernst & Blazak (1985) conducted an *in vivo* rat bone marrow cytogenetic assay using technical grade propachlor (95.6% pure) at dose levels of 0, 0.05, 0.2 and 1 mg/kg body weight. The results were evaluated for mitotic index (based on at least 1000 cells per animal) and 60 cells per animal were examined for chromosomal aberrations. Chromatid and isochromatid gaps were recorded for each cell, but these were not considered chromosomal aberrations. The results showed that propachlor does not induce chromosomal damage in male or female Fischer-344 rats under the conditions used in this study.

7.5.8 *Acute* in vivo *mouse bone marrow cytogenicity assay*

Pilinskaya et al. (1980) studied the cytogenetic effect of propachlor on the bone marrow of mice treated orally with 10, 50 and 100 mg/kg body weight. The metaphase frequency of aberration at the lowest dose applied was 2.67 ± 0.66 compared with 0.7 ± 0.19 in the control. At this dose level an approximately 4-fold increase in the frequency of chromosome aberrations was observed. No statistically significant changes were found at a dose level of 1 mg/kg.

7.5.9 In vivo/in vitro *hepatocyte DNA repair assay*

Steinmetz & Mirsalis (1986) presented data on the *in vivo/in vitro* hepatocyte DNA repair assay. Propachlor (97.7% pure) was suspended in corn oil and administered by gavage to five groups of male Fischer-344 rats at dose levels of 25, 250, 300, 400 and 1000 mg/kg. A positive control group received 2-acetyl aminofluorene (2-AAF) (50 mg/kg) while a negative one was given corn oil. The results were negative.

7.6 Long-term toxicity and oncogenicity studies

7.6.1 Rat

Propachlor (96% pure) was administered via the diet to four groups of 60 male and 60 female Charles River CD SDBR rats at concentrations of 0, 10, 50 and 500 mg/kg (equivalent to 0, 0.5, 2.6 and 27 mg/kg body weight) (Hamada, 1987a). A complete battery of haematological, clinical chemistry and urinalysis tests was carried out every 6 months for 2 years. No treatment-related effects were noted on survival, incidence of clinical and ophthalmoscopic observations, body weight gain or food consumption. Haematological and clinical chemistry parameters and urinalysis data of treated animals were comparable to control values. Thyroid and liver weights were slightly increased in high-dose males at the 12-month interim sacrifice but not at the end of the study. An increased incidence of liver changes (centrilobular hypertrophy, clear cell cytoplasmic alteration and eosinophilic cytoplasmic alteration) was observed in high-dose males and females. A slightly higher incidence of thyroid c-cell tumours (adenomas and carcinomas) noted in high-dose animals was within the testing laboratories' historical range for such tumours. All other organ weight changes and gross and microscopic pathological findings were comparable to controls. An increase in benign granulosa/theca cell tumours was observed for high-dose females (4/60) compared to controls (0/60). The historical control data for this tumour ranged from 0/80 to 4/96. On the basis of these results, 50 mg/kg diet (2.6 mg/kg body weight) can be considered the no-observed-effect level (NOEL) for rats.

7.6.2 Mouse

When propachlor (96.1% pure) was administered in the diet to male and female CD1 mice at dose levels of 10, 50 and 500 mg/kg (equivalent to 1.6, 8.1 and 81.3 mg/kg for males and 2.0, 10.5 and 104.9 mg/kg for females) for 18 months, no histological changes were noted (Hamada et al., 1987b). The survival of all treated male groups was similar to that of controls. Female survival was lower than that of controls in all treated groups. There was a significant increase in segmented neutrophilic leucocytes in the

500-mg/kg group at 12 months, but this change was not evident at study termination. At the end of the study, ratio of liver (with gall bladder) to body weight was increased in the 50- and 500-mg/kg group females, and the ratio of kidney to body weight was decreased in males of the highest-dose group. The NOEL was considered to be 10 mg/kg (1.6 mg/kg per day).

7.6.3 Dog

In a study by Naylor & Ruecker (1986), propachlor was administered daily via the diet to four groups of six male and six female beagle dogs for 12 months (0, 25, 250 and 1000 mg/kg diet). No mortality occurred during the study. Absolute body weights were lower than those of controls at study termination (approximately 14% for males and 8% for females in the high-dose group and 5% for males in the mid-dose group. A slight increase in emesis and/or stool change was noted in treated dogs. No other changes in clinical and pathological parameters were observed that could be related to treatment. Based on the body weight depression at the high dose, a dietary level of 250 mg/kg (9 mg/kg body weight) was considered a no-observed-adverse-effect level (NOAEL) in this chronic study.

7.7 Miscellaneous studies

Propachlor has a strong inhibitory effect on the proliferation of L1210 mouse leukaemia cells *in vitro* (the ID_{50} for cell proliferation is < 3 x 10^{-7} mol/litre). Propachlor also inhibits significantly the uptake of leucine, thymidine and uridine. The inhibitory effect of propachlor is largely reversible, i.e. cells grown in propachlor and then washed free of the compound return to an almost normal rate of proliferation (Zilkah et al., 1981).

It has been demonstrated that propachlor treatment also causes L1210 cells to accumulate in the G1 phase. This effect is dose dependent; a concentration of 10 μmol/litre causes more than 90% of cells to accumulate in the G1 phase (Zilkah et al., 1985).

The combined effect of propachlor and vibration has been studied. Propachlor was given orally to Wistar rats (20 animals in each group) at doses equivalent to 6, 12 and 60 mg/kg body weight per day for 3 months, and the animals were exposed to low-frequency vibration (15 Hz) during the last 30 days of the study. The results were compared with those obtained from groups of rats subjected to the effect of 15 Hz vibration daily for 30 days, as well as with those of groups of rats dosed only with propachlor. It was found that the combined exposure (with 12 or 60 mg propachlor/kg) caused more severe haemodynamic alterations and degenerative (even necrotic) changes in the epithelial cells of the renal tubules, either in the proximal or distal convoluted tubules (Maleva & Zlateva, 1982).

In a study by Baynova et al. (1978b), groups of 20 white rats were pretreated with oral doses of 4 ml/kg 40% ethanol (one tenth of the LD_{50}), 6 days per week, for 4 months. Propachlor was then given daily at a dose level of 140 mg/kg (one tenth of the LD_{50}), 6 days per week, every other week for a further 4-month period. The controls were subjected to 8 months of treatment with ethanol and 4 months of intermittent (every second week) treatment with propachlor using the same doses as in the combined experiment. Both experiments had untreated control groups. The combined treatment led to a reduction of the hepatotoxic effect. This was probably due to induction of mixed-function oxidases and to a more rapid biotransformation in the hepatocytes. It has also been found that propachlor (140 mg/kg for 6 days) reduces the hexabarbital sleeping time by speeding up its metabolism in the hepatic endoplasmic reticulum as a result of induction of the mixed-function oxidase system in the liver cell microsomes (Nenov & Baynova, 1978).

8. EFFECTS ON HUMANS

8.1 Occupational exposure

There have been few reports dealing with the effects of propachlor on humans.

Von Schubert (1979) reported a case of contact eczema on the palms, wrists and forearms of a 29-year-old agricultural worker who had been in contact with propachlor for 8 days. Once this contact ceased, the skin lesions disappeared.

Iden & Schroeter (1977) patch-tested 17 patients, predominantly farmers, who had been exposed simultaneously to many types of herbicides. Seven showed a positive patch test reaction and five others had an irritant reaction to propachlor. One of these farmers, who was highly sensitive to propachlor, used to develop generalized airborne contact dermatitis each spring when his neighbours used this product. Farkasdy et al. (1976) and Dombay & Farkasdy (1978) examined dermatologically 79 workers manufacturing Satecid 65 WP (65% propachlor). Of these, 19% showed contact dermatitis attributed to propachlor exposure. Patch testing was carried out on 67 workers of this group, 12 of whom showed monovalent and bivalent hypersensitivity reaction to propachlor. Photosensitization tests were negative in 28 of the cases tested. Three years later, the same authors examined 108 workers who were continuously exposed to Satecid in the same factory without finding any sign of sensitization.

Jung et al. (1989) patch-tested 19 allergic cases and one irritative case with occupational contact eczema, who were exposed to different types of herbicides. Two of them showed positive testing to Satecid 65 WP. One of these two was only exposed to the substance for 10 days and the other for 6 months.

8.2 General population exposure

No reports on general population exposure are available.

9. EFFECTS ON OTHER ORGANISMS IN THE LABORATORY AND FIELD

9.1 Microorganisms

9.1.1 Soil

The effects of propachlor with regard to changes in numbers of four types of soil bacteria (aerobic nitrogen-fixing, aerobic cellulose-decomposing, ammonifying and nitrifying) was studied by Helmeczi (1977). The studies were carried out using pseudomycelial chernozem soil with maize plants. For the purpose of the microbial examinations, samples from the field were taken three times a year (after spraying propachlor in spring, summer, and autumn at a rate of 8-10 kg/ha) from the upper 20-cm layer of the soil. Sampling was carried out under sterile conditions and samples were collected in sterile vessels. The nitrifying bacteria had the greatest sensitivity to propachlor, their number decreasing considerably from 2720 to 610 per g soil in 1974 and from 4510 to 1920 per g soil in 1975. The aerobic cellulose-decomposing bacteria were the least sensitive, their numbers, with respect to the control bacteria, increasing to a small extent.

Long-term studies in smolnista and alluvial soils have been carried out to establish the effects of propachlor on useful soil microorganisms and the processes of nitrification (Bakalivanov & Kostov, 1981). These studies were conducted under laboratory conditions at 20 °C and 60-70% soil moisture for a period of 10 days. The concentration of propachlor used was 80 mg/kg soil. The results showed an inhibitory effect on nitrification and weaker effect on soil microorganisms (bacteria, actinomycetes and microscopic fungi). High adsorption of propachlor to clay minerals reduced the toxic effect on microorganisms.

Rankov & Velev (1976) studied the effect of propachlor on the biological activity of soil microorganisms and showed that inhibition was greater at a temperature of 2 to 4 °C than at 20 to 22 °C.

9.1.2 Water

The acute toxicity of propachlor to *Selenastrum capricornutum* Printz has been assessed in two studies. In the first (Richards & Kaiser, 1984), the 96-h EC_{50} for growth in algae was calculated to be 0.029 mg/litre with 95% confidence intervals of 0.021-0.038 mg/litre. The no-observed-effect concentration (NOEC) was calculated to be 0.01 mg/litre. In the second study (Zschaler & Jonas, 1990), the 72-h EC_{50} for growth was 5.3 mg/litre and the NOEC 1.9 mg/litre for a propachlor formulation containing 65% active ingredient. The differences in toxicity observed between the two studies may be either because the 65% formulation is less toxic than technical propachlor or because the duration of the second study was 24 h shorter.

9.2 Aquatic organisms

9.2.1 *Aquatic invertebrates*

Thompson & Forbes (1979a) determined a 24-h LC_{50} of 11 mg/litre and a 48-h LC_{50} of 7.8 mg/litre for the water flea *Daphnia magna*. The NOEC in this study was < 5.6 mg/litre. A 48-h LC_{50} of 6.9 mg/litre in the same species was reported by Mayer & Ellersieck (1986). The same authors reported a 48-h LC_{50} of 0.79 mg/litre for the midge larva *Chironomus plumosus*. Another midge larva *Chironomus riparius* was reported to show a 24-h LC_{50} of 5.2 mg/litre and a 48-h LC_{50} of 1.8 mg/litre (Buhl & Faerber, 1989).

The effects of propachlor on daphnia reproduction was assessed in a 21-day life-cycle study (Thun, 1990a). In this study, there was decreased reproductive performance at concentrations from 0.29 to 2.6 mg/litre; the NOEC for reproduction was considered to be 0.097 mg/litre.

9.2.2 *Fish*

Thompson & Forbes (1979b) determined 24-h, 48-h and 96-h LC_{50} values for rainbow trout (*Onchorynchus mykiss*) of 0.75, 0.28 and 0.17 mg/litre, respectively. Thun (1990b) conducted a 21-day study on rainbow trout and found that fish died at concentrations between 0.11 and 0.3 mg/litre. No deaths related to exposure occurred at concentrations between 0.009 and 0.075 mg/litre. The NOEC was considered to be 0.019 mg/litre. Mayer & Ellersieck (1986) reported a 96-h LC_{50} of 0.23 mg/litre for the channel catfish (*Channa punctatus*).

9.3 Terrestrial organisms

9.3.1 Terrestrial invertebrates

The toxicity of propachlor to earthworms was assessed in a 14-day study (Thun et al., 1991). Propachlor (97.8% pure) was added to the soil at five concentrations ranging from 100 to 1000 mg/kg, and 40 worms were added to the soil at each concentration. Worms were removed from the soil at 7 and 14 days and examined for any adverse effects. Body weights were measured at the beginning and end of the test. The LC_{100} was 560 mg/kg and the LC_0 218 mg/kg; the NOEC was 100 mg/kg.

The contact LD_{50} of propachlor for honey bees was reported to be 311 μg/bee (Kenaga, 1979).

Under laboratory conditions, Tanke & Franz (1978) studied the side effects of propachlor on some beneficial insects by measuring the reduction of the beneficial capacity of three enthomophagous insects. The egg parasite *Trichogramma cacoeciae* March reacted very strongly in laboratory as well as in field conditions to the effects of the herbicide. Contact toxicity tested using residues of propachlor on glass plates (residue level not stated) caused a reduction of the degree of parasitization leading to total mortality of the population in contaminated cages. In a study on the contact toxicity of the spray deposit on single leaves as well as on whole plants, the parasitization of *Trichogramma* was reduced by 100 and 83%, respectively. The direct toxic effect should be distinguished from a repellent effect, which is probably more important in the field. In addition to this direct contact effect of spray deposits, systemic application also caused an effect after transport of the herbicide through the soil and the plant. This was demonstrated by a reduction of the degree of parasitization compared with untreated controls.

Propachlor does not seem to have any influence on *Chysopa carnea* Steph larvae. No effect was visible either in tests of contact toxicity or contaminated sandy soil, in choice studies on a repellent action of the residue or after topical application of the preparation. After oral application through an artificial food chain, no influence could be demonstrated. Only overdosage increased the mortality rate of the test larvae. No repellent effect of the herbicide on adults was demonstrated (Tanke & Franz, 1978).

The syrphid *Epistrophe balteata* DeG was more sensitive. Both in contact toxicity studies and in studies for a possible repellent effect, an influence of propachlor on the larval stages was shown. Oral intake through an artificial food chain did not have an effect on the larvae. When the herbicide was sprayed directly on the plant, an increase in larval mortality was observed. Adults of this syrphid also showed reactions to herbicides; during egg deposition, females avoided surfaces previously treated (Tanke & Franz, 1978).

The potential toxicity of a 65% formulation of propachlor to *Aleochara bilineta* Gyll was assessed by Pietrzik (1991). The imagos were dug into moist sand and the test substance was added at recommended use rates (8 kg in 400 litres/ha water). For the assessment of parasitical capacity, pupae of *Delia antiqua* were dug into the sand. At the termination of the test, the sum of hatched *Aleochara* larvae in the pupae was determined. These were compared to the number of control organisms treated with tap water. The parasitic capacity of the test beetles was decreased by 11.4% when compared to controls.

9.3.2 Birds

Palazzolo (1964) reported data for pheasants indicating an acute oral LD_{50} of 735 mg/kg body weight. Increased respiration, loss of reflexes, mydriasis, salivation and intermittent tonic/clonic convulsions were found among birds receiving dose levels of 900 and 1350 mg/kg. The onset of symptoms occurred approximately 15 min following dosing and persisted until death 3-5 h later. Kenaga (1979) reported an LD_{50} of 512 mg/kg for Mallard duck and Beavers & Fink (1979) reported an LD_{50} for Bobwhite quail of 137 mg/kg body weight for a 65% propachlor formulation.

When propachlor was administered in the diet to quail or Mallard ducks for five consecutive days, the LC_{50} for both species of birds was more than 5620 mg/kg diet (Beavers & Fink, 1983a,b). For the quail, a dietary level of 5620 mg/kg is approximately equivalent to a dose of 1400 mg/kg per day. The data presented above indicate that the quail is more susceptible to exposure to propachlor via stomach tube than via the diet.

10. CONCLUSIONS AND RECOMMENDATIONS FOR PROTECTION OF HUMAN HEALTH

10.1 Conclusions

- Under conditions of normal use, the general population is not likely to be exposed to propachlor.

- Those occupationally exposed to propachlor should take adequate safety and hygienic precautions in order to protect the skin, eye and respiratory tract.

- Propachlor is rapidly degraded in the environment under most conditions. It persists longer in cold dry environments. The conjugated *N*-isopropylaniline metabolite persists longer than the parent compound. Propachlor does not bioconcentrate or biomagnify.

- Propachlor is highly toxic to some aquatic organisms. Exposure of aquatic organisms under conditions of normal use is low, the maximum expected concentrations being several orders of magnitude lower than the no-observed-effect concentrations. Direct contamination of water courses will kill aquatic organisms and should be avoided. Propachlor poses a low hazard to birds, earthworms and honey-bees.

10.2 Recommendations for protection of human health

Workers should be educated about the hazards of propachlor and systematically trained to practice safety and personal hygiene and to use protective equipment.

11. FURTHER RESEARCH

- The results of the existing animal studies on mutagenicity are inconclusive and more research is needed.

- Studies should be performed in laboratory animals to determine the potential neurotoxic effects of propachlor.

- Only validated analytical methods for residues of propachlor should be used.

- Epidemiological studies on occupationally exposed workers are needed.

- There is a need to develop methods of biological monitoring for evaluating human exposure to propachlor.

- Research is needed to clarify the exposure of workers in the production and agricultural use of propachlor. Studies should also include examination of health effects at the measured exposure levels.

12. PREVIOUS EVALUATIONS BY INTERNATIONAL BODIES

In the WHO recommended classification of pesticides by hazard, technical propachlor is classified in Class III as slightly hazardous in normal use (WHO, 1990). A data sheet on propachlor has been issued (WHO/FAO, 1989).

Neither the FAO/WHO Joint Meeting on Pesticide Residues (JMPR) nor the International Agency for Research on Cancer (IARC) has so far evaluated propachlor.

REFERENCES

Aschbacher PW & Struble CB (1987) Evidence for involvement of non-biliary excretion into the intestine of the formation of methyl-sulphonyl containing metabolites of 2-chloro-N-isopropylacetanilide (propachlor) by swine and rats. Xenobiotica, **13**(2): 115-126.

Auletta CS (1983) A propachlor dermal sensitization study in guinea-pigs (Project No. 4236-83). East Millstone, New Jersey, Bio/dynamics Inc. (Unpublished proprietary report submitted to WHO by Monsanto International Services, Brussels).

Auletta CS (1984) Eye irritation study with propachlor in rabbits (Project No. 5050-84). East Millstone, New Jersey, Bio/dynamics Inc. (Unpublished proprietary report submitted to WHO by Monsanto International Services, Brussels).

Auletta CS & Rinehart WE (1979) Acute dermal toxicity study in rabbits (Project No. 4892-77). East Millstone, New Jersey, Bio/dynamics Inc. (Unpublished proprietary report submitted to WHO by Monsanto Agricultural Services, Brussels).

Auletta CS, Erickson J, & Webb M (1984a) A closed-patch repeated insult dermal sensitization study in guinea-pigs (modified Buehler method) (Project No. 4946-84). East Millstone, New Jersey, Bio/dynamics Inc. (Unpublished proprietary report submitted to WHO by Monsanto International Services, Brussels).

Auletta CS, Erickson J, & Webb M (1984b) A closed-patch repeated insult dermal sensitization study in guinea-pigs (modified Buehler method) (Project No. 4540-83). East Millstone, New Jersey, Bio/dynamics Inc. (Unpublished proprietary report submitted to WHO by Monsanto International Services, Brussels).

Bakalivanov D & Kostov O (1981) Soil microbiological assessment of toxicity of alkanoate, amide, and other herbicides. Acta microb Acad Sci Hung, **28**: 141-146.

Baker JL (1980) Agricultural areas as non-point sources of pollution. In: Overcash MR & Davidson JM ed. Environmental impact of non-point source pollution. Ann Arbor, Michigan, Ann Arbor Science Publishers, pp 275-310.

Baker JL & Laflen JM (1979) Run-off losses of surface applied herbicides as affected by wheel tracks and incorporation. J Environ Qual, **8**(4): 602-607.

Baker JL, Laflen JM, & Hartwig RO (1982) Effects of corn residue and herbicide placement on herbicide run-off losses. Trans Am Soc Anal Eng, **25**(2): 340-343.

Bakke JE, Gustafsson JA, & Gustafsson BE (1980) Metabolism of propachlor by the germ-free rat. Science, **210**: 433-435.

Bakke JE & Price CE (1979) Metabolism of 2-chloro-N-isopropylacetanilide (propachlor) in the rat. J Environ Sci Health, **B14**(4): 427-441.

Bakke JE, Davison KL, & Larsen GL (1990) Evidence for the absence of cysteine S-conjugate N-acetyltransferase activity in the metabolism of propachlor, naphthalene, and dichlobenil in calves. Xenobiotica, **20**: 801-807.

Bakke JE, Rafter J, Larsen GL, Gustafsson JA, & Gustafsson BE (1981a) Enterohepatic circulation of the mercapturic acid and cysteine conjugates of propachlor. Drug Metab Dispos, **9**(6): 525-528.

Bakke JE, Rafter J, Lindeskog P, Feil V, Gustafsson JA, & Gustafsson BE (1981b) Metabolism of 2-acetamido-4-(chlormethyl) thioazole in germ-free and conventional rats. Biochem Pharmacol, **30**(13): 1831-1844.

Bakke JE, Larsen GL, Aschbacher PW, Rafter J, & Gustafsson JA (1981c) Role of gut microflora in metabolism of glutathione conjugates of xenobiotics. In: Rosen JD, Magee PhS, & Casida JE ed. Sulfur in pesticide action and metabolism. Washington, DC, American Chemical Society, pp 165-178 (ACS Symposium Series No. 158).

Balinova AM (1981) Investigations in the residues of some herbicides in plant production in view of its hygienic evaluation. Sofia, University of Sofia (Dissertation).

Balinova A & Konstantinov K (1975) Investigations on residues of several herbicides in vegetables. In: Proceedings of the COMECOM Symposium on Residues of Herbicides in Plants and Soils, Vrozlav, 1973, pp 111-116.

Barrows ME & Macek KJ (1974) Exposure of fish to ^{14}C-Ramrod^{TM}: Accumulation, distribution and elimination of ^{14}C-residues. Wareham, Massachusetts, Bionomics, E.G. & G. Inc., 18 pp (Unpublished proprietary report submitted to WHO by Monsanto International Services, Brussels).

Baynova A, Burkova T, & Michailova A (1977) [Determination of dermal toxicity of Ramrod.] Gig Zdraveopazvane, **20**(3): 234-240 (in Russian).

Baynova A, Burkova T, & Michailova A (1978a) [Comparative study on intermittent and monotonous effects of the herbicide Ramrod.] Gig Zdraveopazvane, **21**: 568-573 (in Russian).

Baynova A, Krastev L, Dikova M, & Michailova JA (1978b) Effect of alcohol on acute and chronic intoxication with the herbicide Ramrod. Acta med Bulg, **2**: 36-41.

Beavers JB & Fink R (1979) Acute oral LD_{50}-Bobwhite Quail. Propachlor report No. WL-79-026. Easton, Maryland, Wildlife International Ltd (Unpublished proprietary report submitted to WHO by Monsanto International Services, Brussels).

Beavers JB & Fink R (1983a) Eight-day dietary LC_{50} - Bobwhite Quail propachlor. Easton, Maryland, Wildlife International Ltd (Unpublished proprietary report No. WL-83-90, submitted to WHO by Monsanto International Services, Brussels).

Beavers JB & Fink (1983b) Eight-day dietary LC_{50} - Mallard Duck propachlor. Easton, Maryland, Wildlife International Ltd (Unpublished proprietary report No. WL-83-89, submitted to WHO by Monsanto International Services, Brussels).

Bechtel CL (1991) Acute inhalation study of propachlor Technical (Project No. ML-91-2). Newstead, St. Louis, Monsanto Environmental Health Laboratory (Unpublished proprietary report submitted to WHO by Monsanto International Services, Brussels).

Beestman GB & Deming JM (1974) Dissipation of acetanilide herbicides from soils. Agron J, **66**: 306-311.

Blaszcak DL (1988) A comparative acute oral toxicity study in Sprague-Dawley and Fischer rats (Project No. 4359-87). East Millstone, New Jersey, Bio/dynamics Inc., 37 pp (Unpublished proprietary report submitted to WHO by Monsanto International Services, Brussels).

Bleeke MS, Carr KH, & Elliot RC (1987) Propachlor metabolism in the laying hen (Project No. MSL-6217). St. Louis, Missouri, Monsanto Agricultural Company, 134 pp (Unpublished proprietary report submitted to WHO by Monsanto International Services, Brussels).

Branch DK, Stout LD, & Folk RN (1982a) Acute oral toxicity of Ramrod® 4L flowable herbicide for rats (Project No. ML-81-182). Newstead, St. Louis, Monsanto Environmental Health Laboratory (Unpublished proprietary report submitted to WHO by Monsanto International Services, Brussels).

Branch DK, Stout LD, & Folk RN (1982b) Primary skin irritation of Ramrod® 4L flowable herbicide to rabbits (Project No. 810096). Newstead, St. Louis, Monsanto Environmental Health Laboratory (Unpublished proprietary report of Monsanto Agricultural Company, submitted to WHO by Monsanto International Services, Brussels).

Braun WG (1979) Rabbit eye irritation study (Project No. 4889-77). East Millstone, New Jersey, Bio/dynamics Inc., 4 pp (Unpublished proprietary report of Monsanto Agricultural Company, submitted to WHO by Monsanto International Services, Brussels).

Braun WG & Rinehart E (1978) Acute dermal toxicity study in rabbits (Project No. 4888-77). East Millstone, New Jersey, Bio/dynamics Inc., 4 pp (Unpublished proprietary report, submitted to WHO by Monsanto International Services, Brussels).

Braun WG, Heenehan PR, & Rinehart WE (1979a) Primary dermal irritation study in rabbits (Project No. 4890-77). East Millstone, New Jersey, Bio/dynamics Inc. (Unpublished proprietary report of Monsanto Agricultural Company, submitted to WHO by Monsanto International Services, Brussels).

Braun WG, Heenehan PR, & Rinehart WE (1979b) Primary dermal irritation study in rabbits (Project No. 4898-77). East Millstone, New Jersey, Bio/dynamics Inc. (Unpublished proprietary report of Monsanto Agricultural Company, submitted to WHO by Monsanto International Services, Brussels).

Braun WG, Heenehan PR, & Rinehart WE (1979c) Primary dermal irritation study in rabbits (Project No. 4894-77). East Millstone, New Jersey, Bio/dynamics Inc. (Unpublished proprietary report of Monsanto Agricultural Company, submitted to WHO by Monsanto International Services, Brussels).

Brightwell BB & Rueppel ML (1976) Lasso® and Ramrod®: physical properties and their relationship to the environment. St. Louis, Missouri, Monsanto Agricultural Company (Unpublished report No. 443, submitted to WHO by Monsanto International Services, Brussels).

Brightwell BB, Malik JM, & Wong SC (1981) The environmental fate of propachlor [2-chloro-N (1-methyl)-N-phenyl-acetamide] in soil and water. St. Louis, Missouri, Monsanto Research Laboratory, 1300 pp (Unpublished proprietary report No. MSL-1900, submitted to WHO by Monsanto International Services, Brussels).

Buhl KJ & Faerber NL (1989) Acute toxicity of selected herbicides and surfactants to larvae of the midge *Chironomus riparius*. Arch Environ Contam Toxicol, **18**: 530-536.

Caverly DJ & Denney RC (1978) Determination of substituted ureas and some related herbicide residues in soils by gas chromatography. Analyst, **103**: 368-374.

Daly I & Knezevich A (1984) Four-week toxicity study in dogs (Bio/dynamics Inc. Project No. 84-2798). Unpublished proprietary report of Monsanto Agricultural Company, submitted to WHO by Monsanto International Services, Brussels.

Davison KL (1991) Propachlor-s-glutathione metabolism by kidneys and ureters of calves. J Anim Sci, **69**: 1116-1121.

Davison KL, Bakke JE, & Larsen GL (1988) A kidney perfusion method for metabolism. Studies with chickens using propachlor as a model. Xenobiotica, **18**(3): 323-329.

Davison KL, Bakke JE, & Larsen GL (1990) Metabolism of the glutathione conjugate of propachlor by *in situ* perfused kidneys and livers of rats. Xenobiotica, **20**(4): 375-383.

Dombay Z & Farkasdy J (1978) [Problems of safety technique and of occupational safety as related to propachlor and its formulations.] In: [Conference on Safety Technology in the Application of Agricultural Chemicals], Budapest, Technoinform, pp. 49-58 (in German).

Eisenbeis SJ, Lynch DL, & Hampel AE (1981) The Ames mutagen assay tested against herbicides and herbicide combinations. Soil Sci, **131**(1): 44-46.

Ernst L & Blazak F (1985) An assessment of the mutagenic potential of propachlor utilizing the acute *in vivo* rat bone marrow cytogenetics assay (Project No. SR-84-180). Menlo Park, California, Stanford Research Institute, 39 pp. (Unpublished proprietary report, submitted to WHO by Monsanto International Services, Brussels).

FAO (1982) Second Government Consultation on International Harmonization of Pesticide Registration Requirements, Rome, 11-15 October 1982. Rome, Food and Agriculture Organization of the United Nations.

Farkasdy J, Horvath A, & Meszleri E (1976) [Occupational dermatitis caused by the selective herbicide Satecid 65WP.] Borgyogy venerol Sz, **52**: 112-118 (in German).

Feil VJ, Bakke JE, & Larsen GL (1981) A new metabolite of propachlor isolated from germ-free rat excreta. Biomed Mass Spectrom, **8**(1): 1-4.

Fletcher WW & Kirkwood RC (1982) Herbicide and plant growth regulators. London, Toronto, Sydney, New York, Granada.

Flowers LJ (1984) Salmonella mutagenicity assay of propachlor. Newstead, St. Louis, Monsanto Environmental Health Laboratory, 18 pp (Unpublished proprietary report No. MSL-1694, submitted to WHO by Monsanto International Services, Brussels).

Flowers LJ (1985) CHO/HGPRT gene mutation assay with propachlor. Newstead, St. Louis, Monsanto Environmental Health Laboratory, 9 pp (Unpublished proprietary report No. ML-84-237, submitted to WHO by Monsanto International Services, Brussels).

Frank R, Sirons GJ, Paik NJ, & Valk M (1977) Fate of propachlor applied to onions and organic soils. Can J Plant Sci, **57**: 473-477.

Gentille JM, Wagner ED, & Plewa MJ (1977) The detection of weak recombinogenic activities in the herbicides alachlor and propachlor using a plant activation bioassay. Mutat Res, **48**: 113-116.

Gustafson DI (1989) Groundwater ubiquity score: A simple method for assessing pesticide leachability. Environ Toxicol Chem, **8**: 339-357.

Hamada NN (1987a) Combined chronic toxicity and oncogenicity study in rats with propachlor (Study No. HL-83-350/241-169). Vienna, Virginia, Hazleton Laboratories America Inc., 2452 pp (Unpublished proprietary report submitted to WHO by Monsanto International Services, Brussels).

Hamada NN (1987b) Oncogenicity study with propachlor in mice (Study No. HL-83-349/241-159). Vienna, Virginia, Hazleton Laboratories America Inc., 520 pp (Unpublished proprietary report submitted to WHO by Monsanto International Services, Brussels).

Heenehan BS, Rinehart WE, & Braun WG (1979) Acute oral toxicity study in rats (Project No. 1895-77) (Unpublished proprietary report submitted to WHO by Monsanto International Services, Brussels).

Heise H, Mattheus A, & Pushkeiler TH (1983) [The irritant and allergic effect of the herbicidal agent propachlor.] Z Gesamte Hyg, **29**(11): 675-677 (in German).

Helmeczi B (1977) The effect of herbicides on soil bacteria belonging to certain physiological groups. Acta phytopathol Acad Sci Hung, **12**(1-2): 41-49.

Humburg NE, Colby SR, Lym RG, Prasad R, Hill ER, Kitchen LM, & McAvoy WJ (1989) Herbicide handbook, 6th ed. Champaign, Illinois, The Weed Science Society of America.

Iden DL & Schroeter AL (1977) Allergic contact dermatitis to herbicides. Arch Dermatol, **113**(7): 983.

Ivanova-Chemishanska L, Vergieva T, & Mirkova E (1975) Embryotoxic and teratogenic effects of some pesticides. Exp Med Morfol, **14**(1): 29-33.

Jung HD, Honemann W, Kloth C, Lubbe D, & Pambor M (1989) Contact eczema caused by pesticides in East Germany. Dermatol Monatschrift, **175**: 203-214.

Kaempfe BS (1991) Acute inhalation study of MON 15606 (Project No. ML-91-48). Newstead, St Louis, Monsanto Company Environmental Health Laboratory. (Unpublished proprietary report of Monsanto Agricultural Company, submitted to WHO by Monsanto International Services, Brussels).

Kenaga EE (1979) Acute and chronic toxicity of 75 pesticides to various animal species. Down Earth, **35**(2): 25-31.

Kofman IS & Nishko P (1984) Determination of micro-quantities of herbicides from a group of acetylanilides by thin-layer chromatography. Physiol Biochem Cult Plant, **16**(3): 290-292.

Kolesnikov VA, Abramova KA, & Grip OK (1979) Use of herbicides on white cabbage. Khim Sel'skom Khoz, **17**(10): 27-31.

Kolesnikov VA, Karetskaia NA, & Petuchova VI (1980) Efficacy of herbicides in garlic crop. Khim Sel'skom Khoz, **18**(8): 38-40.

Lamoureux GL & Davidson KL (1975) Mercapturic acid formation in the metabolism of propachlor, CDAA and Flurodifen in the rat. Pestic Biochem Physiol, **5**: 497-506.

Lamoureux GL & Rusness DG (1989) Propachlor metabolism in soybean plants, excised soybean tissues, and soil. Pestic Biochem Physiol, **34**: 187-204.

Lamoureux GL, Stafford LE, & Tanaka FS (1971) Metabolism of 2-chloror-N-isopropyl-acetanilide (propachlor) in the leaves of corn, sorghum, sugar cane, and barley. J Agric Food Chem, **19**(2): 346-350.

Lapina TV, Grigorenko NV, Morgun V, Logvinenko VF, & Merjinskii JG (1984) Study of the mutagenic effect of the herbicides Treflan, Ramrod, and Banvel on corn. Tsitol i Genet, **18**(2): 119-122.

Larsen GL & Bakke JE (1979) Studies on the origin of the methylsulfonyl-containing metabolites from propachlor. J Environ Sci Health, **B14**: 427.

Larsen GL & Bakke JE (1981) Enterohepatic circulation in formation of propachlor (2-chloro-N-N-isopropylacetanilide) metabolites in the rat. Xenobiotica, **11**(7): 473-480.

Larsen GL & Bakke JE (1983) Metabolism of mercapturic acid-pathway metabolites of 2-chloro-N-isopropylacetanilide (propachlor) by gastrointestinal bacteria. Xenobiotica, **13**(2): 115-126.

Larsen GL, Larsen JD, & Gustafson JA (1983) Cysteine conjugate beta-lyase in the gastrointestinal bacterium *Fusobacterium necrophorum*. Xenobiotica, **13**(11): 689-700.

Lee JK, Minard RD, & Bollag JM (1982) Microbial metabolism of propachlor in soil suspension. J Korean Agric Chem Saf, **25**(1): 44-53.

Lehotzky K, Szeberenyl JMS, & Tatrai E (1979) On the local and systematic toxic effects of the herbicide propachlor (Satecid 65WP) in experimental animals. Egeszegtudomany, **23**: 89-96.

Li AP & Meyers CA (1987) *In vitro* cytogenetics study of propachlor (Study No. MSL-6939), 24 pp (Unpublished proprietary report submitted to WHO by Monsanto International Services, Brussels).

Lottman CM & Cowell JE (1986) Propachlor residues in processed sorghum grain applications following pre-emergent applications of Ramrod 4L herbicide (Project No. MSL 6091) (Unpublished proprietary report of Monsanto Agricultural Company, submitted to WHO by Monsanto International Services, Brussels).

Lottman CM & Cowell JE (1987) Propachlor residues in processed corn grain fractions following pre-emergent applications at Ramrod 4 h herbicide (Study No. MSL-6260) (Unpublished proprietary report submitted to WHO by Monsanto International Services, Brussels).

Magnusson B & Kligman AM (1969) The identification of allergens by animal assay. The guinea-pig maximalization test. J Invest Dermatol, **52**: 268-276.

Maleva E & Stereva M (1977) [Biochemical investigation on changes of gonads of male white rats under combined action of low frequency vibrations and intoxication with

Ramrod. I. Changes in the content of protein.] In: [Proceedings of the National Scientific Session of Chemists with Medical Direction, Part 2], pp. 306-313 (in Bulgarian).

Maleva E & Zlateva M (1982) Histomorphological changes in kidneys of experimental animals under the combined effect of low-frequency vibration and intoxication with Ramrod herbicide. Hig Zdraveopazvane, **25**(3): 244-249.

Malik JM (1982) Bioconcentration of propachlor in channel catfish under static conditions. Columbia, Missouri, Analytical Biochemistry Laboratories, 144 pp (Unpublished proprietary report No. 24242, submitted to WHO by Monsanto International Services, Brussels).

Malik JM (1986) Metabolism of propachlor in rats (Project No. 7815). St. Louis, Missouri, Monsanto Agricultural Company, Research Department (Unpublished proprietary report submitted to WHO by Monsanto International Services, Brussels).

Markus JR & Puma B (1973) Pesticide analytical manual. Volume II: Methods for individual pesticide residues. Springfield, Virginia, US Department of Commerce, National Technical Information Service, pp 1-7.

Martin CD, Baker JL, Erbach DC, & Johnson HP (1978) Wash-off of herbicides applied to corn residue. Trans Am Soc Anal Eng, **21**(6): 1164-1168.

Mayer FL Jr & Ellersieck MR (1986) Manual of acute toxicity: Interpretation and data base for 410 chemicals and 66 species of freshwater animals. Washington, DC, US Department of the Interior, Fish and Wildlife Service (Resource Publication 160).

Medved LI (1977) [Manual of pesticides.] Kiev, K. Urojai (in Russian).

Melnikov NN, Novojilov KV, Belen SP, & Pilova TN (1985) [Manual of pesticides.] Moscow, M. Khimia (in Russian).

Menges RM & Tamez S (1973) Effect of soil incorporation on selectivity, movement, and persistence of herbicides in onion plantings. J Am Soc Hortic Sci, **98**(4): 390-393.

Mirkova E (1975) Embryotoxic and teratogenic action of pesticides Basfungin and Ramrod. Sofia, University of Sofia (Dissertation).

Molnar J & Paksy KA (1978) Acute inflammation of rat membranes evoked by eye-instillation and inhalation of pesticide formulations containing propachlor and TMTD. Egeszsegtudomany, **22**: 393-397.

Nadeau RG & Pantano LK (1986) Metabolism study of synthetic $^{13}C/^{14}C$-labelled plant metabolites of propachlor in lactating goats. Part II: Identification characterization and quantification of metabolites (Project No. MSL-5909), 119 pp (Unpublished proprietary report submitted to WHO by Monsanto International Services, Brussels).

Naylor MW & Ruecker RW (1986) One-year dog study with propachlor (Study No. ML-84-379). Newstead, St. Louis, Monsanto Environmental Health Laboratory (Unpublished proprietary report of Monsanto Agricultural Company, submitted to WHO by Monsanto International Services, Brussels).

Nenov P & Baynova A (1978) Ramrod (propachlor) effect on the activity of rat hepatic microsomal enzymosystems. Acta med Bulg, **5**(2): 44-52.

Nesterova OA, Popova VV, & Kolesnikova OP (1980) [Accumulation of semeron, mesoranil, and Ramrod in the soil and cabbage during long-term use.] Sibirski Vestn S-Kh Nauki, **10**(4): 19-21 (in Russian).

Njagi GDE & Gopalan HNB (1980) Mutagenicity testing of some selected food preservatives, herbicides, and insecticides. II. Ames test, Bangladesh. J Bot, **9**(2): 141-146.

Njagi GDE & Gopalan HNB (1981) Mutagenicity testing of herbicides, fungicides, and insecticides. I. Chromosome aberrations in *Vicia faba*. Cytologia, **46**: 169-172.

Novick NJ & Alexander M (1985) Co-metabolism of low concentrations of propachlor, alachlor, and cycloate in sewage and lake water. Appl Environ Microbiol, **April**: 737-743.

Novick NJ, Mukherjee R, & Alexander M (1986) Metabolism of alachlor and propachlor in suspensions of pretreated soil and in samples from ground water aquifers. J Agric Food Chem, **34**: 721-725.

Palazzolo RJ (1964) Acute oral toxicity study on CP 31393 in Golden Ring-necked pheasants. Northbrook, Illinois, Industrial Biotest Laboratories (Unpublished proprietary report No. BLT-64-3, submitted to WHO by Monsanto International Services, Brussels).

Panshina TN (1973) [Materials about toxicology of new herbicide Ramrod.] Gig Primen toksikol pestic klin otravlenni, **1973**: 301-303 (in Russian).

Panshina TN (1976) [Hygienic aspects of the use of certain herbicides in agriculture and toxicology.] Gig i Sanit, **7**: 38-41 (in Russian).

Panshina TN (1977) Establishment of maximum permissible concentrations and approximately safe levels of action exerted by herbicides of haloid-substituted carboxylic acid anilides in the air of a production sector. Gig Tr Prof Zabol, **12**: 30-33 (in Russian).

Panshina TN (1985) IRPTC scientific reviews of Soviet literature on toxicity and hazards of chemicals No. 83: Propachlor (Ramrod). Moscow, Centre of International Projects, GKNT, 19 pp.

Pantano LK & Anderson KS (1987) The metabolic fate of propachlor [2-chloro-N-(1-methylethyl)-N-Phenylacetamide] in sorghum foliage and grain (Project No. MSL-5412). St. Louis, Missouri, Monsanto Agricultural Company (Unpublished proprietary report submitted to WHO by Monsanto International Services, Brussels).

Pekas JV, Larsen GL, & Feil VJ (1979) Propachlor detoxication in the small intestine: cysteine conjugation. J Toxicol environ Health, **5**: 653-662.

Pietrzik J (1991) [Laboratory determination of side effects of Ramrod 65WP on the short-winged beetle *Aleochara bilineata* Gyll (Project No. 112/01-AB).] Niefern-Öchselbronn, Austria, GAB Biotechnologie GmbH (Unpublished proprietary report of Monsanto Agricultural Company, submitted to WHO by Monsanto International Services, Brussels) (in German).

Pilinskaya M, Kurinny AI, & Ivova TS (1980) [The primary evaluation of cytogenetic activity and potential mutagenic hazard of 22 pesticides.] Cytol Genet, **14**(6): 41-46 (in Russian).

Plewa MJ, Wagner ED, Glenda G, & Gentille JM (1984) An evaluation of the genotoxic properties of herbicides following plant and animal activation. Mutat Res, **136**: 233-245.

Pressley TA & Longbottom JE (1982) The determination of organochlorine pesticides in industrial and municipal waste water. Cincinnati, Ohio, US Environmental Protection Agency, Environmental Monitoring and Support Laboratory, Office of Research and Development.

Rafter JJ, Bakke J, Larsen G, Gustafson B, & Gustafson JA (1983a) Role of the intestinal microflora in the formation of sulfur-containing conjugates of xenobiotics. Rev Biochem Toxicol, **5**: 387-408.

Rafter JJ, Gustafson JA, Bakke J, Larsen G, Norin KE, & Gustafson BE (1983b) Studies on the re-establishment of the intestinal microflora in germ-free rats with special reference to the metabolism of N-isopropyl-alpha-chloracetanilide (propachlor). Xenobiotica, **13**(3): 171-178.

Rankov V & Velev B (1976) Effect of temperature on the interaction between the metribuzin and propachlor herbicides and soil microorganisms. Agrokhimiya, **11**(5): 100-105.

Rankov V & Velev B (1977) Detoxication of the herbicide propachlor by certain microscopic fungi. Acta phytopathol Acad Sci Hung, **12**(1-2): 67-72.

Rao KS (1981) Two-generation dietary reproduction study with propachlor in rats (Study No. HET-K-077810(8)). Midland, Michigan, Dow Chemical Company, Health and Environmental Science, Toxicology Research Laboratory, 171 pp (Unpublished proprietary report submitted to WHO by Monsanto International Services, Brussels).

Rejtö M, Saltzman S, & Acher AJ (1984) Photodecomposition of propachlor. J Agric Food Chem, **32**: 226-230.

Reyna MS & Ribelin WE (1984a) Three-month feeding study of propachlor to albino rats (Study No. 83037). Newstead, St. Louis, Monsanto Environmental Health Laboratory (Unpublished proprietary report submitted to WHO by Monsanto International Services, Brussels).

Reyna MS & Ribelin WE (1984b) Three-month feeding study of propachlor to albino mice (Study No. 820061). Newstead, St. Louis, Monsanto Environmental Health Laboratory (Unpublished proprietary report of Monsanto Agricultural Company, submitted to WHO by Monsanto International Services, Brussels).

Richards C & Kaiser FE (1984) Acute toxicity of propachlor (AB 83-367) to *Selenastrum capricornutum* Printz. Columbia, Missouri, Analytical Biochemistry Laboratories, 39 pp (Unpublished proprietary report No. 31348, submitted to WHO by Monsanto International Services, Brussels).

Ritter WP, Johnson HP, & Lovely WG (1973) Diffusion of atrazine, propachlor, and diazinon in silt loam soil. Weed Sci, **5**: 381-384.

Roberts HA, Walker A, & Bond W (1978) Persistence of chlorthaldimethyl activity in soil. In: Proceedings of the British Crop Protection Conference: Weeds. Croydon, British Crop Protection Council, pp 87-92.

Schardein JW (1982) Teratology study in rabbits. Mattawan, Michigan, International Research and Development Corporation, 47 pp (Unpublished proprietary report No. IR 81-224, submitted to WHO by Monsanto International Services, Brussels).

Schardein JW & Wahlberg A (1982) Teratology study in rats. Mattawan, Michigan, International Research and Development Corporation, 81 pp (Unpublished proprietary report No. IR 81-264, submitted to WHO by Monsanto International Services, Brussels).

Shirko ST & Belova VL (1982) [Level of Ramrod, semeron, and mesoranil in the soil and cabbage plants in relation of dose of nitrogen and potassium.] Khim Sel'skom Khoz, **20**(I): 51-53 (in Russian).

Sjovall J, Rafter J, Larsen G, & Egestad B (1983) Lipophilic ion exchange for group separation of conjugated metabolites of xenobiotics. J Chromatogr, **276**: 150-156.

Spalding RF & Snow DD (1989) Stream levels of agrochemicals during a spring discharge event. Chemosphere, **19**(8/9): 1129-1140.

Steen WC & Collette TW (1989) Microbial degradation of seven amides by suspended bacterial populations. Appl Environ Microbiol, **55**(10): 2545-2549.

Steinmetz L & Mirsalis C (1984) Evaluation of the potential of propachlor to induce unscheduled DNA synthesis in the primary rat hepatocyte cultures (Project No. LSC-7538). Menlo Park, California, Stanford Research Institute, 8 pp (Unpublished proprietary report submitted to WHO by Monsanto International Services, Brussels).

Steinmetz L & Mirsalis C (1986) Evaluation of the potential of propachlor to induce unscheduled DNA synthesis in the *in vivo- in vitro* rat hepatocyte DNA repair assay (Project No. LSC-2021). Menlo Park, California, Stanford Research Institute, 37 pp (Unpublished proprietary report submitted to WHO by Monsanto International Services, Brussels).

Stereva M & Maleva E (1977) [Biochemical studies on changes in gonads of male white rats under combined action of low frequency vibrations and intoxication with Ramrod. II. Dynamic in changes of 5-nucleotidase activity.] In: [Proceedings of the National Scientific Session of Chemists with Medical Direction, Part I], pp 133-139 (in Bulgarian).

Strateva A (1974a) [Hygienic-toxicologic study on Ramrod aiming its hygienic standardization in water.] Sofia, University of Sofia (Dissertation) (in Bulgarian).

Strateva A (1974b) [Amid preparations with herbicide action. Experimental data on the acute oral toxicity of propachlor (Ramrod).] Exp Med Morphol, **13**(2): 123-129 (in Russian).

Strateva A (1975) [On some toxicologic properties of Ramrod and their significance on its hygienic standardization in waters.] Hyg Zdraveopazvane, **18**(4): 401-405 (in Russian).

Strateva A (1976) [The experimental determination of MAC of Ramrod in water.] Gig i Sanit, **4**: 85-87 (in Russian).

Strateva A, Velisarov A, & Georgiev A (1974) [Morphological and enzymohistochemical investigations on some internal organs of experimental animals under the effect of Ramrod in acute experiment.] Hyg Zdraveopazvane, **17**(3): 283-286 (in Russian).

Struble CB (1991) *In situ* intestinal absorption of 2-chloro-N-isopropylacetanilide (propachlor) and non-biliary excretion of metabolites into the intestinal tract of rats, pigs and chickens. Xenobiotica, **21**: 85-95.

Tanaka FS, Wien RG, & Mansager ER (1981) Survey for surfactant effects on the photodegradation of herbicides in aqueous media. J Agric Food Chem, **29**: 227-230.

Tanke W & Franz JM (1978) [Side effects of herbicides on economically useful insects.] Entomophaga, **23**(3): 275-280 (in German).

Thompson CM & Forbes AD (1979a) Acute toxicity of propachlor to *Daphnia magna*. Columbia, Missouri, ABC-Laboratories Inc., 40 pp (Unpublished proprietary report No. 24708, submitted to WHO by Monsanto International Services, Brussels).

Thompson CM & Forbes AD (1979b) Acute toxicity of propachlor to Rainbow trout *Salmo gairdneri*. Columbia, Missouri, ABC-Laboratories Inc., 40 pp (Unpublished proprietary report No. 24019, submitted to WHO by Monsanto International Services, Brussels).

Thun S (1990a) Propachlor 21-day reproduction test in *Daphnia* (Project Number XX-89-126). Walsrode, Germany, IBR Forschung GmbH (Unpublished proprietary report of Monsanto Agricultural Company, submitted to WHO by Monsanto International Services, Brussels).

Thun S (1990b) Prolonged fish toxicity test in the rainbow trout (*Salmo gairdneri*) (Project Number XX-89-163). Walsrode, Germany, IBR Forschung GmbH (Unpublished proprietary report of Monsanto Agricultural Company, submitted to WHO by Monsanto International Services, Brussels).

Thun S, Lemke G, & Fulst S (1991) Acute toxicity in earthworms according to OECD 207. (Project Number IB-90-566). Walsrode, Germany, IBR Forschung GmbH (Unpublished proprietary report of Monsanto Agricultural Company, submitted to WHO by Monsanto International Services, Brussels).

US EPA (1984a) Guidance for the registration of pesticide products containing propachlor (019101) (EPA Case number 17). Washington, DC, US Environmental Protection Agency, Office of Pesticide Programme.

US EPA (1984b) Health and environmental effects profile for propachlor. Cincinnati, Ohio, US Environmental Protection Agency (600/X-84/335).

US EPA (1988) Propachlor. Washington, DC, US Environmental Protection Agency, Health Advisory Office of Drinking-Water.

Vasilev NV (1982) [Residual quantity of Ramrod in soil and fodder rurabages.] Khim Sel'skom Khoz, **20**(6): 51-53 (in Russian).

Villarreal DT, Turco RF, & Konopka A (1991) Propachlor degradation by a soil bacterial community. Appl Environ Microbiol, **57**(8): 2135-2140.

Von Schubert H (1979) [Allergic contact dermatitis caused by propachlor.] Dermatol Monatsschr, **165**: 495-498 (in German).

Walker A & Brown PA (1982) Effects of soil on the activity and persistence of propachlor. In: Proceedings of the British Crop Protection Conference: Weeds. Croydon, British Crop Protection Council, pp 171-177.

Walker A & Brown PA (1985) The relative persistence in soil of five acetanilide herbicides. Bull Environ Contam Toxicol, **34**: 143-149.

Warholic DT, Gutenmann WH, & Lisk DJ (1983) Propachlor herbicide residue studies in cabbage using modified analytical procedure. Bull Environ Contam Toxicol, **31**: 585-587.

WHO/FAO (1989) Data sheets on pesticides No. 78: Propachlor. Geneva, World Health Organization, 7 pp (WHO/VBC/DS/87.78).

WHO (1990) The WHO recommended classification of pesticides by hazard and guidelines to classification 1990-91. Geneva, World Health Organization, 39 pp (WHO/PCS/90.1).

Worthing CR & Hance RJ (1991) The pesticide manual, 9th ed. Croydon, British Crop Protection Council.

Yu Ching Chien, Booth GM, Hansen DJ, & Larsen JR (1975) Fate of alachlor and propachlor in a model ecosystem. J Agric Food Chem, **23**(5): 877-878.

Zhukova PS & Shirko TS (1979) [Herbicide residues in soil and vegetables.] Khim Sel'skom Khoz, **17**(6): 46-50 (in Russian).

Zilkah S, Osband ME, & Mccaffrey RP (1981) Characterization of the inhibitory effects of the phytotoxic agent propachlor on L1210 cell proliferation. Cancer Lett. (Irel), **13**(3): 241-248.

Zilkah S, Osband ME, Mccaffrey RP, & Shapiro H (1985) The effect of the plant cell inhibitor propachlor on the cell cycle of LI210 cells as evaluated by flow cytometry. Life Sci, **6**: 2111-2115.

Zimdahl RL & Clark SK (1982) Degradation of three acetanilide herbicides in soil. Weed Sci, **30**: 545-548.

Zlateva M & Maleva E (1978) [Late changes in the gonads of male white rats upon combined treatment with low frequency vibrations and Ramrod intoxication.] Med Fizkult, pp 85-91 (in Bulgarian).

Zlateva M & Maleva E (1979) Disorders in the processes of division and differentiation of seminiferous epithelium in case of chronic intoxication with Ramrod. Exp Med Morphol, **18**(1): 35-39.

Zlateva M, Maleva E, & Stareva M (1978) Changes of adenosine triphosphatase activity in the testes of albino rats under combined influence of low-frequency vibration and intoxication with the herbicide Ramrod. Rev Toxicol Eur Res, **6**(78): 375-378.

Zschaler R & Jonas W (1990) Growth inhibition test with algae (Project No. NC-90-592). Hamburg, Natec Institut für Naturwissenschaftlich-technische Dienste GmbH. (Unpublished proprietary report of Monsanto Agricultural Company, submitted to WHO by Monsanto International Services, Brussels).

RESUME ET EVALUATION

1. Identité, modalités d'utilisation, propriétés physiques et chimiques, méthodes d'analyse

Le propachlor est un herbicide dérivé de l'acétanilide qu'on utilise depuis 1965 en traitement de pré-levée et en traitement précoce de post-levée. Il est principalement formulé en poudre mouillable, liquide (concentré en suspension) et granulés. On l'utilise en agriculture pour détruire les graminées annuelles et certaines adventices à feuilles larges dans des cultures comme le maïs, le sorgho, les potirons, le lin et les fleurs.

Le propachlor est légèrement soluble dans l'eau et facilement soluble dans la plupart des solvants organiques. Il est peu volatil, non inflammable et stable au rayonnement ultra-violet. La méthode d'analyse la plus pratique est la chromatographie en phase gazeuse avec détection par capture d'électrons après extraction et purification par des méthodes appropriées.

2. Transport, distribution et transformation dans l'environnement

Le propachlor ne semble pas subir de dégradation photochimique à la surface du sol. Il se volatilise en présence de vent lorsque la surface du sol est encore humide.

Il n'est que modérément adsorbé aux particules du sol et aux matières organiques, d'où un risque de lessivage à travers le sol jusqu'aux eaux souterraines. Toutefois toutes les études montrent que ce risque est faible en pratique. Il faut des précipitations très importantes pour que les résidus se déplacent de 30 cm à l'intérieur du sol. Selon la plupart des auteurs, la majorité des résidus demeurent à moins de 4 cm de profondeur. Les caractéristiques du sol influent beaucoup sur la mobilité du composé. Le lessivage se produit surtout dans des sols sableux pauvres en matières organiques.

On a étudié en laboratoire et sur le terrain l'entraînement du propachlor par ruissellement. Une des études a montré que la présence de matières organiques dans le sol réduisait de 7 à 1 % de la quantité appliquée, la concentration de l'herbicide dans l'eau de ruissellement. L'incorporation de propachlor dans le sol réduit également les pertes par ruissellement (de 3 à 0,8 % selon une étude).

En ce qui concerne la réduction de la concentration de propachlor dans le sol et dans l'eau, le facteur de loin le plus important est sa dégradation par les micro-organismes. On a montré que bactéries et champignons étaient responsables de la dégradation de ce composé. Peu de bactéries sont apparemment capables d'utiliser le propachlor comme seule source de carbone. On a également isolé des bactéries qui sont en mesure d'utiliser des métabolites telluriques du propachlor.

Les principaux métabolites qui se forment dans le sol sont des acides oxaniliques et sulfoniques solubles dans l'eau. Il peut se former un grand nombre d'autres métabolites mais ils ne représentent qu'une faible proportion du total.

Le propachlor disparaît rapidement du sol et on a fait état de demi-vies allant jusqu'à trois semaines. La plupart des études indiquent une dégradation pratiquement complète en moins de six mois. Les conditions écologiques influent sur la vitesse de dégradation qui est favorisée par une température élevée et une forte humidité du sol. Les résultats qui indiquent une persistance élevée du propachlor dans le sol ont été obtenus à basse température et dans des sols secs. La présence de nutriments en quantité suffisante dans le sol est également nécessaire à la dégradation du propachlor.

Un des métabolites, la *N*-isopropylaniline conjuguée est beaucoup plus persistante que le composé initial. On a retrouvé des résidus de ce métabolite jusqu'à deux ans après l'épandage de propachlor à titre expérimental à des doses plus élevées que celles que l'on utilise normalement en agriculture.

Dans les conditions normales d'utilisation, le propachlor ne devrait pas être entraîné à travers le sol par lessivage jusqu'aux nappes souterraines et ne demeure pas dans le sol. Des conditions exceptionnelles (température très basse ou sécheresse) peuvent prolonger la persistance du propachlor et de ses métabolites.

Dans les conditions normales, le propachlor ne subit pas de dégradation photochimique importante dans l'eau. Cependant, en présence de photosensibilisateurs, cette dégradation photochimique peut se produire. Le propachlor est stable à l'hydrolyse. Il est peu probable qu'il se volatilise à partir de l'eau du fait de sa forte solubilité dans l'eau et de sa faible tension de vapeur.

Comme dans le sol, c'est principalement par dégradation biologique que le propachlor s'élimine de l'eau. Sa vitesse d'élimination est donc liée à la population microbienne. Une étude effectuée sur de l'eau contenant peu de bactéries a permis d'obtenir une demi-vie d'environ cinq mois. Une autre étude a montré qu'au bout de six semaines, il n'y avait toujours pas d'ouverture du cycle. Des études de laboratoire portant sur des modèles d'écosystèmes ont montré que le propachlor était presque complètement dégradé en l'espace de 33 jours.

Plusieurs études portant sur différentes espèces végétales ont montré que le propachlor était rapidement métabolisé par les plantes intactes ainsi que par des tissus végétaux excisés. Les voies métaboliques se sont révélées analogues chez tous les végétaux étudiés, tout au moins pendant les six à 24 premières heures, conduisant à des métabolites hydrosolubles. On n'a pas observé de décomposition métabolique du reste *N*-isopropylaniline. Seule une très faible proportion (< 1 % selon une étude) des métabolites a été retrouvée dans les fruits de ces végétaux; ils étaient concentrés en grande majorité dans les racines et les feuilles. Les principaux métabolites produits par les plantes sont identiques à ceux qui prennent naissance dans le sol. On sait que ces métabolites peuvent être fixés à partir du sol et un certain nombre d'études ne permettent pas de déterminer avec certitude si les métabolites analysés proviennent de la plantes ou du sol.

Bien que, d'après le coefficient de partage octanol/eau, ce composé ait une tendance modérée à la bioaccumulation, on a montré qu'il n'y avait ni bioconcentration ni bioamplification chez les êtres vivants.

3. Concentrations dans l'environnement et exposition humaine

Les rapports d'analyse du propachlor dans l'air au cours de l'épandage sont rares et insuffisants.

Aux Etats-Unis d'Amérique, la concentration du propachlor dans les eaux de surface et les eaux souterraines est toujours faible, les maxima atteignant 10 μg/litre dans les eaux de surface et 0,12 µg/litre dans les eaux souterraines. Le concentration la plus forte enregistrée lors d'une étude sur les eaux de ruissellement était de 46 µg/litre.

Les résidus de propachlor dans les denrées alimentaires sont généralement inférieurs à la limite de détection de la méthode d'analyse (0,005 mg/kg). L'expérimentation a permis de retrouver des résidus de l'ordre de 0,005 mg/kg dans des tomates, des poivrons, des oignons et des choux.

Le dosage du propachlor dans l'atmosphère de la zone de travail de conducteurs de tracteur pendant l'épandage du composé a donné des résultats allant de 0,1 à 3,7 mg/m^3.

4. Cinétique et métabolisme

Chez les mammifères, le propachlor peut être absorbé au niveau des voies respiratoires, des voies digestives et de la peau. Il ne s'accumule pas dans l'organisme et devient indétectable au bout de 48 heures.

La plupart des espèces animales (rats, porcs, poulets) métabolisent le propachlor par la voie de l'acide mercapturique (MAP). Il se forme des conjugués de cystéine par conjugaison avec le glutathion et on a avancé que ces conjugués jouaient le rôle d'intermédiaires dans la formation métabolique des acides mercapturiques. La métabolisation du conjugué cystéinique du propachlor se poursuit, notamment sous l'action de la C-S lyase bactérienne qui intervient également dans la formation des métabolites terminaux contenant le groupement méthylsulfonyle, métabolites qui sont principalement excrétés dans l'urine (68 % de la dose initiale de propachlor) et, sous forme de résidus insolubles, dans les matières fécales (19 %). La C-S lyase du propachlor est sans action chez les rats axéniques.

On a montré qu'il y avait un certain nombre de différences dans le métabolisme du propachlor chez le rat et le porc. La bile est la principale voie d'élimination des métabolites mercapturiques chez le rat, mais on a montré qu'il existait une voie métabolique extra-biliaire chez le porc.

Des études de métabolisme effectués sur des veaux ont montré que ces animaux pourraient être incapables de former de l'acide mercapturique à partir des conjugués du glutathion, ce qui les rendrait plus sensibles à l'intoxication par le propachlor.

5. Effets sur les animaux d'expérience et les systèmes d'épreuves *in vitro*

Le propachlor est légèrement toxique en cas d'exposition aiguë par voie orale (la DL_{50} pour le rat varie de 950 à 2176 mg/kg de poids corporel). Les signes d'intoxication aiguë proviennent principalement d'effets sur le système nerveux central (excitation et convulsions suivies d'une dépression). Chez des rongeurs, la toxicité aiguë par inhalation est faible (CL_{50} = 1,0 mg/litre). Le propachlor provoque de graves irritations des yeux et de la peau.

Des rats, des souris et des chiens ont été soumis à une exposition de longue ou de courte durée au propachlor. Les organes cibles sont le foie et les reins. Chez le chien, la dose sans effet nocif observable a été de 45 mg/kg de poids corporel lors d'une étude de trois mois où l'animal était exposé par la voie alimentaire. Lors d'une étude d'une année sur des chiens, la dose sans effet nocif observable a été estimée à 9 mg/kg de poids corporel (200 ppm dans la nourriture). Lors d'une étude sur des rats exposés de la même manière pendant 24 mois au propachlor, la dose sans effet observable a été évaluée à 50 mg/kg de nourriture (2,6 mg/kg de poids corporel). Lors d'une étude semblable effectuée sur des souris pendant 18 mois, on a évalué à 1,6 mg/kg de poids corporel (10 ppm) la dose sans effet observable.

Le propachlor ne s'est révélé cancérogène ni pour la souris ni pour le rat. Dans la plupart des systèmes d'épreuve mammaliens, sa réponse mutagène est négative tout en étant positive dans quelques autres cas. Les données expérimentales disponibles de fournissent pas une preuve suffisante de son pouvoir mutagène.

Administré en dose unique (675 mg/kg) à des rats et à des souris, le propachlor a donné lieu à des signes d'embryotoxicité. On a également observé des effets embryotoxiques lors d'études où du propachlor avait été administré à plusieurs reprises (35,7 à 270 mg/kg). Toutefois, lors d'une autre étude sur des rats, où les doses variaient de 20 à 200 mg/kg, aucun effet embryotoxique n'a été observé.

Aux doses respectives de 12 et 60 mg/kg de poids corporel, le propachlor (en poudre mouillable) a entraîné une réduction de la teneur en protéines et un accroissement de l'activité de l'ATPase et de la 5-nucléotidase dans des homogénats de testicules de rats, provoquant également une dégénérescence du tissu testiculaire. Lors d'une étude de reproduction portant sur deux générations, on n'a pas véritablement obtenu la preuve d'effets indésirables.

6. Effets sur l'homme

On a signalé quelques dermatites de contact et dermatites allergiques chez des agriculteurs et des ouvriers de production exposés au propachlor (Ramrod et Satecid). Des tests cutanés ont été effectués parmi un certain nombre d'entre eux, avec un résultat positif, qui révèle une réaction d'irritation et une hypersensibilité mono- et bivalente.

On n'a pas eu connaissance de symptômes ou de maladies, soit chez des personnes exposées de par leur profession, soit dans la population générale - à part les quelques cas d'effets cutanés chez les ouvriers professionnellement exposés.

7. Effets sur les êtres vivant dans leur milieu naturel

Des études portant sur la microflore terricole ont montré que les bactéries nitrifiantes constituaient le groupe le plus sensible aux effets inhibiteurs du propachlor, leur nombre étant réduit d'un facteur 3 à 4 après épandage de 8 à 10 kg de propachlor par hectare. Ce sont les bactéries décomposant la cellulose qui étaient les moins sensibles. La forte adsorption du propachlor aux particules d'argile présentes dans le sol et une température élevée sont deux facteurs qui réduisent les effets inhibiteurs.

Chez l'algue *Selenastrum capricornutum*, on a fait état d'une CE_{50} à 96 heures de 0,02 mg/litre (pour la croissance) et d'une concentration sans effet observable de 0,01 mg/litre. D'après une deuxième étude portant sur une formulation de propachlor et menée pendant 72 heures, le risque pour cette même algue serait nettement moindre.

Pour la daphnie *Daphnia magna*, on donne des CL_{50} de 7,8 ou 6,9 mg/litre et une concentration sans effet observable inférieure à 5,6 mg/litre. La concentration sans effet observable sur la reproduction était de 0,097 mg/litre. Pour des larves de deux espèces de moucherons, on a obtenu pour la CL_{50} des valeurs respectives de 0,79 et 1,8 mg/litre.

Chez la truite arc-en-ciel la CL_{50} à 96 heures est de 0,17 mg/litre et la concentration sans effet observable sur 21 jours, de 0,019 mg/litre.

Le propachlor est considéré comme modérément à fortement toxique pour les organismes aquatiques.

Le propachlor n'est pas toxique pour les lombrics aux concentrations présentes dans le sol par suite d'un usage normal (la concentration sans effet observable est de 100 mg/kg de terre). La DL_{50} par contact pour les abeilles (311 μg/abeille) montre que le propachlor ne constitue pas un danger pour ces insectes. En revanche, des études menées en laboratoire et sur le terrain montrent que des parasites utiles peuvent souffrir des effets du propachlor.

Le propachlor est plus toxique pour les oiseaux lorsqu'on l'introduit directement dans l'estomac que lorsqu'on l'administre dans la nourriture. La DL_{50} aiguë varie de 137 à 735 mg/kg de poids corporel pour différentes espèces. Quant à la CL_{50} lors d'une exposition par voie alimentaire, elle dépasse 5620 mg/kg de nourriture chez les oiseaux.

Le propachlor ne constitue pas un danger pour les oiseaux dans la nature, même sous forme de granulés.

RESUMEN Y EVALUACION

1. Identidad, modalidades de uso, propiedades físicas y químicas y métodos analíticos

El propacloro es un herbicida derivado de la acetanilida utilizado desde 1965 que actúa en las plantas antes de nacer o poco después. Las principales formulaciones son de polvo humectable, líquido fluido (concentrado en suspensión) y gránulos. Se aplica en la agricultura a la lucha contra las gramíneas anuales y algunas malas hierbas de hoja ancha en varios cultivos, como los de maíz, sorgo, calabaza, lino y flores ornamentales.

El propacloro es ligeramente soluble en agua y se disuelve fácilmente en la mayoría de los disolventes orgánicos. Su volatilidad es escasa, no es inflamable y es estable a la radiación ultravioleta. El método más práctico de análisis es la cromatografía de gases con detección por captura de electrones, después de aplicar procedimientos apropiados de extracción y purificación.

2. Transporte, distribución y transformación en el medio ambiente

Según la información disponible, el propacloro no se fotodegrada sobre la superficie del suelo. El producto se volatiliza cuando hay viento y la superficie del suelo está todavía mojada.

La adsorción sobre las partículas del suelo y la materia orgánica es sólo moderada. Debido a esto, es posible la lixiviación a través del perfil del suelo hacia el agua subterránea. Sin embargo, todos los estudios indican que en la práctica es poco probable que esto ocurra. Se requiere una precipitación muy abundante para hacer descender los residuos 30 cm en el perfil del suelo. La mayoría de los autores señalan que la mayor parte de los residuos se mantienen en una capa superficial del suelo de 4 cm. Las características del suelo influyen mucho en el desplazamiento del producto. La lixiviación se produce en su mayor parte en suelo arenoso con poca materia orgánica.

Se ha estudiado el arrastre del propacloro por el agua tanto en el laboratorio como sobre el terreno. En un estudio, la materia orgánica del suelo redujo el arrastre del herbicida aplicado del 7%

al 1%. Su incorporación al suelo también redujo la pérdida por arrastre del agua (del 3% al 0,8% en un estudio).

El factor que más contribuye, con diferencia, a reducir los niveles de propacloro en el suelo y el agua es la degradación por los microorganismos. Se ha comprobado que en la degradación de la sustancia intervienen tanto bacterias como hongos. Son pocas las bacterias que parecen tener capacidad para usar el propacloro como única fuente de carbono. También se han aislado bacterias que pueden utilizar los metabolitos del propacloro presentes en el suelo.

Los metabolitos predominantes entre los que se forman en el suelo son los ácidos oxanílico y sulfónico, solubles en agua. Pueden formarse otros muchos metabolitos, pero representan una proporción pequeña del total.

El propacloro desaparece con rapidez del suelo, habiéndose registrado semividas de hasta tres semanas. En la mayoría de los estudios se señala que la degradación es casi completa en menos de seis meses. Las condiciones del medio ambiente influyen en la velocidad de degradación, que se ve favorecida por los valores elevados de la temperatura y el contenido de humedad del suelo. Los estudios en los que se describía una permanencia más prolongada del propacloro en el suelo se realizaron en condiciones de baja temperatura o suelo seco. También es necesaria una cantidad suficiente de nutrientes en el suelo para la degradación.

El metabolito conjugado *N*-isopropilanilina es mucho más persistente que el producto del que procede. Se han encontrado residuos de este metabolito hasta dos años después de la aplicación experimental de dosis de propacloro más altas de las que se utilizan normalmente en la agricultura.

Con el uso normal no es previsible que el propacloro llegue por lixiviación a través del suelo hasta el agua subterránea, y no se mantiene mucho tiempo en el suelo. En condiciones excepcionales de baja temperatura o sequedad, el propacloro y sus metabolitos pueden permanecer más tiempo en él. En condiciones normales, el propacloro no sufre una fotodegradación significativa en el agua. En presencia de fotosensibilizadores puede fotodegradarse. El propacloro es estable desde el punto de vista hidrolítico. No es probable la volatilización a partir del agua, debido a la elevada solubilidad en ella y la baja tensión de vapor del producto.

Al igual que en el suelo, la principal ruta de pérdida de propacloro del agua es la degradación biótica. La velocidad de desaparición del propacloro del agua depende, pues, de la población microbiana. En un estudio realizado con un pequeño número de bacterias presentes en el agua se obtuvo una semivida de unos cinco meses. En otro estudio, a las seis semanas no se había roto el anillo. En estudios de laboratorio con modelos de ecosistemas se observó una degradación casi completa en un período de 33 días.

En varios estudios con distintas especies vegetales se vio que el propacloro se metabolizaba con rapidez tanto en las plantas intactas como en tejidos vegetales extirpados. Las rutas metabólicas eran análogas en todas las plantas estudiadas, por lo menos durante las primeras 6-24 horas, produciendo metabolitos hidrosolubles. No se observó degradación metabólica del fragmento de la *N*-isopropilanilina. En los frutos de las plantas solamente se encontró una proporción muy pequeña (< 1% en un estudio) de los metabolitos; en su mayor parte estaban en las raíces y el follaje. Los principales metabolitos producidos en las plantas son idénticos a los que se forman en el suelo. Se sabe que las plantas absorben esos metabolitos del suelo, y en algunos estudios había dudas acerca de si los metabolitos medidos procedían de la planta o del suelo.

Aunque del coeficiente de reparto en octanol y agua parece deducirse un potencial moderado de bioacumulación, los estudios realizados indican que no hay ni bioconcentración ni bioamplificación en los organismos.

3. Niveles medioambientales y exposición humana

Las mediciones descritas de la concentración del propacloro en el aire durante la aplicación son pocas e inadecuadas.

Las concentraciones en el agua superficial y subterránea en los Estados Unidos fueron siempre bajas, con un máximo de 10 μg/litro en la superficial y de 0,12 μg/litro en la subterránea. La mayor concentración registrada en el agua en un estudio del arrastre fue de 46 μg/litro.

Los residuos de propacloro en los alimentos suelen ser inferiores al límite de detección del método analítico (0,005 mg/kg). En estudios experimentales se han identificado concentraciones de residuos del orden de 0,05 mg/kg en tomates, pimientos, cebollas y coles.

Las concentraciones de propacloro en el aire de la zona de trabajo de los conductores de tractores que aplicaban la sustancia oscilaban entre 0,1 y 3,7 mg/m^3.

4. Cinética y metabolismo

Los mamíferos pueden absorber el propacloro por los tractos respiratorio y gastrointestinal, así como a través de la piel. El producto no se acumula en el organismo, en el que no es detectable a las 48 horas.

La mayoría de las especies animales (ratas, cerdos, pollos) metabolizan el propacloro siguiendo la vía de los ácidos mercaptúricos. Mediante conjugación con el glutatión se forman productos conjugados de cisteína, que se han señalado como posibles intermediarios en la formación metabólica de ácidos mercaptúricos. La C-S liasa bacteriana participa en el ulterior metabolismo del sistema conjugado del propacloro con la cisteína y en la formación de los metabolitos finales con metilsulfonilo, que se excretan sobre todo en la orina (68% de la dosis de propacloro), y de residuos insolubles, que se excretan en las heces (19%). La propacloro C-S liasa es inactiva en ratas sin microorganismos.

En los estudios realizados se observaron algunas diferencias en cuanto al metabolismo entre las ratas y los cerdos. La bilis es el principal camino de eliminación de los metabolitos de la vía de los ácidos mercaptúricos en las ratas, pero se ha demostrado que en los cerdos existe una vía metabólica extrabiliar.

En estudios metabólicos con terneros se observó que pueden ser incapaces de formar ácidos mercaptúricos a partir de los productos conjugados del glutatión, por lo que pueden ser más susceptibles a la intoxicación.

5. Efectos en los animales de experimentación y en sistemas de prueba *in vitro*

El propacloro es ligeramente tóxico en la exposición oral aguda (la DL_{50} en ratas va de 950 a 2176 mg/kg de peso corporal). Los signos de intoxicación aguda son predominantemente efectos sobre el sistema nervioso central (excitación y convulsiones, seguidas de depresión). La toxicidad aguda por inhalación en roedores es baja (CL_{50} = 1,0 mg/litro). El propacloro produjo efectos graves de irritación en los ojos y la piel.

El propacloro se ha ensayado en estudios de exposición de corta y larga duración en ratas, ratones y perros. Los órganos sobre los que actuaba eran el hígado y los riñones. En un estudio de administración con los alimentos a perros durante tres meses, el nivel sin efectos adversos observados (NOAEL) fue de 45 mg/kg de peso corporal. En otro estudio de un año, también en perros, el NOAEL fue de 9 mg/kg de peso corporal (250 ppm en la dieta). El nivel sin efectos observados (NOEL) en un estudio de alimentación de ratas durante 24 meses fue de 50 mg/kg de la dieta (2,6 mg/kg de peso corporal). En un estudio en el que administró el producto a ratones con los alimentos durante 18 meses, el NOEL fue de 1,6 mg/kg de peso corporal (10 ppm).

No se encontraron efectos carcinogénicos del propacloro en ratones y ratas. En la mayoría de los sistemas de prueba de mamíferos la respuesta mutagénica fue negativa, obteniéndose resultados positivos en un pequeño número de ensayos. Los datos experimentales disponibles no aportan suficientes pruebas de su potencial mutagénico.

En pruebas de dosis única (675 mg/kg) con ratones y ratas se demostró la embriotoxicidad del propacloro. También se detectaron efectos embriotóxicos en tratamientos con dosis repetidas (35,7-270 mg/kg). Sin embargo, en otro estudio en ratas, con una gama de dosis de 20-200 mg/kg, no se observó embriotoxicidad.

Con niveles de 12 y 60 mg/kg de peso corporal, el propacloro (polvo humectable) provocó una disminución del contenido de proteínas y un aumento de la actividad de la ATPasa y la 5-nucleotidasa en un homogeneizado de testículo de rata y cambios degenerativos en los testículos. En un estudio de reproducción de dos generaciones no se obtuvieron pruebas definitivas de efectos adversos.

6. Efectos en la especie humana

Se ha descrito un pequeño número de casos de dermatitis de contacto y alérgica en agricultores y trabajadores expuestos al propacloro durante la producción (Ramrod y Satecid). En algunos de ellos se efectuaron pruebas del parche y la reacción fue positiva, con irritación e hipersensibilidad monovalente y bivalente.

No se han notificado casos de síntomas o enfermedades entre las personas expuestas profesionalmente o en la población general, salvo un pequeño número de informes de sus efectos cutáneos en trabajadores expuestos profesionalmente.

7. Efectos en los seres vivos del medio ambiente

En varios estudios sobre los microorganismos del suelo, las bacterias nitrificantes fueron el grupo más sensible a los efectos inhibidores del propacloro, reduciéndose su número a la tercera o cuarta parte tras la aplicación de 8-10 kg/ha de propacloro. Las menos sensibles fueron las bacterias celulolíticas. La adsorción elevada sobre las partículas de arcilla del suelo y la temperatura alta reducen los efectos inhibidores.

En el alga *Selenastrum capricornutum* se ha registrado una CE_{50} a las 96 horas de 0,02 mg/litro para el crecimiento y una concentración sin efectos observados (NOEC) de 0,01 mg/litro. De un segundo estudio de 72 horas realizado con una formulación, parece desprenderse que el peligro es mucho menor para este mismo organismo.

Se ha informado de unos valores de la CL_{50} para *Daphnia magna* de 7,8 y 6,9 mg/litro y una NOEC de < 5,6 mg/litro. En las larvas de dos especies de moscas enanas, los valores registrados de la CL_{50} fueron de 0,79 y 1,8 mg/litro.

La CL_{50} para la trucha arcoiris a las 96 horas es de 0,17 mg/litro, y la NOEC en un estudio de 26 días fue de 0,019 mg/litro.

Se considera que el propacloro tiene una toxicidad entre moderada e intensa para los organismos acuáticos.

La exposición a las concentraciones de propacloro que cabe prever en el suelo no es tóxica para las lombrices de tierra si la aplicación es normal (la NOEC es de 100 mg/kg de suelo). La DL_{50} por contacto para las abejas (311 μg/abeja) demuestra que el propacloro no representa un peligro para estos insectos. En estudios de laboratorio y de campo se han detectado efectos adversos del propacloro en algunos insectos parasitarios beneficiosos.

El propacloro es más tóxico para las aves cuando se administra mediante sonda gástrica que cuando se incorpora a la dieta. Los valores de la DL_{50} aguda para distintas especies de aves oscilan entre 137 y 735 mg/kg de peso corporal. Los valores de la CL_{50} en la administración con los alimentos fueron superiores a los 5620 mg/kg de la dieta.

El propacloro no representa un peligro para las aves en el campo, ni siquiera con la formulación granulada.